Hospital Bureaucracy

A Comparative Study of Organizations

Wolf Heydebrand

Foreword
by
Paul F. Lazarsfeld

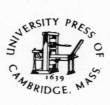

DUNELLEN

New York

To Gitry

Contents

List of Tables and Figures

Foreword

In 1955 I was co-editor of a collection of empirical studies. The purpose was to bring out methodological implications. One section dealt with statistical analysis of collectives. I then mentioned with regret that little work had been done studying large sets of organizations. And most of all we couldn't find any study where more than two variables at a time had been taken into consideration.

Since then the situation has radically changed. Funds became available to study on a comparative basis colleges, government agencies, business organizations, hospitals, etc. These in turn greatly increased the number of variables which were suggested for the description of organizations. By 1961 my colleague Allen Barton was able to publish a systematic collection called "Organizational Measurement". Computers became available and so multivariate analysis could be applied to sets of organizations by using the same techniques which survey analysts had developed for the analysis of interviews and questionnaires obtained from individual respondents.

Mr. Heydebrand, the author of this book, first came to my attention through an interesting article on "The Study of Organizations", *Social Science Information* VI (1967), a Journal of the International Social Science Council. He had taken advantage of material which had appeared subsequent to Barton's monograph.

His article showed great insight into the methodological problems of organizational research and he announced that his ideas would be applied to a forthcoming study of hospitals.

He now presents his analysis. To my knowledge it is the broadest approach to one single type of organization in at least four respects: the number of units covered; the number of organizational characteristics considered; the explicitness by which empirical indicators and conceptual notions are linked; and, finally, the number of variables simultaneously taken into account. This preface is a welcome occasion to review the elements which make up the comparative analysis of organizations. The author himself stresses the unavoidable complexity of his presentation. I am confident that the book will be highly valuable for college teachers in both graduate and undergraduate teaching. I shall try to enhance this value somewhat by a kind of methodological guide to some of its contents.

I shall divide my comments into two parts: the kind of empirical data Mr. Heydebrand had available and their relations to conceptual ideas; and then his analytical procedures and the interpretation of his findings.

The core of the author's information are official surveys on the labor force in practically all American hospitals, their functional and departmental organization, and occasionally some data on workload, equipment and similar information on the hospitals' objective activities. As he wanted to work with practically all American hospitals he obviously had no general knowledge of the attitudes of the staff, nor their concrete interaction with each other and with the patients. His first problem was, therefore, to use his raw material in such flexible combinations that they would support a large variety of conceptual ideas.

Let us quickly run down the numerical combinations which appear in the book. There are first straight counts. Thus, for instance, the author has established a list of 39 occupations which hospitals may provide. But not all hospitals provide all of them. The proportion of jobs actually in operation is used as an indicator of "functional specialization" (chapter 3, p. 48). Or, a hospital can vary according to the humber of medical services performed (internal medicine, surgery, pediatrics) and that provides one of several indicators of how complex its task structure is (p. 235). In the community at large hospitals can be affiliated with other institutions and belong to a variety of associations; here again a straight count provides an indicator of "external relations" (p. 131).

Then, of course, there are ratios. Some of them are well known in organizational research, like, for instance, the proportion of the labor force concerned only with administration; this is used as an indicator of conventional bureaucratization. Other ratios are more subtle. Thus, for instance, nurses are divided according to whether they have or have not a specialized degree. But the latter group is further divided to establish the proportion of graduate nurses who have also administrative functions in the hospital. This ratio is used as the indicator of a concept very basic to Mr. Heydebrand's analysis, the bureaucratization of professionals (p. 220).

Probably the most distinctive feature of organizational research is the study of distribution between vertical hierarchic levels or across horizontal departmental divisions. Here the author has chosen as his basic measure the so-called Gini index which he explains carefully in different parts of his text. The basic idea is easily grasped. The investigator is faced with a given classification of skills or authority among occupations such as technicians (chapter 6) or nurses (chapter 8). In a second type of application one faces various departments such as nursing, technical services, clerical work, etc. (chapter 7). The problem is always to show how the labor force is divided over these various divisions. (In the latter case the index indicates "departmental specialization", while the job count mentioned above is called functional specialization.) While the Gini index always has the same statistical meaning, its interpretation will differ greatly according to the context in which it is used. Thus in chapter 10 the index applied to departmental divisions is interpreted in terms of communication and interaction between various specialities. In chapter 6 where the same index refers to the hierarchy among technicians it is used to indicate the extent to which authority is delegated.

When dealing with his most crucial variables, Mr. Heydebrand goes to great length to explain his operational decisions. He feels that the professionalization of hospitals is best gauged by looking at the skill structure of the nursing staff which, in some hospital types, makes up more than 50 per cent of the total personnel. Furthermore, nurses have closer and more continuous contact with the patients than do the physicians. He justified his decision in several extensive and instructuve discussions, for instance, pages 52 and 204. This kind of argumentation is an important part of the author's work due to the nature of his data. When in chapter 6 he talks about medical technology, for example, he does have some information on the facilities and services available in these hospitals. But his main source is inferential: the type, frequency and hierarchy of technical personnel available from the tables of organization. This makes for a considerable distance between the empirical data and the concepts, which leaves room for flexibility as well as for controversy. The gap is open both ways. Thus, for instance, the notion of "size" could be indicated by the number of employees or the capital resources of the hospital. Inversely, a large ratio of employees per hospital bed may indicate good patient care or great task complexity.

In the type of organizational analysis represented by this book there is then no one-to-one relation between the statistical material and the author's conceptual map. To appreciate this point fully I have a suggestion for the reader's strategy. He might want to get a rough idea of the author's basic concepts and their translation into indicators by reading chapter 3. Then he might want to sample part II by looking at some of the empirical findings. He will not easily remember the basic terminology of chapter 3. But by moving back and forth between part II and chapter 3 he will slowly get acquainted with the author's analytical world. He will then be prepared to understand the crucial role of chapter 2 where a "hierarchy of variables" really explains the whole organization of the book. He will then be ready to delve into part III. Here he will also find the most complex relation between data and concepts. Notions like professional coordination or delegation of authority are no longer directly linked to statistical evidence. They emerge as generalizing formulae derived from a large variety of relations between his basic variables.

The final chapters of the book broaden the traditional theory of organization as it is described in chapter 4. The new ideas grow out of the need to integrate such large amounts of empirical observations on organizations in which professionals play an important role. In such organizations the need is for a network of coordinations: some of it must come from the top, but other forms result from the self-directing norms of the professional groups themselves. The mixture of these elements in turn depends upon the size of the hospital and its substantive specialization. It is interesting to follow some of the "dialectic" moves of thought by which the author traces the various alternatives. But departmental divisions provide also positive chances for contact and exchange. Chapter 10 developed this more optimistic line and its possible use for avoiding too much regulation. Chapter 11 in turn raises the possibility that a subdivision could break off from an organization which has become too large for its own stability. The balance of authoritarian and professional coordination and the mediating role of delegation is the main theme toward which the data and the discussions of the whole book converge.

Ultimately, Mr. Heydebrand provides a rather firm scaffolding within which many of his ideas can be placed. He selects four of his indicators to construct four "modes of coordination" (p. 280): two are taken from the skill level of the nursing staff and their involvement in administrative work: the other two are taken from the department organization of the hospitals and the relative size of the purely administrative staff. For all 12 original hospital groups he computes the weight these "ingredients" of coordination have in the total picture.

By a clever combination of factors he forms 6 major hospital types, each has its own pattern depending upon which of his four modes prevail. Table 4 and figure 9 in chapter 10 are the guides to a vivid verbal description of these six abstract types and the concrete group of hospitals in which they can be found. Not being acquainted with the operating problems of hospitals I have nothing to add to this final analysis. But I am greatly impressed by Mr. Heydebrand's decision not to stop at this point. He has the courage in his final chapter to make concrete recommendations as to what he considers an ideal hospital. I am sure that his ideas will be controversial but any basic research which can lead to practical recommendation deserves special attention.

I now turn to the second purpose of this introduction, giving some guidance to the use of multivariate analysis. This technique has been most elaborately developed in survey analysis where the statistical units are individual people and their characteristics. This tradition is by now well known and I shall begin by comparing it with what one might call survey analysis of organization. One begins usually with a small number of pivotal variables around which the rest of the analysis is organized. Mr. Heydebrand uses for this purpose the organizational complexity of a hospital (the initial indicator is the presence or absence of a teaching function), the specificity of its medical goal, indicated by a distinction between psychiatric and general hospitals, and the type of control—whether it is voluntary, under Federal supervision or established by a state or city government. The importance of this 3-dimensional typology is made abundantly clear through numerous tables throughout the text. It would help the reader if we select a single row from one of these tables and put it into terms familiar in the survey literature. In row 4, table 23, Mr. Heydebrand describes the proportion of nurses who have no duties other than to direct patient care in 12 types of hospitals:

Table 1

	Voluntary		Local		Federal		
Psychiatric	.14		.05		.16		Nonteaching
		.18		.11		.17	Teaching
General	.34		.25		.39		
		.43		.33		.41	

A mere inspection shows that all three pivotal distinctions play a basic role. The largest average difference is accounted for by a comparison of general and psychiatric hospitals, that is to say, by one aspect of complexity; its other aspect, teaching, is still clearly discernible but less marked because type of control has the smallest effect on the dependent variable. However, the three dimensions do not act independently from one another. In federally controlled hospitals (see the last column) teaching accounts for only a one or two percent difference; under the other two types of control the difference in the diagonal within each square is considerably larger.* Such a finding is usually called a contextual proposition. The relation between the teaching function and the composition of the nursing staff is affected by the type of external control under which a hospital operates. In statistical parlance we speak of an interaction between outside controls and educational goals in their functional effect upon the type of nurses required. (A possible interpretation is that in federal hospitals this teaching function plays a lesser role because staff appointments are more dependent upon central civil service regulations.) Incidentally, it is remarkable how important the three pivotal variables are, if considered jointly. The proportion of nurses concerned only with patient care is 43 per cent in privately owned general teaching hospitals and 5 per cent in psychiatric hospitals which have no teaching function and are controlled by local government.†

*The reader is advised to transcribe some of the rows in some of the tables into this form. It will help him to follow the text which accompany the figures in this book.

† The importance of variates considered individually or combined can statistically be expressed by the so-called F-ratio which the author uses with some tables. This measure has the advantage of providing a compact summary although it does not enable one to follow the rich details of a full multivariate tabulation.

Notice that we deal here with four variables and we have already devised a special trick to present the results in a 2-dimensional page of paper. When we deal with more variables the complexity of the patterns becomes so great that one has to organize one's thinking. Instead of the conventional effect of a few independent variables upon one "dependent" one, we have to study the effect upon the correlation between *two* dependent variables.

This means developing further the notion of contextual propositions. The reader will be helped by following this development in three steps. In the first row of table 15, for instance, the figures can again be organized into a multivariate table such as the one given above. But the entries there are no longer single dependent variables. They are instead correlations between the proportion of salaried physicians and qualified technicians. This means that the finding includes five different variates. The text's interpretation of this table shows that the result becomes understandable if one draws in additional factors, such as size, for interpretation. Sometimes this extension can itself be established numerically as can be seen Table 34. Here the "dependent phenomenon" is the relation b tween the degree of professionalization and the relative size of tl administrative staff. The main finding, very important for tl argument of the whole book, is the fact that if within hospit... groups, nurses have a high skill standard, less administra⁺ e machinery is needed to coordinate their activity. But to bring .iis out clearly, a number of additional variables have to be "kept constant" by partial correlation techniques.

The main finding of table 34 covers, in fact, eight variates simultaneously. In this kind of result, organizational research by far surpasses traditional survey analysis. The explanation is not difficult to find. The use of partial correlation techniques is based on the use of continuous quantitative data. They become available in organizational research because of the ample use of ratios and proportions. Questionnaires addressed to individuals usually cannot provide such data. Surely we can use scales there but they would require so many single items that a questionnaire would become unmanageable.

Not all tables show as smooth a pattern as the one I chose for didactical purposes. Here another parallel to conventional survey analysis appears: deviant case analysis. Thus, for instance, in table 14 row 5, the proportion of technical personnel is reported for the twelve basic types. One figure is surprising: psychiatric non-teaching hospitals have a large number of technicians. Mr. Heydebrand surmises from his general knowledge that this is due to the prevalence of occupational therapists in this type of hospital. What he does is to refine the variate "technicians," which one usually associates with personnel handling physical equipment such as electrocardiograms, x-ray machines, and/or blood tests. But sometimes deviant case analysis does not simply respectify variates; it can also suggest the need to introduce additional ones. The author has provided a number of such possibilities at the end of chapter 5. Beginning on page 120 he reports a variety of correlates for his 3 pivotal variates. They can be drawn upon wherever the standard tables show unusual patterns.

There is an abundance of literature dealing with hospitals, and the author has found two ways to weave it into the fabric of his own work. Quite a number of studies have used similar variates, and the author utilizes such cases for corroboration. But, because he has such a large number of units and such a flexible set of indicators, he is often able to combine special findings of other works into a more integrated set of propositions. A remarkable example can be found in chapter 10, page 273. Two authors have reported findings which seem to be contradictory. Mr. Heydebrand shows that they are compatible if one introduces, as a specifying variate, the task complexity of the hospitals. Other studies have used questionnaires answered by staff members or observations on their activities and interrelations. Because this kind of material was not available to Mr. Heydebrand, it is very helpful to see how he used the findings of his colleagues to interpret and make more understandable his own objective data. (Good examples can be found on pages 271 and 231.) Finally, I wish to draw attention to the places where Mr. Heydebrand has made fine use of historical material (pages 153 and 251).

In the past, sociologists have been concerned with where to place their bets: quantification vs. case studies, micro- vs. macro-sociology, conceptual analysis vs. empirical propositions. Such controversies become more and more uninteresting. The plane on which mutual understanding develops most rapidly is the comparative study of organizations. This book is a fortunate example of this trend and I hope it will be beneficial for other substantive areas as well.

Paul F. Lazarsfeld

July, 1972
Columbia University
New York, New York

Preface

This book is one of the first large-scale systematic analyses of organizations in general, as represented by one of their most interesting species: the modern hospital. In fact, the hospital today is not just the extreme point on a continuum of task complexity and professional performance; it finds itself at the intersection of various dimensions of organizational structure.

The hospital is, therefore, a prototype of modern work organizations. Rather than adjusting to more traditional models of business organization and bureaucratic structure, modern hospitals have become organizational models in their own right. They serve as ideal types for work organizations that make the solution of complex and variable, hence never fully predictable, tasks their routine business. This does not mean that hospitals are above and beyond organizational problems; nor does it mean that the challenge to maintain life or restitute health always calls forth the highest quality of care and the utmost in technical, professional, and human performance. But considering the frequent urgency and delicate nature of medical judgment, the advanced technology available for its implementation, and the vast array of specialized service and functions that are to be coordinated for a common purpose, it is certainly amazing that the modern hospital functions at all, let alone at a high level of effective goal-attainment.

To be an organizational model in its own right, an organization must exemplify or strive toward the achievement of an agreed-upon standard of performance. But even if the standard is agreed upon and explicit, other elements of the model may not be visible or even be known. The proof of this assertion lies in the fact that there is a broad spectrum of efforts to find a viable organizational form and a corresponding variability of organizational structure. Hospitals vary so much along different dimensions and criteria that the term "hospital," designating a variety of broad basic functions, is hardly more than a label.

Thus, one may well have the 100-bed community general hospital in mind when one speaks of a hospital. To another, it may mean a state mental institution with 5,000 patient-inmates, its staff trying, against many odds, to change from a custodial to a therapeutic orientation; or it may mean the modern medical center containing specialized hospitals, clinics, and services and resembling more a cluster of swarming bees than a formal organization. The hospital may be viewed primarily as an institution established for the training of medical interns and residents, or as an exclusive, private institution owned by a group of businessmen-doctors and operated for profit. It may be thought of as an institution designed for the needs of a particular patient population, such as veterans or children; or, for complicated social, economic, and political reasons, as an abode for low-income patients. For each of these "hospitals," we may identify a different structural type.

It is the purpose of this book to develop and describe a number of dimensions common to all of these different types of organizations called hospitals. Furthermore, the book is an attempt to define hospitals in terms of basic general characteristics of organizations and to learn something in the process not only about hospitals but about organizations in general. In other words, it is an attempt to locate the organizational model of which the modern general hospital is the prototype.

Such an objective calls for a comparative analysis of a large number of hospitals in terms of general organizational variables, for an examination of the results in the light of organizational theory, and for a reorientation of organizational analysis toward a broader, more comprehensive approach to the realities of modern organizations.

If the book realizes its objectives, then it is, first of all, directly relevant to anyone concerned with the complex task of "running a hospital." In particular, chapter 5 (on organizational autonomy and task structure), chapters 8 to 10 (on the problem of coordination), and chapter 11 (on the uses and limits of bureaucracy) will be of special interest to hospital administrators and students of administration in such areas as nursing, medicine, welfare, education, and research. Nurses, in particular, might be interested in chapters 2, 8, 9, and the discussion in Ch. 10 of the transition from 'generalists' to 'specialists'. Medical and medico-technical specialists may find chapter 6 to be of special interest to them. Organizational methodologists and researchers may want to look at chapters 2 and 3, the discussion of the Gini index in chapters 3 and 10, the relative skewness index of the organizational hierarchy in chapter 9, the general design of the study and the use of multivariate techniques of analysis, and the list of empirical generalizations in Appendix G. Finally, the social policymaker in the health and welfare field might find chapters 1, 2, 5, and 11 directly relevant to some of the current concerns with improving the quality and availability of hospital-based health services.

More generally, the book should show the structural variability and complexity of modern organizations so that anyone concerned with administration and management may find that he can translate a given hospital type into a different, but corresponding, structural type. More specifically, the analysis of the conflict between professional and bureaucratic requirements experienced by professional nurses who assume administrative and supervisory duties may illuminate similar conflicts and pressures afflicting the chemist or engineer promoted to division head, the group worker who is an agency executive, the teacher-professor who becomes principal or dean, the skilled worker promoted to foreman, the research scientist turned scientific advisor or consultant, etc. Further, the problems of effectiveness and quality that arise from the growth of mental hospitals beyond a certain size have obvious parallels in the implications of the 25,000-student multiversity campus for the quality of higher education, of "mass production" for product quality, of efficiency measures for morale, of the quantity of exposures for the quality of treatment.

Finally, and basically, the book should be of some interest to sociologists, not only to those specializing in the field of formal organization, but also to those concerned with problems of structural change and processes of interdependence, exchange, and conflict.

At the heart of this enterprise lies a concern with a fundamental dilemma of all human social organization, namely the tension between what is to be done and how it is to be done. There are various ways of expressing this tension, and I will discuss a number of them at different points in this book. Perhaps its most rational expression is given in the relation between means and ends. Yet this relationship is frequently unstable. Means may become ends in themselves. Ends may be adjusted to limited means. The means employed may not be consistent with the desired ends, neither morally nor economically nor in terms of plans, designs, or anticipated outcomes. These and other possibilities illustrate the precarious balance between means and ends. Posing this dilemma in terms of sociological concepts means to deal with the problem of coordination in relation to organizational goals and tasks.

Broadly speaking, coordination refers to the process of how given goals are attained, after they have been defined and agreed upon. Coordination is understood as the necessary and sufficient condition, other conditions being equal, for the effective functioning of an organization. Thus, as a general condition for the effective realization of organizational goals, coordination includes the patterned relationship and adjustment of the parts to each other and to the whole. In other words, coordination is used here as a generic concept which has reference to all integrative aspects of the social structure called "organization." However, any attempt to achieve set goals, to accomplish defined tasks and, generally, to routinize and institutionalize solutions to complex problems generates new questions and forces. These new questions move the established pattern in the direction of an increasing inconsistency between means and ends, and thus toward the redefinition of old goals or the setting of new ones. It is this tension between goal-setting and goal-attainment that, on a general intellectual level, underlies the present attempt to understand an organizational model in which this tension is of paramount significance: the modern professional organization.

The tension between what is to be done and how it is to be done in hospitals is important not only from the vantage point of life vis-a-vis death. It is also significant from the point of view of finding viable organizational solutions to basic human, social, and political problems, and yet to avoid stagnating in the process of "getting things done," rationalized as it may be.

If any organization is an example of how to survive between the need to routinize emergencies and the need to constantly improve and maximize the preservation of human values about life and health, it is the modern hospital. Therefore, it is also one of the fastest changing organizations, rendering today's life-saving innovation obsolete tomorrow. While considerations of efficiency and economic rationality become increasingly dominant in today's hospital technology and management, they can never fully explain nor justify the always slightly precarious character of hospital operations, the constant adjustments to variable work loads, and the need to deal reasonably yet responsibly with uncertainty and critical situations.

By the same token, the research operations involved in a comparative analysis of almost 7,000 hospitals cannot do justice to understanding the intricate functioning of any one of them. Why, then, has this project been undertaken at all? What is to be gained from such relatively crude, abstract comparisons?

While there are a number of systematic answers that must and can be given to these questions, the most important one is that comparative, quantitative organizational research is the only way to advance our knowledge of organizations beyond that of a single case or type. Any experienced hospital administrator knows his hospital and its problems better than anybody else. What he may not know is that there are recurrent patterns and problems associated with the general category of hospitals of which he is operating one specimen, rather than with the individual history of his organization. The scope of his insight is, therefore, comparable to that of the psychological therapist who ascribes a person's problem to the peculiarities of his individual history, whereas a comparative study of such persons may reveal that the problem is a situational or group characteristic rather than an individual idiosyncrasy. Both therapist and administrator may deal successfully with the problem, but they do not necessarily do so in terms of an explanation or a program of prevention. Problem-solving remains on the level of "muddling through," with all its implications of avoiding radical change.

Stated positively, problem-solving within and through organizations can and should go beyond the "reasonableness" of short-term adjustments by planning on the basis of present or future knowledge, i.e., research, and on the basis of a concern for the common good. The introduction of Medicare and Medicaid, for example, although a result of compromise, nevertheless can be seen as a response to deeply felt needs and widely experienced gaps in the distribution of high quality health care. Many hospitals had already been moving toward different forms of inter-organizational cooperation such as medical centers, multiservice clinics, community health care systems, and inter-community or regional care and referral systems. Now, these developments are becoming mandatory in view of the need for centralized facilities providing the whole spectrum of specialized services at an adequate level of quality and cost. At the same time, public involvement in the provision of health care is likely to increase, both at the level of planning and the mobilization of resources and at the level of auditing hospital operations and insuring the public accountability of hospitals. This may not necessarily take the form of patients refusing to take medicine or engaging in demonstrations, but it is likely to lead to greater patient participation in medical decision-making and, consequently, to a reduction of the unquestioned professional authority of physicians and other hospital personnel. The operation of patient councils in some mental hospitals can perhaps be seen as a step in this direction.

In short, there is both increasing pressure and slow but visible change in the direction of creating institutions of health care geared to the idea of health as a fundamental right, rather than to a conception of health as a personal or class privilege to be purchased in the market place. The reorganization of health care with a view toward the common good has been a major element in many recent policies issuing from the U.S. Public Health Service, the Department of Health, Education and Welfare, and even from the presidential level. The traditional hospital is changing under the influence of ideas such as combining public and private medical systems; providing integrated networks of hospitals, clinics, and other institutional arrangements, including group practice, to serve the entire community; and, generally, rationalizing and improving the provision and administration of health care.

While government policies and programs are not in and of themselves necessarily better or more rational than those formulated by responsible health professionals, federal involvement is usually a response to inadequacies on the local level which have harmful consequences for the public good (e.g., the handling of riots, unemployment, discrimination in housing and education, the fragmentation of metropolitan government, etc.). For this reason, the centralization of functions under delegated authority may be an optimal response to the continuing problems of health care organization.

The research reported here can be no more than a small contribution to the larger goal of social progress. But it is hoped to be such a contribution.

Furthermore, and on technical grounds, I believe that research based on a comparative-quantitative analysis of a large number of organizations and of a number of significant characteristics for each case will enable the social scientist to improve the power of existing theories of organizations and, if necessary, to develop new and more adequate ones. This book is therefore not directed at organizational problem-solving, but at identifying the general conditions underlying different organizational solutions extant among modern hospitals. It is thus an attempt to examine the joint outcome of evolution and planning of hospital organization, and by implication and extrapolation to say something about the future direction of these processes.

The research on which this book is based was conceived in 1961 and completed in 1965. The original plan was to compare empirically different types of organizations, such as hospitals, universities, business organizations, government agencies, and other "bureaucracies" in terms of general sociological and organizational concepts. However, the task of dealing with a large number of cases and variables simultaneously became technically so overwhelming and involved that it was necessary to limit the initial research effort to one basic organizational type. This decision, in turn, made it desirable and feasible to study structural variations within that type. The choice fell on hospitals partly because they are among the most interesting formal organizations I have encountered, partly because the variations among hospitals permit the systematic study of many theoretically important attributes of professional organizations, and partly because data were available on a large number of cases. Moreover, the raw data did lend themselves to the construction of various operational indicators amenable to multivariate statistical analysis.

The original plan for the research reported here called for a two-step strategy, i.e., an analysis of the available hospital statistics followed by an interview survey of a sample of hospitals. Thus, new questions and lines of investigation emerging from the analysis of the statistical data were to become the focus of a more detailed study based on interviews with key informants, e.g., the hospital administrator, the director of nursing, and the chief of the medical staff in each of the hospitals. In this way it was hoped to maximize the gains of the quantitative analysis and to supplement it by a more qualitative and focused inquiry into the processes of decision-making and innovation. This second part of the research scheme was not carried through for hospitals due to limitations of time and funds. But the general strategy of combining the analysis of published statistical data with those from a direct survey of organizations proved to be a useful idea. Thus, the substantive results and theoretical implications drawn from the general approach developed in the present study led to the consideration and planning of a series of similar comparative studies. These studies were to focus on different types of organizations within a common theoretical and comparative framework, thus implementing the original idea of comparative organizational research which also underlies the conception of the present study. In the summer of 1964, the National Science Foundation, under Grant GS-553, provided funds for the establishment of a comprehensive organizational research program with Peter Blau and myself as principal investigators. The Comparative Organization Research Program which had been established at the University of Chicago can be seen as a direct outgrowth of the ideas, methods, and mistakes discussed in this book. It was thus not without pride that I witnessed the continuity of research already established before this book was completed.

The book contains four major parts. Part I deals with the relation between sociological theory and organizational analysis. Chapter 2 in particular presents the principal conceptual and theoretical dimensions of this study. Chapter 3 deals with the operationalization of these concepts. Chapter 4 provides the theoretical background for the relationships between autonomy, task complexity, division of labor, and coordination. It represents an attempt to integrate the ideas of Durkheim, Weber, and the classical and neo-classical organization theorists. This chapter concludes with a statement of the major hypotheses of this study.

Part II deals with the analysis of hospitals as prototypes of modern work organizations. Chapter 5 deals with the basic comparative design which classifies hospitals according to the degree of organizational autonomy and task complexity. In Chapter 6, the structure of medical technology is analyzed, together with a historical comparison using 1935 Public Health census data on hospitals as a baseline. Chapter 7 discusses the interrelations between organizational size and the division of labor, using for the first time empirical data in the comparative-quantitative analysis of a large number of organizations.

Part III is concerned with the problem of coordination in hospitals and in modern professional organizations in general. Building on the analysis of structural variation among hospitals presented in Part II, Part III deals with the patterns of bureaucratic and non-bureaucratic administration that are developing in response to different kinds and degrees of task complexity. Chapter 8 discusses the role of professionals in organizations, with particular emphasis on the role of nursing in modern patient care. Chapter 9 represents an analysis of the bureaucratic modes of administration, i.e., administrative specialization and hierarchical differentiation, again using historical data for comparative purposes. Chapter 10 deals with certain nonbureaucratic modes of coordination, notably the effect of professionalization and departmentalization on each other and on the modes of bureaucratic administration.

Finally, Part IV is an epilogue on the uses and limits of bureaucracy. Chapter 11 deals with the consequences of viewing hospitals as organizational models in their own right for the theoretical conception of organizations in general and for the future development of hospitals in particular.

I am happy to acknowledge the many debts I have incurred in undertaking this work. For their generous advice and support at various stages of this work, as well as for their comments on parts of the manuscript, I want to thank especially Odin Anderson, Peter Blau, George Bugbee, Robert Crain, James Davis, Jack Feldman, Louis Pondy, Jack Sawyer, Arthur Stinchcombe, Seymour Warkov, Harrison White, and Mayer Zald. For an especially valuable critical reading of the entire manuscript, I want to thank Dennis Magill, Jay Noell, and Stanley Udy.

During the period between 1961 and 1967, a number of organizations gave financial support to this study. Acknowledgment of support is due to:

The Ford Foundation for providing a Fellowship in Organization Research in 1961 and a Research Grant in 1962;

The Kellogg Foundation for a Fellowship in 1962-63;

The Health Information Foundation for a Research Grant in 1963-64;

The National Science Foundation for Grant GS-553, 1964-67.

The use of computer facilities was supported by the Biological Sciences Computation Center, University of Chicago, under USPHS Grant FR-00013 from the Division of Research, Facilities and Resources of the National Institutes of Health, and also by the IBM 7094 Computation Center, University of Chicago, under a grant from the National Science Foundation.

I also want to acknowledge the support of USPHS Grant CH-00024 under the auspices of the Medical Care Research Center and its Executive Director, Dr. Rodney Coe, at Washington University. In particular, I want to thank Mrs. Irene Brown, Mrs. Lee Drifon, Miss Mary Peters, Mrs. Freda Sofian, and Mrs. Marcella Waddell for their help in preparing the manuscript.

Wolf Heydebrand

1

Introduction: The Changing Nature of Organizations

To treat the hospital as the prototype of modern work organization is to acknowledge, paradoxically, that it is a rapidly changing type of organization. The change itself has many sources, elements, and consequences. Examples are the continuous changes in technology, in the skill structure, and, generally, in the internal division of labor of the modern hospital. Increasing complexities in the nature of the tasks to be performed and in the internal division of labor have far-reaching consequences for the bases of legitimacy, the structure of authority, and the modes of coordination and control. Changing definitions of patient care impose new demands for competence and expertise on hospital personnel. New goals and changing conceptions of the functions of medical care in hospitals have an impact on what can legitimately be expected of doctors, patients, hospital administration, and personnel. Perhaps the central element of all these changes is the increasing diversification, heterogeneity, and even fragmentation of activities which, though separate and specialized, ultimately contribute in some fashion to the realization of the avowed purposes of the organization.

The changing nature of organizations makes it difficult to define precisely what an organization is and to distinguish it from other types of social structure. Besides, it may not be useful to treat an organization as a phenomenon sui generis if the aim of the analysis is to generalize from hospitals to other kinds of organizations and from organizations to other kinds of social structure.

Thus, rather than following a rigorous and formal definition of what an organization is, it will simply be assumed here that a hospital is a kind of social structure which is formally established to serve a number of specific purposes. "Social structure," in turn, is viewed as a network of relationships based on the recurrent interactions among individuals, groups, and sets of groups. This use of the term "social structure" differs from others in that it is not solely conceived as a normative-cognitive or prescriptive-model in terms of which interactions will occur and recur; nor is it conceived as an equilibrium-seeking and boundary-maintaining action system. It also differs from other conceptions in that it subordinates technology and other aspects of the man-made world to the definitions and realities of interacting individuals and groups. The hospital is thus not seen as "having" a technology, a social structure, and a formal organization, but as a cluster of social relationships, some of which involve the use of machines and are formally arranged.

The idea of social structure as a normative theoretical model comes closest to the sociological concept of institution, an expected way of doing things, a value pattern that has become embodied in a certain social arrangement. This normative model, i.e., an institution, is not to be confused with the actual, empirical character of organizations as formally established groups or social structures. Definitions of organizations range from Barnard's informal "composition of cooperative acts"[1] to Weber's rationally planned and operated bureaucracy. More generally, most definitions contain the idea that organizations are formally established for the explicit purpose of achieving specific objectives. It is this latter notion of planned, formally defined relationships which underlies a constitution, a set of by-laws, or an organization chart. Conceptually, then, "constitution" ties together the idea of organization, community, and national society. While a constitution is also a kind of model of an organization, it is so in the sense of a formal charter. Thus, it remains the empirical object of analysis rather than becoming a theoretical model, i.e., a system of analytical concepts used to describe the object in the first place.

In the following, I will outline some of the problem areas in modern organizations where the nature of change appears to be most critical. This discussion will also serve to identify some of the substantive theoretical questions which have stimulated the research underlying this book. Next, I will indicate the aims and objectives of this study as well as its limitations. Finally, I will briefly discuss the data and methods used in this research.

Critical Areas of Change in Organizations

The fact that modern organizations are changing entities does not mean that all organizations are changing equally rapidly, nor that all aspects of organizational life are equally involved in this change. Among hospitals, for example, psychiatric hospitals tend to be more immune to change than general ones, and nonteaching hospitals more than teaching hospitals. This statement can be generalized to the effect that multi-functional and diversified organizations are more likely undergoing change than unifunctional, nondiversified ones. A corollary of this generalization is that the more complex a system is, the more open it is for change; and the more open it is, the more it will be under pressure to change. The causal sequence here is, of course, not entirely unidirectional. Diversification and the proliferation of goals may simply be indicators of adaptation to changing conditions, while at the same time generating internal inconsistencies, making the organizational boundaries more permeable, and opening the whole structure to external influences.

While the question of causality, in the strict sense, must await further quantitative-comparative study of organizations over time, it is possible to identify certain processes which continue to have a crucial impact on organizational life and on traditional conceptions of organizational structure. In particular, I want to refer to three of these processes of change: the modification of the basis of legitimacy and authority by changes in the complexity of the task structure and in the requisite technology; the development of coordination involving both functional centralization (e.g., the use of computers) and nonbureaucratic forms of administration (e.g., the use of "generalist" professional practitioners or craftsmen for certain complex sub-tasks, or the establishment of joint committees and other horizontal channels of communication for purposes of lateral coordination and mutual regulation among different hierarchies); and the transformation of the role of salaried professionals working in an organizational context.

The hierarchical structuring of authority as embodied in an organizational pyramid has long been viewed as a sine qua non of administrative efficiency, especially insofar as it reflects the operation of an integrated system of legitimate values and authoritative goal-attainment. However, the present study suggests that the relevance of hierarchical coordination may be limited to conditions of low task complexity and high routinization of work. Even where complex problem-solving is capable of routinization, standardization, and "seriability," by design or by default, hierarchical administrative patterns may, indeed, be more effective and therefore more prevalent, as in large mental hospitals. But where the task complexity is generated by multiple and diverse objectives, nonbureaucratic, "associational" forms of administration involving lateral coordination will predominate. Examples are general teaching hospitals, as documented in the present study, or pre-industrial work organizations with diffuse, multiple objectives.[2]

Weber has dealt with these nonbureaucratic forms of administration partly in terms of the principle of collegiality. Collegial authority limits or modifies monocratic authority by virtue of one or more of the following arrangements: separation of powers, consultation among experts, cooperation among a plurality of individuals or advisory collegial bodies, mutual veto powers, and voting.[3] However, Weber believed that the prevalent value orientations of his time and society as well as economic interests in efficiency would lead to a preference for a monocratic type of organization. Although the concept of collegial authority has been applied in empirical studies mainly to the structure of medical professional authority,[4] it is clearly relevant also to the patterns of administration in modern work organizations such as hospitals, welfare organizations, research institutes and universities, modern military units, and business corporations, especially the larger diversified industrial conglomerates.

In short, it has been shown by a number of students of organizations that monocratic, hierarchical authority is not a necessary element of complex task administration, and may actually impede it or simply be inefficient. By the same token, it has been suggested that alternative or additional modes of coordination are operating under conditions of complex task performance, including the use of market and price mechanisms as well as various types of social and symbolic incentives. The emergence of new, competing bases of legitimacy and the operation of multiple modes of coordination are invariably tied to the complexity, variability, and change of the organizational goal and task structure, and to the related changes in technology, skill level, and division of labor.

Gouldner, for example, develops the distinction between representative and punishment-centered bureaucracy from his comparative analysis of work arrangements in the gypsum mine and

4

of the surface operations. The more complex and more dangerous situation in the mine proves to be a powerful determinant of the "representative" pattern.[5]

Similarly, Janowitz has shown that changes in the goal structure as well as in the technology of the modern military establishment lead to far-reaching changes in traditional conceptions and practices involving the role of hierarchical authority in military command. Thus, the increasing complexity of military technology, division of labor, and task structure lead to the emergence of multiple hierarchies and competing lines of authority. Organizational pyramids are being transformed into diamond-shaped forms, with the middle levels of the hierarchies bulging with technical specialists as well as managerial, service, and clerical job categories. The exercise of direct military rank authority is supplemented, if not supplanted, by cooperation and lateral coordination among technically specialized units. The emphasis in the control-compliance nexus shifts from domination to manipulation.[6]

In modern hospitals, similar changes are visible. The effect of technical skill and specialized expertise on the work process and on discretionary decision-making at the work level suggests that the professionalization of the hospital labor force tends to modify and replace bureaucratic coordination. Nevertheless, both professional and bureaucratic modes of coordination may be subsumed under the concept of rational administration.[7]

The present study shows that both professional and bureaucratic coordination may coexist in the same organization and that both may, in turn, be modified by the nature of the internal division of labor, especially by the extent of departmental specialization. Thus, the interrelation between division of labor, professionalization, and coordination has an important further implication. The results of this study suggest that the characteristics of professional work are not impermeable to change and transformation under the influence of a changing division of labor. In distinguishing between two conceptions of professional (person-specialized) work, namely a client or person-oriented form of general practice and a task-oriented, specialist form, one may assume that an organizational setting provides both context and purpose for the increased technical specialization of professionals. But as professional work becomes functionally more specific, it contributes relatively less to organizational coordination. This situation, in turn, increases the need for the coordination of specialists. One may speculate that once this process has advanced to the point where professionals are highly job-specialized, the development of differentiated subunits and departments around these specialized functions will lead to an increased interdependence between them, and hence to still other forms of coordination and integration, including, paradoxically, delegation and hierarchization among specialists within subunits, but also teamwork, ad hoc functional task groups, and other types of cooperative work organization.

In sum, it is my thesis that the nature of organizational control has been profoundly altered by the increasing complexity in the goal and task structure of modern organizations, by the emergence of multiple bases of legitimacy, by nonbureaucratic modes of coordination such as the use of generalist professions and lateral mechanisms of coordination, and by the professional's own transformation of his role from generalist practitioner to technical specialist.

Objectives and Limitations of This Study

This study has four objectives: to develop a theoretical framework for the analysis of formal organizations; to devise appropriate methodological procedures which are applicable primarily where organizations as a whole are chosen as the unit of analysis; to test the usefulness of both the theory and the methods by applying them to data on U.S. hospitals; and to draw substantive conclusions as to the present structure and future development of modern hospitals.

Theoretically, this study is an attempt to integrate certain perspectives on the division of labor and the problem of coordination and control in complex social structures. Let me briefly indicate what I mean by "theory" and "theoretical". In sociology, the term "theory" refers to a variety of different intellectual operations, as Paul Lazarsfeld has pointed out. Following his lead, the term "theory" is used in this study in a relatively broad sense and refers to a series of what Lazarsfeld calls "analytical procedures". This felicitously broad notion of theory makes it easier to understand and accomodate the process of systematic reflexion in sociology.[8]

Among the basic assumptions reaching into the conceptual apparatus of this study, I want to single out two which are particularly important to me. The first is that social and organizational change are seen as continuous processes. In the study of organizations this perspective implies an emphasis on the formation, persistence, and resistance to change of social and organizational structures, be they private enterprises, semi-public service systems, or the governmental bureaucracies of nation-states. Rather than assuming organizations to be stable systems, the conditions of their stability are taken as problematic.

Secondly, it is assumed that all forms of social organization involve, and perhaps require, some integration and coordination of activities, but that the form and mode of coordination is problematic. To raise the question of social integration in this form, however, points up two fundamental dimensions of social organization which are not—and perhaps never can be—entirely compatible. The two dimensions are best formulated in terms of a series of alternatives or antinomies; they could even be conceived analytically as the horizontal and the vertical dimensions of a coordinate system in which the phenomena of the empirical social world are located. Thus, human social behavior can be described variously in terms of free-floating interaction vs. socialization into a common culture, interests vs. values, association vs. normative integration, and the definition of new goals vs. the attainment of given goals. While these analytical elements can be conceived as phases of a dialectical process, certain corresponding social structures may result and become objectified, such as society vs. the state, private vs. public law (the law of coordination vs. the law of subordination), the economic vs. the political dimension of organizations and institutions, work vs. authority, cooperation vs. conflict, exchange vs. power, and division of labor vs. coordination.

It should be apparent from this list that there is a tendency in sociology, and perhaps in Western cultures, to equate the horizontal dimension with differentiation, division, heterogeneity, pluralism, opposition, conflict, and anarchy, and the vertical dimension with integration, unity, homogeneity, consensus, control, and order. But it is my purpose here to explore also those variations of these dimensions which, on the one hand, reveal the integrative, associational possibilities of horizontal diversity and the divisive, alienating aspects of vertical differentiation.

Translated into operational concepts and applied to organizations, this approach implies that functional and hierarchical differentiation are taken not as the constants of a type or model, but as variables; not as givens of a "realistic" view of the world, but as problematic; not as principles of bureaucratic-organizational efficiency, but as instruments of rational planning in the midst of continuous social change.

In short, there is nothing "inevitable" and "diabolic" about the nature of large-scale, complex, formal organizations. They are neither purely evolving and adaptive natural-organic systems, nor robot-like, mechanical feedback systems beyond human control.

Seen from this perspective, the differences between such "natural" system models as that of Parsons and "rational" system models as that of Simon are more apparent than real.[9] Whether natural or rational, the very notion of a system implies a conception of organizations as unitary structures, integrated in terms of over-arching (cognitive or normative) symbols of legitimation.

The approach taken here implies, further, that various attributes of social structure can and should be studied independently of the attributes of individuals, but without relinquishing the claim that human social organization is the result of human purposes and actions. It implies that structural attributes are variable and measurable, and that the relationships between them may vary themselves along different dimensions.

Finally, this approach assumes that the coordination of social structural elements may take more than one form and, specifically, that in formal organizations it may take forms which are non-bureaucratic or nonhierarchical, or which supplement the more traditional bureaucratic modes of administration.

The following are the main structural variables involved in this analysis:

1. *Organizational Autonomy*: the extent to which an organization is independent of an external locus of decision-making, including the limitations of the organization's financial, political, and legal status.

2. *Complexity of Task Structure:* scope, specificity and stability of objectives and size of task, reflecting the underlying goal structure; the degree to which the task structure is differentiated in terms of the number and diversity of objectives; multiple bases of legitimacy and separate hierarchies; and the degree of uncertainty and variability in task structure.

3. *Complexity of Organizational Environment:* the degree to which the social, economic, ecological, and demographic environment of the organization is itself organizationally differentiated; and the types and rates of interaction across organizational boundaries.

4. *Organizational Size:* the size of the organizational labor force; in some situations this variable can be defined in terms of the size of the task, or size of resources, subsuming both under task complexity.

5. *Technological Complexity:* the degree of mechanization and automation of the work process; the extent of use of machines, technical facilities and equipment, and nonhuman sources of energy, and the extent of employment of technical personnel.

6. *Internal Division of Labor:*
   a. *Functional Specialization:* the total amount of division of labor among specific work functions.
   b. *Departmental Specialization:* the degree of differentiation among departments or organizational components.

7. *Professionalization:* the formal training and technical expertise of the nonmanagerial labor force, i.e., of subordinates; and the level of "generalist" and "specialist" professional skill of the organizational production component or of personnel on the operating level.

8. *Bureaucratization:*
   a. *Bureaucratic Hierarchy:* within a given hierarchy, the number and relative size of hierarchical levels in terms of which organizational authority is structured; the proportion of supervisors and managers; and the average span of control.
   b. *Administrative-Clerical Specialization:* the relative size of the administrative-clerical staff.

9. *Organizational Effectiveness:* the extent of goal-attainment per time unit; volume and quality of output; availability of skills and resources, and efficiency and quality of service.

These structural variables are conceived, first of all, as basic, general characteristics of formal organizations. They are based on existing theory as well as previous empirical research and permit the exploration and testing of theoretical relationships within a comparative (cross-structural) framework through the use of multivariate statistical analysis.

While these structural variables are not all on the same level of generality, taken together they provide the conceptual underpinning of a theoretical framework for the empirical analysis of different types of organizations. The operational definitions of these variables and their interrelations will be discussed in the next chapters.

The basic research design of this study aims at the systematic comparison of twelve hospital types. These types are the result of a three-way classification of hospitals in terms of medical service (general vs. psychiatric), teaching status (teaching vs. nonteaching), and external control (federal Veterans' Administration, state, and local governmental—or, in short, "public"—and voluntary non-profit—or "private—hospitals). Moreover, the determination of technological and structural differences between the hospital types makes it possible to develop a number of organizational types representing specific constellations of teaching, service, and control as well as simple and complex internal division of labor.

In order to investigate the variation of structural characteristics *between* the twelve different organizational types separately from the variation occurring *within* types, two kinds of analyses were employed. They yielded essentially different kinds of results.

The analysis of structural differences (the between-group analysis) leads us to understand a range of different types of organizations regardless of the fact that they happen to be called "hospitals." This analysis demonstrates the relative prevalence of certain organizational characteristics, such as the professionalization of the labor force or the bureaucratization of professionals. By the same token, it is possible to investigate and compare the prevalence of organizational characteristics in government agencies, welfare agencies, business corporations, etc. under various external conditions.[10]

By contrast, the analysis of structural relationships within the different types of organizations results in statements about the functioning of any one type of organization. In this case, then, it is assumed that elements of organizational structure and coordination stand in a relation of mutual dependence and causal influence, and that changes in one element of organizational structure will bring about changes in others. Obviously, it is feasible under this assumption to investigate the similarity of the characteristics of a given organizational type to possible system-properties of the organization.

By using the between-group analysis as a prerequisite for the within-group analysis, i.e., by developing organizational types and then looking at the relationships within each type, it is possible to combine and integrate the methodology as well as the results of both the comparative and the structural-functional analysis of organizations.

Perhaps the most important single conclusion from this study is that an understanding of organizational structure cannot be obtained from the correlation of any two characteristics alone. While the relationships between size, complexity, division of labor, professionalization, bureaucratization, and other variables have been studied before, it is the *patterns* of their *interrelations* which constitute the central concern of this study.

Yet, at the same time, it becomes clear that statements about processes of organizational development and change are not possible without taking into account the relations between the organization and other organizations in its environment. The concept of an organizationally differentiated environment is intended to avoid the notion of external influences as residual, and to convey the idea of a structured context which may be just as variable as the organizational structure itself. For these reasons, the two kinds of analysis used in this study constitute a minimum methodological requirement for relating intra-organizational to inter-organizational analysis.

In sum, this study aims at advancing the analysis of organizations beyond the case-study approach. While the use of a random sample of organizations might have been sufficient for answering certain kinds of questions, the possibility of using practically the universe of American hospitals made it feasible to deal with a broad scope of theoretical issues and substantive hypotheses. This fortunate circumstance also enabled me to perform certain crucial comparisons in a systematic fashion, such as between different types of organizational autonomy, as well as between different types and degrees of task complexity.

An analysis of the kind undertaken here offers not only advantages; it also has certain limitations. Among the most important ones are the relatively high level of abstraction and the problem of simplification. Both problems are involved insofar as we are dealing with many organizations, rather than one or two, and with multivariate relationships, rather than a concrete "gestalt" of familiar experiences. Both of these limitations have contradictory implications for interpreting and communicating the results of research.

As far as the level of abstraction is concerned, it derives mainly from the fact that this study focuses on structural relationships in organizations, i.e., on the covariation among general organizational characteristics. Although the raw data are based on census-type hospital statistics, their transformation and adaptation for the purpose of constructing operational variables as indicators of the underlying theoretical concepts makes them less accessible to intuitive understanding. The multiple statistical relationships between such abstract variables are, indeed, difficult to communicate, especially when it is necessary to keep several different relationships in mind simultaneously.

As to the second difficulty, simplification, it must first be said that it is inevitable in any scientific endeavor; that is to say, the very process of conceptualizing and abstracting aspects of the empirical world involves simplification. Looking at an individual hospital as a historical, unique, complex organization is one thing. Some famous case-studies of hospitals give the reader a sense of that complexity.[11] Another point of contact with that complex reality is the overwhelming, fascinating, and confusing experience many persons have as participants in the ongoing processes of hospital life, be it as patients or staff members.

But to analyze a large sample of hospitals in terms of a small set of variables is quite another thing. It implies a kind of regression to a cruder level of insight, just as Durkheim's "Suicide" or most modern survey research implies the simplification of complex social and individual phenomena. It implies imposing an arbitrarily simple model on situations which, from the point of view of everyday individual experience and common sense, cannot be simplified. Thus, while simplicity is a goal of scientific description and explanation, its results battle against one's sense of wholeness, detail, and richness of experience. Consequently, an attempt to describe hospitals as large, complex, formal, professional organizations makes it difficult to do justice to the need for concrete understanding, intuitive insight, and literary detail.

But the description of complex relationships, if based on a large number of cases, also enables the researcher to take a broader approach to the problem of organizational analysis. Moreover, it is claimed here that such an approach is a necessary condition for building a theory of organizations.

Although it is my personal predilection and style to look at the complexity of an issue rather than its simple, immediate appearance, it will at times be necessary to talk about its simplified, abstract, underlying structure. For these reasons it is hoped that the reader will bear in mind the difficulty of achieving a balance between the two sides of this dilemma.

Data and Method

The data for this research were collected by the American Hospital Association (A.H.A.) as part of a routine questionnaire survey of their member hospitals in 1959. These survey data represent about 7,000 U.S. hospitals. This is not the complete universe of American hospitals since questionnaires are mailed only to those hospitals listed with the A.H.A., with a return rate of over 90 per cent. Listing is voluntary. Hospitals accepted for listing must meet certain requirements, the most important of which are as follows:

The hospital shall have at least six beds for the care of patients who are nonrelated, who are sick, and who stay on the average in excess of 24 hours per admission.

Only doctors of medicine or osteopathy shall practice in hospitals listed by the A.H.A.

Records of clinical work shall be maintained by the hospital on all patients.

Registered nurse supervision and such other nursing service as is necessary for patient care around the clock shall be available; further, there should be surgical and obstetrical facilities and complete diagnostic and treatment facilities for medical patients.[12]

Hospitals not listed by the A.H.A. are either those that would qualify but have not applied, or have applied and are awaiting a decision, or do not meet the listing requirements. In general, according to A.H.A. tabulations, "unlisted hospitals are small and have a relatively small number of patient-days."[13]

The data used for this study were collected in 1959, covering the twelve-month period ending September 30, 1959. Questionnaires were sent to 6,920 hospitals and returned by 6,470. Thus, the initial response rate was 93.5 per cent. Through follow-up mailings as well as through pressure exerted on the delinquent hospitals by the respective State Hospital Associations, a total of 6,845 hospitals returned questionnaires. After eliminating those hospitals for which data were incomplete, the final total used in the present study was 6,825.

An unusual feature of the 1959 survey is its detailed classification of occupations and personnel available for individual hospitals. This information serves as the basis for the construction of a number of variables, such as functional and departmental specialization, professionalization, hierarchical differentiation, the relative size of the administrative-clerical staff, and certain aspects of technological complexity.

The quality of these data and the extent to which they can be considered valid is discussed in Appendix A.

A crucial step in preparing the data for analysis was the transformation of the raw data into variables. The technical aspects of that operation are discussed in Appendix B.

As indicated earlier, the data represent all listed U.S. hospitals in a given classification (except a few cases eliminated because of insufficient reporting), and they are therefore not subject to sampling error. Nevertheless, they are treated as if they were, in fact, sampled from a larger universe. Statistically, the major emphasis is on the analysis of variation and covariation rather than on the prediction of relationships on the basis of regression analysis. Therefore, generalizations about properties of hospitals qua hospitals refer only to the groups of hospitals under study. Generalizations about characteristics of hospitals qua formal organizations are qualified according to context and type of analysis from which they derive.

Summary

In this introductory chapter, I have sought to outline some of the problem areas common to complex professional organizations, typified by the modern hospital.

Summarizing the main points, from a slightly different perspective, the following may be argued.

Professional services, in general, can be seen as strongly influenced by a change in the "supply and demand" structure, due to a continuing trend of rising educational standards in a more or less affluent society.

In very simple terms, this change has created a more informed and "knowledgeable" public that is concerned with the availability and quality of specialized service. On the other hand, the hospital, as an organization, must implement goals that seem to become more and more contradictory. It must provide the setting or framework in which the principles and practices of modern business and technology can be successfully related to the standards and imagery of "helping people" as derived from ethical precepts, social and psychological insights, and medical practice.

Thus, an affluent and sophisticated public demands a great variety of services from an organization that responds by employing highly trained specialists who, in turn, and for a price, cater to an almost endless number of "human needs" with the latest devices and formulas of modern science and technology. It is these interacting forces that have drastically changed the structure and organization of the hospital.

Three issues, in particular, shape the administration of complex professional service. One is the emergence of *multiple* bases of legitimacy and authority as a consequence of changes in the goal and task structure of professional organizations. The second issue, resulting primarily from higher educational standards, concerns the increasing prominence of nonbureaucratic modes of coordination, especially the professionalization of the nonmanagerial labor force and the development of lateral paths of communication and coordination. Finally, the role of professionals in organizations is still in flux, and several patterns can be delineated. All of them are based on the interpenetration of professional and organizational roles, while the transformation of professionals from general practitioners to specialists is continuing.

In terms of research objectives, this study tries to use a comparative-quantitative approach in the study of hospitals as formal organizations. This requires that a theoretical framework and an appropriate methodology for organizational analysis must be developed, and that their usefulness is tested and explored on the basis of the data collected from about 7,000 American hospitals.

Notes

1. Chester I. Barnard, *Organization and Management* (Cambridge, Mass.: Harvard University Press, 1948), p. 118.
2. Stanley H. Udy, Jr., *Organization of Work* (New Haven, Conn.: Human Relations Area File Press, 1959), p. 40.
3. Max Weber, *The Theory of Social and Economic Organization*, tr. A.M. Henderson and Talcott Parsons, ed. Talcott Parsons (New York: Oxford University Press, 1947), pp. 392-407; Max Rheinstein, ed., *Max Weber on Law in Economy and Society*, tr. Edward A. Shils and Max Rheinstein (Cambridge, Mass.: Harvard University Press, 1954), pp. 322-348.
4. Mary E.W. Goss, "Patterns of Bureaucracy Among Hospital Staff Physicians," in Eliot Freidson, ed., *The Hospital in Modern Society* (Glencoe, Ill.: The Free Press, 1963), pp. 170-194.
5. A.W. Gouldner, *Patterns of Industrial Bureaucracy* (Glencoe, Ill.: The Free Press, 1954), pp. 105-154.
6. Morris Janowitz, *Sociology and the Military Establishment* (New York: Russell Sage, 1959), pp. 24-43, 83-100; see also *The Professional Soldier* (Glencoe, Ill.: The Free Press, 1960), pp. 21-37, 54-78.
7. Arthur L. Stinchcombe, "Bureaucratic and Craft Administration of Production: A Comparative Study," *Administrative Science Quarterly*, IV (1959), 184-187.
8. Paul F. Lazarsfeld, *Qu'est ce que la sociologie?* Paris: Gallimard, 1970, pp. 76-77.
9. A. W. Gouldner, "Organizational Analysis," in Robert K. Merton et. al., eds., *Sociology Today* (New York: Basic Books, 1959), pp. 400-429; Talcott Parsons, "An Outline of the Social System," in Talcott Parsons et al., eds., *Theories of Society* (New York: The Free Press, 1961), Vol. I, pp. 30-79; Herbert A. Simon, *Administrative Behavior* (2nd ed; New York: Macmillan, 1957), and *Models of Man* (New York: Wiley, 1957); Tom Burns and George M. Stalker, *The Management of Innovation* (London: Tavistock, 1961).
10. For a discussion of some examples of this type of comparative research, see Wolf V. Heydebrand, "The Study of Organizations," *Social Science Information*, VI,5 (1967), 59-86.
11. Temple Burling et al., *The Give and Take in Hospitals* (New York: Putnam, 1956); Alfred H. Stanton and Morris F. Schwartz, *The Mental Hospital* (New York: Basic Books, 1954); William Caudill, *The Psychiatric*

Hospital as a Small Society. (Cambridge, Mass.: Harvard University Press, 1958).

12. *Hospital Accreditation References* (Chicago: American Hospital Association, 1961), p. xi.

13. "Hospitals," *Journal of the American Hospital Association,* XXXIV (1960), Guide Issue, Part II, 413.

Part I: Sociological Theory and Organizational Analysis

2   Hospital Bureaucracy: A Theoretical Framework

If the purpose of organizations is to achieve specific objectives according to some kind of plan or design, one may well try to understand their structure and functioning in terms of the component parts of such a plan. In a given society organizations with similar objectives might be expected to represent, or approximate, an underlying collective design, assuming limited resources and rationality of decision-making. There may be cultural differences as to what resources are available, and how they are utilized, i.e., according to what schedule of priorities they are allocated. But also within a given culture or macro-economic system, one may assume a certain degree of variation of such broad external factors. Hence, attention must be focused on the structural variation within a given cultural, macro-economic, political context, as well as on the variable and conflicting elements of that context itself.

Viewed from this perspective, the problem of organizational analysis may be paraphrased in terms of Lasswell's definition of politics.[1] Applied to organizations, Lasswell's question reads: who *does* what, why, and how? In shorthand form, this question draws attention to variables which would constitute a minimum conceptual baseline in any comparative organizational analysis. Thus, to answer the "who does what, why, and how" of organizations requires information on their identity, boundaries, and autonomy, their socio-environmental context, their goal and task structure, including size and some measure of goal-attainment, their technology and division of labor, and their control structure.)

In this chapter, then, let us first look briefly at the external and internal determinants of hospital organization in order to illuminate the interrelation of these major structural characteristics. There is, of course, no single or absolutely valid procedure for doing so.

The inherent limitation of the scientific method in terms of assumptions about causality forces the process of inquiry into a continuous interplay between inductive and deductive reasoning. The empirical "grounding" of theory is therefore just as dependent on certain prescientific categorical and causal assumptions as "axiomatic theory" is on empirical observation and certain factual givens.[2] Needless to say, the casual structure is imposed on the underlying reality; some might argue it is the only reality we can see. In that sense, any causal structure represents a model of that segment of reality under study, with a greater or smaller degree of "goodness of fit."

Tracing causal relationships can be done in two ways: proceeding from the more general, determining conditions to the specific outcome of a given set of dynamically related factors and forces; or vice versa, proceeding from the specific event, phenomenon, or problem to the general causes. In each case, there are likely to be multiple levels of factors, the intermediate causes often being referred to as "intervening variables."

The following outline may be seen as a first step toward a suggested causal ordering of the variables involved. After such a general overview of the relationships between the major dimensions, the remainder of this chapter will be concerned with the elaboration of these relationships in more specific theoretical terms.

Determinants of Hospital Bureaucracy: A Causal Scheme

Proceeding first from the general to the specific factors, the following picture of the determinants of hospital organization emerges.

The major purposes and objectives of hospitals have changed greatly during the course of historical development. From alms-houses and pesthouses, orphanages, and shelters for the aged, infirm, and insane, hospitals have developed into agencies of medical care, research, and education, directly and indirectly benefiting almost all members of the modern community. The task, once circumscribed by the need to provide custody, to protect the community, and to conform to norms of charity, has developed into a complex network of services, made possible by advances in medical science and technology and at the same time demanded by an increasingly critical clientele. It is not necessary here to trace the history of the American hospital. This development is well and widely documented.[3] But is is important to stress that the modern hospital is the result of the intricate interplay of many factors, ranging from scientific and technological change to social and economic, demographic and regional-geographic, religious and political factors to the dynamics of professional development and organizational differentiation. Nor should it be overlooked that not all of these factors have unequivocally favored the development of the modern hospital. Thus, considerations of status and tradition, convenience and profit, and values and dogma did often have an impeding and retarding influence.[4]

Definitions of the goals and objectives of hospitals almost always include references to patient care, staff training, and medical research. The distinction between curative and preventive medicine enters less frequently into such a definition, and the distinction between different treatment goals is made only with respect to psychiatric hospitals.[5] Since most studies of hospitals are case studies, focusing moreover on intra-organizational factors and the influence of the hospital setting on interpersonal relationships and on the therapeutic goal, the question of uniformity or variations in task structure, size, and autonomy is seldom raised explicitly or on a comparative or quantitative basis. Thus, knowledge about hospitals is largely based on the descriptions of specific types such as the small private psychiatric hospital,[6] the large state mental hospital,[7] the small community hospital,[8] and the community general hospital.[9] In addition, there is, of course, a wealth of studies of different aspects of hospitals such as wards, departments, personnel groups, administration, interpersonal relations, and patient subculture, to name only a few categories.

It is possible to describe the hospital's task structure in a variety of terms. Thus, a broad description of the hospital as a "multipurpose institution" may include the following functions: economic enterprise, provision of medical care, professional decision-making, that of a social agency (which nevertheless is subject to the "test of financial solvency" like a business enterprise), educational enterprise (this role being "among the most diverse purposes of the hospital" and "much more than a sideline activity"), research, that of a religious institution (especially when spiritual care is seen as an additional responsibility in church-affiliated hospitals), community enterprise, and public enterprise (because hospital costs are of public concern).[10]

This list of major purposes is essentially a description of hospital functions with respect to the larger social system. The functions described here are not mutually exclusive nor do they focus specifically on the hospital as an organization with specific objectives. However, such a list serves to point to the interdependence between hospitals and the surrounding environment and the need for a contextual and relational analysis of organizations in general.

It is typical of most general descriptions of hospitals to emphasize the "voluntary" character of the organization and to view its efficiency and viability as subject to the test of financial solvency. This emphasis tends to be related to the view that health is a commodity to be purchased on a more or less open market and that any interference with the autonomy of the hospital can only depreciate the product: the care and cure of the patient. By the same token, it is widely believed that the modern hospital is "the result of evolutionary adaptation rather than rational planning." [11] Since, however, a relatively large proportion of hospitals are planned, built, and operated under some form of public control, whether local governmental, state, or federal, it seems obvious that variations along the dimension of type of control or degree of autonomy may significantly influence the structural characteristics of hospitals. The recent introduction of Medicare and Medicaid further underscores the important influence of public policy through governmental agencies and legal provisions.

In other words, both the nature of the task as well as the patterns of hospital ownership and control are defined and determined by the needs, standards, and resources of the larger organized environment they serve. Moreover, both managerial control and task structure influence each other and interact in their determination of the patterns of hospital organization. One way of looking at this interaction between managerial and task factors is through the manner in which basic policy decisions are affected by power constellations reaching inside the organization. These constellations, which in hospitals have changed historically from the predominance of doctors to that of the board and finally the administrator,[12] may persist in one form or another as dyads or triangles of power where the board of directors competes with the medical staff and hospital administration for the exercise of effective authority.[13]

The prominence of the two major organizational elements of autonomy and task complexity in the present approach has a further significance beyond delimiting the coordinate system of vertical (normative) and horizontal (relational) dimensions. Both autonomy and task complexity, in my view, constitute independent determinants of organizational processes. While the influence of task complexity can ultimately be traced to the assumptions of technological determinism, the effect of organizational autonomy could probably be reduced to some form of managerial determinism so prominent in the world of business administration.[14]

But the sociological importance of organizational autonomy lies in the fact that the ownership-management dimension has undergone a pervasive historical transformation.[15] Thus, modern organizational autonomy is to a large extent rooted in the relative independence of an increasingly professionalized form of managerial decision-making. Insofar as this independence has developed in the public sector of modern nations, i.e., in public agencies and organizations, it constitutes an unprecedented potential for rational problem-solving and social change.[16]

Paradoxically, then, publicly managed organizations will have formally a lower degree of autonomy than private ones. But, due to public accountability and the specification of standards of quality and performance, decisions emanating from public agencies play a crucial role as pace-setters and models for the rest of the spectrum of local-governmental and communal, and even for semi-private and proprietary, organizations. This, at least, is very much the case for organizations like hospitals, where federal institutions far outrank other types in terms of a variety of quality-indicators.

Thus, the various relevant characteristics of the organizational environment, together with ownership-control and task structure, represent a crucial first set of independent variables which define and determine much of the organizational patterns of hospitals, their size and internal structure, and quite possibly their quality and ultimate effectiveness. For, if we know that a voluntary, nonprofit community hospital provides a certain number of medical services (one of the criteria of a general hospital), we also know that it will tend to be small to intermediate in size (60 to 100 patients) and to have a relatively short average length of patient stay, say, six or seven days. If, on the other hand, it is a one-specialty (e.g., psychiatric) state hospital, it will tend to be large (more than 1,000 patients) and to have a long average length of stay (one to two years). All of these factors indicate the likely prevalence of custodial care for predominantly chronic patients, as well as a limited budget.

If we know a hospital provides facilities for the training of medical students, interns, and residents (one of the definitions of a teaching hospital), we also know that it must have certain medical specialists on its staff for purposes of training the younger members of the medical profession. It must have a certain minimum size and thus tends to be larger on the average than nonteaching hospitals. It must have an autopsy rate of at least 25 per cent, preferably higher so as to indicate to potential interns and residents an organizational readiness to provide a certain minimum quality in the scientific orientation of its medical staff and an optimal learning environment.

The "Hierarchy" of Variables

We can now identify the "levels" of factors describing and influencing the patterns of hospital organization. (See Figure 1.)

The diagram in Figure 1 basically represents the general working hypothesis of this study, which is composed of a series of more specific hypotheses. It is a schematic representation of the basic parameters of organizational structure and their interrelation. That structure is conceptualized as extending between the characteristics of the organizational environment, i.e., beyond the organizational boundaries, on the one hand, and the highly specific elements of the internal structure, on the other. On the most general level, and external to the organization itself, one may discern three kinds of more or less independent influences: the size and structure of the surrounding community, the interests and power of the medical and other health professions and their accrediting bodies, and the authority and policies of governmental and legal agencies.

The complexity of the task structure, including size, and the degree of organizational autonomy constitute the second level in this hierarchy of variables. At both of these levels we are confronted with the operation of both historical and structural factors, i.e., with the results of long-term developments as well as ongoing processes and current constellations and structures.

I want to make clear that the structure of the community, its cultural traditions, its health and welfare policies must, for the purposes of this study, be treated largely as residual variables. However, by considering accreditation and approvals as well as comparing public and private ownership and control, two aspects of that residuum are singled out. The first, accreditations and approvals, reflects the joint policies, judgments, and interests of various organized health professions. These groups, in turn,

Figure 1
The "Hierarchy" of Variables

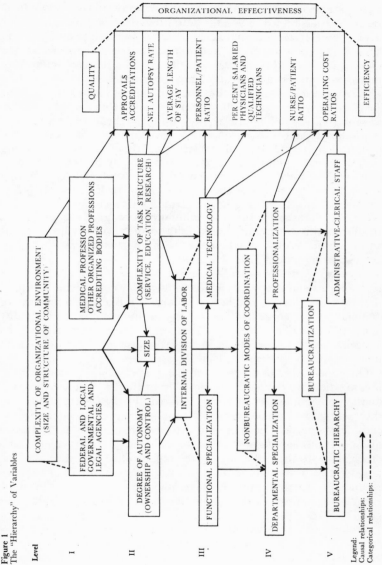

Legend:
Causal relationships: ⟶
Categorical relationships: ----------

25

represent, to a degree, the basic orientations of the community toward matters of health and the definition of health needs.

The second element, public vs. private ownership and control, reflects the political, legal, and administrative arrangements the community is making to deal with its health needs as defined, to allocate resources, and to implement general health and welfare policies in terms of specific objectives and organizational tasks. For these reasons, it is significant to study the separate effects of private, or semi-public, and public responsibility for health services.

Similarly, the organizational task structure must be seen as the result of long-term historical and structural developments. Thus, the diversification of hospital objectives signified by the emergence of teaching hospitals is related to underlying social and legal norms which determine much of the organizational reality. Hospitals are not accredited as teaching hospitals unless they conform to certain rules and standards, such as minimum size and autopsy rates. Insofar as this is true and conformity to such rules is insured, the nature of the task (viz. teaching) can in this particular case be said to determine minimum size or quality.

Once accredited, size and quality of the hospital may attract new technologies and specialists which in turn may change the nature of the task by setting higher standards, initiating research, or demanding a reorganization of the hospital: size and quality determine task. The example makes use of intervening factors such as technology and specialists, variables whose operation and effect may or may not be identifiable in all cases.

Once the nature of the task and the goal-setting autonomy of the organization are defined, it is possible to treat technology and the division of labor as factors both "dictated" by the nature and size of the task as well as the result of rational choices and managerial considerations of efficiency and effective goal-attainment. In addition, various aspects of the division of labor will interact with each other and with the technology of the organization. For example, the proliferation of specialized functions is in part a result of changes in technology. At the same time, the requirements for new and formally certified technical skills will foster the "professionalization of labor."[17]

Professional and technical specialties frequently require new administrative arrangements, including the setting up of new departments and the delegation of skills and responsibilities to lower levels in the professional and bureaucratic hierarchies. [18] The presence of professionals may lead to the adoption of technical innovations, the attraction of other specialists in similar and related fields, and the proliferation of new and auxiliary activities and work functions.

While we may speak of processes of mutual causation here, it is nevertheless useful to deal with these variables as if they were part of a nonrecursive chain of "intermediate" causes, or at least to deal with them on different levels. Thus, technology and functional specialization will be treated on a separate level of our hierarchy of variables, with professionalization and departmental specialization on still another one (see Figure 1). The main reason is that I will argue that professionalization and departmental specialization constitute an aspect both of the division of labor and of coordination at the same time.

In this argument, professionalization, in particular, is assumed to intervene or mediate between the imperatives of technology and job specialization, on the one hand, and the modes of legal-bureaucratic administration, on the other. Professionalization constitutes what could be called a nonbureaucratic mode of coordination. It implies certain regulative and administrative responses to the functional division of work.[19]

The argument for the coordinative and regulative implications of departmental specialization are based on a somewhat different premise. It assumes essentially that certain kinds of division of labor, i.e., those which imply the development of blocks or groups of interdependent functions rather than separate, isolated, or atomized activities, require new modes of coordination.

Thus, departmental specialization and interdependence are assumed to give rise to nonbureaucratic modes of coordination through mutual adjustment and lateral communication among departments and subunits. In classical social theory, this phenomenon has been described by Durkheim in terms of "organic solidarity."[20] In modern political sociology, it has been dealt with in terms of the socio-economic determinants of political action, the social basis of democratic political organization.[21]

A suggestive analysis of the phenomenon of structural coordination is given in Coleman's *Community Conflict.*[22] Coleman views the structure of communities as a major element in conflict resolution, or better, conflict absorption and subsumption on structurally higher levels. From a somewhat different perspective, Etzioni has recently made a strong case for the integrative effects of interdependence among nation-states in terms of the formation of supra-units.[23]

The difference between Coleman's and Etzioni's views of the integrative consequences of interdependence appear to lie in a differential emphasis on structural and normative factors. Thus, Coleman argues that the web of social relations, i.e., the very structure of the community, contains cross-ties which bind conflicting groups together, bridge gaps and cleavages, and reduce polarization. This is analogous to the notion that a crystal is more difficult to break than, say, a piece of limestone, the latter being simpler and more homogeneous in structure, the former more heterogeneous and complex.[24]

Etzioni, on the other hand, argues for a conception of legitimacy and consensus as underlying the formation of a supra-structural authority. He is thus advocating a form of structural functionalism which views processes of development and change as guided by a kind of social intelligence. The cognitively "active" social system *anticipates* social changes needed for adaptation and mastery. The conception of "epigenesis" is Parsons' structural differentiation in reverse, since Parsons sees change as a *response* to problems of adaptation and integration.[25]

Integration as a consequence of interdependence thus turns out to be more the result of assumption and definition than hypothesis and observation. The theoretical context of these ideas will be spelled out in more detail in Chapter 4. Suffice it to say here that they have influenced the underlying notion of structural coordination.[26]

The last level in the hierarchy of variables discussed here refers to the two central elements of the ideal-type conception of bureaucracy, viz. the hierarchy of authority and the administrative-clerical staff.[27] In one sense, these two are conceived as dependent variables insofar as it is of interest to determine the structural conditions of bureaucratic modes of administration in organizations. But in another sense, bureaucratic coordination is one instrument among others to achieve certain objectives. From this latter perspective it is assumed that bureaucratic elements will not only interact with nonbureaucratic elements and the division of labor, but will also have to be measured in their effect on the two specific aspects of organizational effectiveness, namely quality of services and efficiency as measured by various kinds of operating cost ratios.[28]

While the measurement of effectiveness in professional organizations providing services to people is grossly underdeveloped, it is still an important—and perhaps the most important—problem to be considered in systematic organizational research.[29]

The issues of quality and efficiency in effective goal-attainment bring us back to the larger question of what the organization is to achieve, i.e. to its goal and task structure as well as its autonomy in goal-setting. In other words, effectiveness is related to the operation of all aspects of the organization. In terms of the hierarchy of variables considered here, this means that criteria of effectiveness can be developed for all levels, although the most important ones cluster around the organizational task structure, as can be seen from Figure 1. This is true especially if we would add such quality control functions as medical audits, the operations of a tissue committee, and the rate of consultations among physicians. Similarly, negative indicators of effectiveness in terms of morale or performance, such as turnover rates, absenteeism, malpractice suits, etc., would be relevant at all levels of the organization, although some are certainly more visible and sensitive than others.

The problem of the effectiveness and quality of hospitals will not be settled by this study; in fact, that is not its major focus. It is interesting to note that any mention of even measuring effectiveness evokes at best responses of pity from hospital administrators, at worst a defensive rejection of the very idea of measuring human service to human beings. The main stumbling block to a clear-cut definition of effectiveness criteria in hospitals may well be the differential assumptions made about patients and hospital personnel. Thus, the performance of hospital personnel is frequently judged to be impersonal and "bureaucratic" in the face of deeply personal problems of health and of life crises. Consequently, administrators, physicians, nurses, and other health personnel will tend to react defensively when the adequacy of their performance is questioned by way of raising the issue of criteria of effectiveness and quality.[30]

Conversely (and perhaps as a dialectical response to this "public relations" problem) patients are frequently judged as self-indulgent, demanding of personal service, critical of procedures, and insensititve to the complexities of running a hospital.[31]   Nevertheless, there are certain technical aspects of medical care and of the broader notion of patient care which can be analyzed in terms of certain salient components of these processes. Besides, the concerns of the "human relations" school of organizational studies are not to be disregarded here. Apart from its focus on productivity and performance, that school has helped raise the more important question of the relative cost, in human and social terms, of the "cult of efficiency."[32]

In many hospitals, the question of the relation of input to output, i.e., of efficiency, is probably still subordinated to the ideal of service. But there are also costs, such as the high turnover rate of graduate professional nurses, which can be traced in part to certain structural strains inherent in the hospital and to the general problems of female labor force participation, the employment of low-skill personnel such as aides for generalized care functions, the lagging wage level in many hospital-based occupations and, generally, the shortages and instabilities of the health manpower labor market.[33]

Suffice it to say here that I will deal with some aspects of the question of quality and effectiveness even though it will be necessary at times to make use of indirect rather than direct measurement.

Summary and Conclusions

In this chapter I have attempted to outline the dynamic interplay between the major factors assumed to influence the organization of modern hospitals. This study is concerned with the interrelation between structural characteristics of hospitals as formal organizations. For this reason, the emphasis is on the patterns of structural relationships rather than the development of historical forms. Nevertheless, it is important for the advancement of organizational analysis and sociological theory to go beyond the description of structural patterns. In other words, rather than getting caught in the vicious circle of trying to account for structure in terms of function, and vice versa, speculating on the consequences of structure, I have attempted to discuss my assumptions about the causal direction of the various relationships. For this purpose, I have arranged the major variables considered in this study in a "hierarchical" order which simply reflects the definition of variables as independent, intervening, and dependent ones.

The main point about this causal ordering of the variables is that it constitutes a first step toward an explanatory framework in terms of which organizations, and specifically hospitals, can be compared and analyzed. Moreover, organizations, however complex, have causes; if we understand the causes, we can change the organization according to the purposes it is to serve, rather than having people, or patients, serve the purposes of the organization. Of course, this statement assumes that agreement on purposes can be reached among the parties concerned. For hospitals, as for most other types of organizations, it is likely that there will be multiple definitions of the goals, objectives, and tasks. Thus patients, the larger community, the medical profession, the board of directors, the administrator, the hospital staff, and other beneficiaries of the "health industry" are factors in the determination of what the hospital is and how it is to operate. Put into the more abstract form as variables, these "determinants" can be identified as the size and structure of the community, the ownership and control of the hospital, and its task structure. The task structure, in particular, can be seen as the result of the interplay of complex forces, among them the health needs of the community, the interests and policies of the organized health professions, and the political and legal-administrative considerations determining the allocation of resources. In other words, both task structure and organizational autonomy are dependent variables from the point of view of the community, its size, structure, and organizational differentiation. But for the purposes of this study, their main analytical status is that of independent variables.

The task structure of a hospital, in turn, determines to a large extent the type and degree of technological complexity, the degree of functional specialization, and the extent of departmental specialization and professionalization. Both of these latter two factors, in turn, are conceived as modifying the effects of functional specialization and technology on the bureaucratic modes of coordination, i.e., the bureaucratic hierarchy and the administrative staff.

All of these levels of variables are determinants of organizational effectiveness. Since criteria of quality and effectiveness must, of necessity, be part of any definition of tasks and objectives, it is not surprising that most criteria amenable to measurement at this point are, in fact, tied to the organizational task structure. But "organizational effectiveness" is not a meaningful term unless it can be shown that subunits and subgoals contribute significantly to that overall effectiveness. It is for this reason that effectiveness and quality must be measured at each level and within each substructure, both analytical and empirical, of the organizational structure.

In the following chapter, the major concepts will be discussed in detail. The general pattern of presentation will be to define each concept in its theoretical context, to give the operational definition and its application to hospitals, and to discuss the relative advantages and limitations of the proposed measures.

Notes

1. Harold Lasswell, *Who Gets What, When, How* (Cleveland, Ohio: The World Publishing Company, Meridian Books, 1958).
2. See, for example, Barney E. Glaser and Anselm L. Strauss, *The Discovery of Grounded Theory: Strategies for Qualitative Research* (Chicago: Aldine, 1967); and Hans L. Zetterberg, *On Theory and Verification in Sociology* (3rd ed.; New York: Bedminster Press, 1965).

3. Commission on Hospital Care, *Hospital Care in the United States* (New York: Commonwealth Fund, 1947); E. H. L. Corwin, *The American Hospital* (New York: Commonwealth Fund, 1946); Nathaniel W. Faxon, ed., *The Hospital in Contemporary Life* (Cambridge, Mass.: Harvard University Press, 1949); Eli Ginzberg, *A Pattern of Hospital Care* (New York: Columbia University Press, 1949); Rufus C. Rorem, *The Public's Investment in Hospitals* (Chicago: University of Chicago Press, 1930); James A. Hamilton, *Patterns of Hospital Ownership and Control* (Minneapolis: University of Minnesota Press, 1961).

4. Richard H. Shryock, *The Development of Modern Medicine* (New York: Knopf, 1947); Michael Davis, *Medical Care for Tomorrow* (New York: Harper, 1955).

5. See, for example, Harvey L. Smith and Daniel J. Levinson, "The Major Aims and Organizational Characteristics of Mental Hospitals," Milton Greenblatt, et al., eds., *The Patient and the Mental Hospital* (Glencoe, Ill.: The Free Press, 1957), pp. 3-8; see also Milton Greenblatt et al., *From Custodial to Therapeutic Care in Mental Hospitals* (New York: Russell Sage, 1955).

6. Alfred H. Stanton and Morris F. Schwartz, *The Mental Hospital* (New York: Basic Books, 1954); William Caudill, *The Psychiatric Hospital as a Small Society* (Cambridge, Mass.: Harvard University Press, 1958).

7. Ivan Belknap, *Human Problems of a State Mental Hospital* (New York: McGraw-Hill, 1956); H. Warren Dunham and S. Kirson Weinberg, *The Culture of the State Mental Hospital* (Detroit, Mich.: Wayne State University Press, 1960); Jules Henry, "The Formal Structure of a Psychiatric Hospital," *Psychiatry*, XVII (1954), 139-151; S. Kirson Weinberg, "Organization, Personnel, and Functions of State and Private Mental Hospitals: A Comparative Analysis," in E. Gartly Jaco, ed., *Patients, Physicians, and Illness*, (Glencoe, Ill.: The Free Press, 1958), pp. 478-491.

8. Henry J. Southmayd and Geddes Smith, *Small Community Hospitals* (New York: Commonwealth Fund, 1944).

9. Temple Burling et al., *The Give and Take in Hospitals* (New York: Putnam, 1956); Basil S. Georgopoulos and Floyd C. Mann, *The Community General Hospital* (New York: Macmillan, 1962).

10. Ray E. Brown, "Evaluating Hospital Administration," *Hospitals*, XXXV (1961), 43.

11. Burling et al., op. cit., p. 6.

12. Charles Perrow, "The Analysis of Goals in Complex Organizations," *American Sociological Review*, 26 (1961), 854-866.

13. Paul J. Gordon, "The Top Management Triangle in Voluntary Hospitals," *Journal of the Academy of Management*, IV (1961), 205-214.

14. See, for example, Leonard R. Sayles and George Strauss, *Human Behavior in Organizations* (Englewood Cliffs, N.J.: Prentice Hall, 1966).

15. A. A. Berle, Jr. and G. C. Means, *The Modern Corporation and Private Property* (New York: Macmillan, 1932).

16. On the implications of knowledge for social action and transformation, see Harold L. Wilensky, *Organizational Intelligence* (New York: Basic

Books, 1967), pp. 8-74, and Amitai Etzioni, *The Active Society* (New York: The Free Press, 1968), pp. 155-196.

17. Nelson N. Foote, "The Professionalization of Labor in Detroit," *American Journal of Sociology*, 58 (1953), 371-380.

18. Everett C. Hughes, *Men and Their Work* (Glencoe, Ill.: The Free Press, 1958), pp. 135-138.

19. Arthur L. Stinchcombe, "Bureaucratic and Craft Administration of Production: A Comparative Study," *Administrative Science Quarterly*, IV (1959), 184-187; James G. March and Herbert A. Simon, *Organizations* (New York: Wiley, 1958); especially their concept of "coordination by feedback," pp. 160-161.

20. Emile Durkheim, *The Division of Labor in Society* (Glencoe, Ill.: The Free Press, 1947), pp. 219-229.

21. Bernard R. Berelson et al., *Voting* (Chicago: The University of Chicago Press, 1954); Seymour M. Lipset et al., *Union Democracy* (Glencoe, Ill.: The Free Press, 1956). See also Seymour M. Lipset, *Political Man* (New York: Doubleday Anchor, 1963), pp. 64-86, 387-432.

22. James S. Coleman, *Community Conflict* (Glencoe, Ill.: The Free Press, 1957), pp. 21-23.

23. Amitai Etzioni, *The Active Society* (New York: The Free Press, 1968), pp. 94-129, 553-578; see also his "The Epigenesis of Political Communities at the International Level," *American Journal of Sociology*, 68 (1963), 476-487; his *Political Unification* (New York: Holt, Rinehart, and Winston, 1965); and *A Comparative Analysis of Complex Organizations* (Glencoe, Ill.: The Free Press, 1961).

24. Note that this argument differs from the utilitarian position that postulates an ultimate outcome of harmonious mutual adjustment of conflicting interests. Such a position has recently been advocated by Charles E. Lindblom, *The Intelligence of Democracy* (New York: The Free Press, 1965).

25. Etzioni, "The Epigenesis," 416-417.

26. Notice also the affinity of this approach to the concepts of coordination and conflict as they are discussed in classical and neoclassical organization theory. See, for example, H. C. Metcalf & L. Urwick, eds., *Dynamic Administration: The Collected Papers of Mary Parker Follet* (New York: Harper, 1940), pp. 30-49, 71-117; March and Simon, op. cit., pp. 113-171.

27. Max Weber, *The Theory of Social and Economic Organization*, tr. A. M. Henderson and Talcott Parsons, ed. Talcott Parsons (New York: Oxford University Press, 1947), pp. 329-341; Max Rheinstein, ed., *Max Weber on Law in Economy and Society*, tr. Edward A. Shils and Max Rheinstein (Cambridge, Mass.: Harvard University Press, 1954), pp. 322-348.

28. For an example of research on the effect of the relative size of the administrative staff on operating costs, see a study of state and local civil service commissions (public personnel agencies) by Peter M. Blau et al., "The Structure of Small Bureaucracies," *American Sociological Review*, 31 (1966), 179-191.

29. A good general review of research on organizational effectiveness is

given by James L. Price, *Organizational Effectiveness: An Inventory of Propositions* (Homewood, Ill.: Dorsey, 1968); see also Mindel C. Sheps, "Approaches to the Quality of Hospital Care," *Public Health Reports,* 70 (1955), 877-886; and Lee ¦ Peterson, "Evaluation of the Quality of Medical Care," *New England Journal of Medicine,* 269 (1963), 1238-1245.

30. See also Jacob J. Feldman, *The Dissemination of Health Information* (Chicago: Aldine Press, 1966); Stanley H. King, *Perception of Illness and Medical Practice* (New York: Russell Sage, 1962); Paul B. Sheatsley, "Report of a Survey of Hospital Administrator Attitudes Toward Use" (Chicago: Health Information Foundation, 1962); Jacob J. Feldman, "What Americans Think About Medical Care" (paper presented to the American Statistical Association, Chicago, 1958); "Patients Speak Out," *Medical Economics,* April 20, 1964, pp. 49-106.

31. See, for example, Rose Laub Coser, "A Home Away from Home," *Social Problems,* IV (July 1956), 3-17; and her *Life in the Ward* (East Lansing: Michigan State University Press, 1962).

32. Fritz J. Roethlisberger and William J. Dickson, *Management and the Worker* (Cambridge, Mass.: Harvard University Press, 1939); William F. Whyte, *Money and Motivation* (New York: Harper, 1955); Chris Argyris, *Personality and Organization* (New York: Harper, 1957); Rensis Likert, *New Patterns of Management* (New York: McGraw-Hill, 1961); Karl Mannheim, *Man and Society in an Age of Reconstruction* (London: Routledge & Kegan Paul, 1940), pp. 39-78, 239-381; Daniel Bell, "Work and Its Discontents: The Cult of Efficiency in America," in his *The End of Ideology* (rev. ed.; New York: The Free Press, 1965), pp. 227-272.

33. See, for example, National Commission on Community Health Services, *Health Manpower,* Report of the Task Force on Health Manpower (Washington D.C.: Public Affairs Press, 1967), pp. 32-34, 94-119.

34

3 Major Concepts of the Organizational Analysis of Hospitals

Any list of concepts and variables can be modified in two directions: analytical specification and synthesizing reconceptualization. The former involves the differentiation and expansion of a given set of concepts by breaking each one down into smaller, analytical components. The latter implies contraction and integration of the original set of concepts, and subsuming them under more general ones. This characteristic relativity of any set of definitions lends them their arbitrariness, and often renders agreement between different taxonomies and categorical schemes difficult. The ten major concepts used in this study are on "intermediate" levels of generality. Such factors as autonomy, task structure, task environment, size, technology, division of labor, professionalization, authority structure, administrative staff, and effectiveness are fairly general, especially if they are used to study a wide variety of organizational types. As I have shown, these concepts can be "generalized" still further by subsuming them under a formula such as "who does what, why, and how," or an even more general scheme such as a systems-model of organizations specifying only a series of input-output functions.

However, it is my intention here to move in the opposite direction, i.e., toward the analytical specification and operationalization of the set of concepts listed above. While the starting point is necessarily arbitrary to some extent, it is hoped that these concepts will acquire some validity and legitimacy in the course of being defined, clarified, specified, and, above all, applied to a group of empirical organizations.

Organizational Autonomy

The problem of organizational autonomy is of great significance both historically and structurally. Historically, the development of sovereignty among nation-states has been associated with the rise of the legal-bureaucratic apparatus of governmental administrations. The state, having a monopoly on the legitimate control of the ultimate means of violence, is assumed to be internally and externally sovereign, based on a unitary system of legitimacy and authority. Autonomy, in this sense, is intimately linked with the notion of rule-making (legislative) and law enforcement and implementation (executive) powers on the assumption that ultimate responsibility requires ultimate authority. Here, the emphasis is on the *normative* component of the concept of autonomy: giving oneself laws and living by them.

Yet there is a second, *relational* component in the concept of autonomy, which emphasizes the autonomy of the individual unit relative to other units. This horizontal-relational aspect of autonomy will be elaborated below in the discussion of "Complexity of Organizational Environment."

In general, the legitimacy necessary for the control of industrial production in private enterprises is derived partially from doctrines of individual liberty and partially from the institutionalization of private property. In the extreme case, the autonomy of the enterprise is limited by its ability to control resources. This basic condition gives inordinate weight to the mobilization of power (outside the question of legitimacy) in the interest of maximizing expected utility and profit. Autonomy, in this sense, is defined in terms of relative competitive advantage in an unstructured situation, with the development of market and exchange mechanisms, regulative norms, and state control of production as progressively limiting the lateral autonomy of the individual enterprise. The movement from ownership to managerial control of large industrial concerns represents the shift of the internal control mechanisms from traditional and personal to modern, impersonal, and legal-public bases of legitimacy.[1] This process parallels the progressive rationalization and "socialization," in the economic *and* sociological sense, of modern industry; i.e., the shift from private to public ownership and control, following similar developments in the areas of utilities, education, welfare, and health.

Operationally, one may define organizational autonomy in terms of the degree of control over policies (external bureaucratization) and/or the degree of control over resources, assuming some rational nexus between the choice of means in relation to ends. Frequently, the legal status of an organization or the extent to which it is "part" of another organization will be useful as an indicator of relative autonomy. Thus, a state government is autonomous relative to any one of its departments; but it may be semi-autonomous in relation to federal government, or not autonomous at all in a corporate national state. More useful and accurate would be indicators of relative decision-making autonomy in various functional sectors, and within these sectors various aspects such as legal and fiscal control. Distinctions between public vs. private ownership and control are useful, especially if it is possible to assess the relative authority of federal regulatory agencies and the influence of other economic and political control factors.

The distinction between public and private control also entails the important further distinction between budgetary economic units and profit-making enterprises, with the widespread intermediate form of budget allocation by a voluntary, nonprofit, independent governing board. Applied to hospitals, organizational autonomy is conceptualized in terms of types of ownership and external control, ranging from proprietary (individual and corporate) hospitals to "voluntary," nonprofit religious as well as nondenominational community hospitals to local governmental (city, county, state, etc.) hospitals to federal governmental hospitals. In the present study, three types of ownership and external control are singled out for comparative purposes: (1) federal hospitals, specifically, the hospitals within the Veterans' Administration; (2) local governmental hospitals; and (3) voluntary, nonprofit hospitals not related to religious institutions. The underlying dimension of organizational autonomy is indicated by the two extremes, with federal hospitals assumed to be least autonomous, and voluntary, nonprofit hospitals being most autonomous. The local governmental hospitals are assumed to occupy an intermediate position. In the relevant context, certain comparative reference will be made to the proprietary hospitals which should be even more autonomous than the voluntary, nonprofit institutions. However, because of limitations in the number of different types of proprietary hospitals, they are not included in the systematic comparative analysis.

The general characteristics of the three types of ownership and control selected for study are described in the first part of Chapter 5. In using the distinction between public and private hospitals as representing an underlying dimension of organizational autonomy, I would like to add a word of caution. There is clearly the danger of stereotyping the different kinds of ownership and control of hospitals by assuming that the greater the degree of governmental control, or the larger and more remote the seat of ultimate authority, the less autonomous is the individual organization. While this may be true in a purely formal sense, one could argue that federal hospitals, for example, operate on the basis of a much broader definition of "good" medical and patient care than, say, proprietary hospitals which are constrained by considerations of economic viability. Furthermore, remoteness of authority may be a factor in de facto decentralization. Viewed from another perspective, there may be a minimal difference between the autonomy of the governing board of a local community hospital and the board or commission running a city, county, or even state hospital. Both types operate within the framework of some kind of budget and are ultimately accountable to the respective communities of which they are a part. The only difference may be not even in the degree of direct accountability and responsibility, but in the respective elites to which they are accountable. Thus, while local governmental hospital authorities are presumably responsive to the realities of the political dimensions of the local power structure, the boards of "private" hospitals are oriented to the socio-economic elites of the community.[2] Given the fact that especially in smaller communities both types of elites—i.e., political and socio-economic—are largely coextensive, it follows that the distinction between different degrees of autonomy as based on public vs. private control must be contextually qualified.

Complexity of Task Structure

The most important characteristic of the task structure of an organization is that it is an indicator of the underlying goal structure. Yet while it is difficult, if not impossible, to define the goals of an organization at any one point in time with a minimum of authoritativeness, it is comparatively easy to identify the actual programs and activities, tasks and priorities in terms of which the organizational objectives manifest themselves, and which define the organization as a going concern.

The difference is similar to that of asking a person what he is going to do, and then observing his actual conduct. Both may coincide; but if they do not, the actual conduct is clearly the more valuable type of information, particularly since stated goals tend to be redefined in terms of actual behavior.

The task structure of an organization may, of course, still be far removed from its actual conduct. A task is a program of action in which the objectives are more or less clearly defined. Obviously, the clarity and specificity of objectives are themselves factors in the complexity of the task. But in defining task complexity, one may begin with more basic elements in the task structure, such as the number of criteria or dimensions in terms of which objectives are specified, and the number of objectives on any one of such dimensions. For example, an industrial conglomerate may manufacture a variety of products for two or three different markets, the number of different markets being a rough measure of the organization's diversification. But, in addition, for each market a number of distinct products may be identified. Both of these elements are an integral part of the task structure of that organization. Its degree of complexity is circumscribed by the multiplicity and diversity of objectives.

A further aspect of the task structure is the volume or size of the task, e.g., the actual number of output units per product during a given time period. Finally, one must consider the variability of the task structure, i.e., the number and types of elements which are unstable over time.[3]

The variability introduced by nonroutine tasks or by predictable (hence routinizable) changes in the task structure, such as variable work loads, seasonal variations, or unsolved problems, is clearly distinct from that introduced by unpredictable or "poorly" predictable (emergent) changes. Only the latter type of variability generates a measure of uncertainty in the task environment, raising the question of the viability and realizability of objectives, in contrast to their operational specificity.

Unpredictable changes may, of course, always occur in the task environment. Examples are changes in markets, resources, the number and type of clientele, etc. From this perspective, it seems clear that the degree to which the underlying organizational goals are realizable is an important contingency that affects the task structure itself. Thus, consideration of the means relative to the ends, the realistic assessment of "operational goals,"[4] the definition of the quality of problem-solving in terms of optimal, satisfactory solutions, rather than maximal ones, all these are contextual aspects of the task structure which say something about the complexity of the underlying goal structure without actually revealing it.

In sum, the complexity of an organization's task structure is seen as a function of the diversity and multiplicity of specifiable objectives, the relative size of the tasks involved, and the number of nonroutine tasks and/or of routine changes in the task structure.

The difference between nonroutine tasks and routine changes in task structure is, of course, one of levels of generality in the problem encountered. Nonroutine tasks may be performed without changes in the higher level task structure of an organization. It is only when nonroutine tasks *cannot* be performed that a change in task structure is called for. But even such changes can be planned for and routinized.

Applying the operational definition of the complexity of the task structure to hospitals entails a classification of hospitals with a high degree of face validity and empirical usefulness. Thus, using as a first criterion the *diversity* of objectives, a fundamental distinction can be made between medical service and medical education and research. Translated into organizational task complexity, the distinction implies that hospitals in which educational and teaching functions are added to the service functions are more diversified, and thus more complex than others in which the potential conflict between teaching and service is not present. In this study, the distinction between teaching and nonteaching hospitals is maintained throughout. Occasionally, reference will be made to medical research as an additional dimension, measured by the affiliation of a hospital with a university or medical school. For most purposes, however, this dimension of diversity is subsumed under the one of teaching.

The second criterion of task complexity used here is the *number* of specific objectives. In a hospital, medical service lends itself to the construction of a continuum of task complexity in terms of the number of medical specialties present, or the number of different diseases treated. As a continuum, it ranges from the treatment of one specific type of disease such as tuberculosis or mental illness on the one hand to various general medical-surgical conditions on the other. The number of different diseases treated in a hospital provides a rough index of the multiplicity of major purposes or objectives along the dimension of medical service. Thus, in a general medical and surgical hospital, there is by definition no limitation of service to any particular specialty or disease, so that the whole range of diseases and specialties may potentially be present. By contrast, in a psychiatric hospital diseases other than mental illness are not expected to be treated on a regular or long-term basis. The essential diagnostic and therapeutic facilities will therefore be limited to those connected with the diagnosis and treatment of mental illness.[5]

While the size of the task is closely related to task complexity, I will deal with this variable separately under the heading of "organizational size."

The variability of the work load as well as other, not fully predictable elements in task performance can be gauged in different ways. One of the most widely used indicators in hospitals is the average length of stay of patients, often used also as a measure of "utilization." Defined as "the average number of days of service rendered to each inpatient discharged during a given period"[6] (usually one year), the average length of stay is clearly related to the complexity of the task structure. Thus, general hospitals have a relatively short average length of stay (about one week) compared to hospitals specializing in the care of mental or chronic illness.

Average length of stay is a function of many factors. Most important among them are the nature and acuteness of illnesses treated which is, in turn, related to other characteristics of the patient population, the complexity and relative efficiency of diagnostic and therapeutic medical technology, and the personnel resources mobilized to meet certain standards of quality of medical and overall patient care. The intensity and quality of care is thus bound up with the technical and organizational arrangements of the hospital, and particularly with its overall task structure. Since, in fact, a large amount of variation in average length of stay can be accounted for in terms of the task structure, such as teaching status and type of medical service, the measure is used mainly for descriptive rather than analytical or evaluative purposes.

In sum, the major indicators of task complexity used here are the teaching status of the hospital and, within the dichotomy of teaching vs. nonteaching hospitals, the distinction between institutions offering many vs. few medical services, viz. general vs. psychiatric hospitals.

Complexity of Organizational Environment

If the complexity of the task structure is an integral *structural* attribute of organizations, the complexity of the organizational environment constitutes a *contextual* attribute. For many types of intra-organizational analysis, it will be sufficient to treat the organizational environment as a set of residual "factors" which are not analyzed further once their joint effect is acknowledged, or even taken into account. This is one reason why many causal schemes in social analysis are not and cannot provide total explanations, but must be content with explaining only part of the variance in the effect variable. Thus, variations in organizational structure may be explained up to a point, with no attempt being made to account systematically for all the factors involved. Nevertheless, it is possible to spell out certain types of factors in the organizational environment. This is especially desirable if it is assumed, as is the case in the present approach, that intra- and inter-organizational analysis are both integral aspects of the same framework of inquiry. In other words, organizational analysis does not stop at the boundaries of the organization, but considers both "internal" and "external" factors, preferably at the same time. Two of the most important elements in the complexity of the environment are its structural differentiation and the kind and degree of interaction of the organization with other organizations.

The degree of environmental differentiation can be analyzed in terms of various dimensions, such as the demographic, economic, and political differentiation of the surrounding community. Thus the degree of urbanization itself, or the size of the community, will provide an important indicator for the complexity of the organizational environment. The environmental unit may, of course, vary from community to state, region, or nation-state; from "networks" of organizations such as markets to associations of organizations, "roof organizations," and whole systems of organizations.[7] But particularly for the characterization of communities as organization environments, measures would figure prominently that involve such factors as population size, composition and change, median educational attainment, per cent of white collar of the labor force, per cent in manufacturing, median family income, degree of industrial diversification, type and structure of government, social differentiation and stratification, and the like.[8]

In the present study, the size of the Standard Metropolitan Statistical Area (SMSA for 1960) in which a given hospital is located is used as a measure of the degree of environmental differentiation (see Appendix C). It is assumed, for example, that the size of the surrounding community has implications for the availability of resources and skills, personnel, and clientele. For certain purposes we will also consider the rate of outpatient clinic and emergency room visits as measures of hospital-environment interaction. But such measures are clearly of limited use short of a comprehensive demographic analysis of the potential and actual patient population.

However, even if an organization is located in a differentiated environment, it may still be isolated or have relatively impermeable boundaries, such as might be expected of a closed or "total" institution.[9] Therefore, a second element to be considered in the complexity of the environment is the type and degree of interaction between the organization and other organizations. Clearly, there are a number of dimensions along which interaction across organizational boundaries may occur, such as competition with other similar organizations, bargaining, negotiation and exchange, coalition formation and cooptation, opposition, and conflict.[10] All of these processes involve transactions which have a certain intensity and frequency and thus can be measured in terms of rates, direction and dominance, variability, and periodicity.

While measures of this sort are not easily available for any one organization short of interviewing key informants or even intensive observation, it is possible to gauge the volume of organizational transactions by counting the number of certain permanent relationships the organization has established with other significant organizations in its environment. For hospitals, such a measure would be the number of affiliations and accreditations, such as the affiliation of the hospital with a medical school, the number and type of AMA-approved residency and internship programs, accreditation by the Joint Commission on Accreditation (which in turn is composed of various professional bodies), the approval of a cancer program, the affiliation with a professional nursing school or the maintenance of a practical nurse training program, membership in the state or regional hospital association, and others.

While such external relationships are defining characteristics both of teaching hospitals and of hospital quality in general, they are nevertheless also indicators of certain continuous transactions performed by a given hospital, as compared with other hospitals.

Theoretically and conceptually then, it is not easy—nor perhaps desirable—to draw a hard-and-fast line between the task structure of an organization and its environment. There is a form of continuity between organization and environment, just as there is between person and group or self and society, and the line between them is always, to some extent, arbitrary, and varies with the purpose of the analysis. But precisely because this study seeks to explore the various aspects and phases of this continuum, an initial distinction has to be made. Therefore, I have suggested to distinguish between task structure and organizational environment as dialectically related points of reference, without assigning fixed and absolute properties to them.

Another, more general indicator of the interaction between a given hospital and its environment is the growth rate of the hospital, measured in terms of changes in bed size, personnel, total expenditures, payroll, technical facilities, and services. Such measures indicate not only the amount of change experienced by the hospital, but also the residual underlying ecological pressures toward adaptation, such as expanding community needs for health services.[11] A crucial contextual variable here is, of course, the total number of hospitals or hospital beds available in the community. This is comparable to the concentration ratio of specific industries except that the reference system is not an aggregate or a market, but a community. Finally, one may consider the age of an organization as a variable specifying organization-environment relationships. Organizational age is clearly relevant, first of all, to the different rates of growth and change discussed above.[12] Since increases in size are sometimes interpreted as growth, it is of some interest to obtain empirical assessments of the relationship between age and size for different types of organizations. Age is also relevant in a broader ecological sense in that it is an indicator of when and where in a given environmental context of existing organizations a new organization enters the stage.[13]

Presumably, older organizations are internally more differentiated and complex than younger ones; older ones should be more stable and have firmer ties to or roots in the external environment, and so on. It must be recognized, of course, that the biological, organic analogy is basically limited to such obvious parallels, especially if it is remembered that formal organizations may be defined as "enacted" rather than "crescive" institutions, their continuous change notwithstanding.[14]

In other words, like models in general, the biological model is a descriptive device but does not, in itself, explain the nature and dynamics of organizational growth insofar as it is linked to age rather than to market conditions, community size and structure, autonomy, task structure, and technology. Organizational age is thus important as an intervening variable which helps to articulate the conditions surrounding organizational change.

As to the measurement of the complexity of the organizational environment, then, the present study relies mainly on size of community and, for teaching hospitals, on the number of affiliations and accreditations, on organizational growth rates between 1950 and 1960, and on "organizational age."

Organizational Size

The role of size as an organizational variable derives from the relatively simple sociological fact that social relationships between people in a group change as the number of people increases. The historical and structural consequences of population growth for the nature of society and the quality of social life have been noted by almost every significant social theorist, among them Durkheim, Weber, and Simmel.[15]

For organizations, the major focus of interest centers on the question to what extent an increase in organizational size gives rise to internal structural change such as increasing division of labor and functional specialization, as well as bureaucratization in the form of proliferation of administrative functions and hierarchical levels. In other words, there are sociological, economic, and political aspects to the question of the effect of size.

On the one hand, it involves the problem of primary relations and informal communication patterns turning into secondary, impersonal, and formal ones as soon as the group becomes larger.[16] An underlying assumption here is that as a group or society becomes larger, it also becomes more differentiated.[17]

On the other hand, the effects of size have been of interest to economists and others concerned with the relation between input and output, i.e., with the problem of overhead, economy of scale, and, generally, the problem of efficiency and economic rationality.[18] Since formalization of roles and rationalization of procedures, impersonal human relations, and standardization are part of a more general concept of bureaucracy, it has long been assumed that both economic savings and social costs are incurred as a result of increasing size and bureaucratization. Finally, there is the question as to what extent the administration of large social structures and mass organizations leads to centralization of control and to the development of nondemocratic government, both within organizations and associations and in the larger society.[19] But if an increase in numbers is a necessary (though not sufficient) condition for structural differentiation, as Durkheim has argued, it is conceivable that "bigness" also involves the delegation of authority, increasing functional autonomy of constituent groups and thus ultimately resulting in decentralization of control.[20] For all these reasons, then, it is of considerable theoretical interest to investigate systematically the effects of size and growth on organizational structure and processes.

Operationally, it is useful to distinguish between various aspects of size, or, at least, to be aware of the implications of how organizational size is defined and measured. There are two ways in which size can be conceptualized: the size of the objectives or tasks, and the size of the labor force or membership. The size of the task, again, can be defined in terms of resources (e.g., budget or assets), and in terms of volume of output or service.

In hospitals, the size of the task is usually defined in terms of the number of beds (service capacity) or the average daily patient census (actual volume of service). Since there is always a slight discrepancy between the number of beds and the number of patients, expressed as the occupancy rate, the average daily patient load can be seen as a measure of "effective" size that represents an aspect of the daily work load of the organization. The occupancy rate increases with hospital size, but seldom reaches unity. Most studies of hospitals use the average daily patient census or the number of beds as a measure of size.

Theoretically, it may seem desirable to measure organizational size in terms of number of personnel or total manhours, rather than in terms of work load, volume of service, or units of output, because of the intervening effects of technology and division of labor on task performance and output. Although in hospitals the correlation between number of patients and number of personnel is high (about $r = .90$), there is a considerable variation in the ratio of these two numbers, i.e., in the personnel/patient ratio or the number of personnel per 100 patients. Thus, while there may be an average of 75 employees per 100 patients in large mental hospitals, the number of employees per 100 patients may climb to 225, or three times as many, in general hospitals.

Insofar as personnel constitutes a resource for the effective provision of hospital services, this ratio would be a rough measure of the magnitude of this resource relative to the size of the task. In the present study, however, the average daily patient census is used as a measure of size. None of the indicators we have discussed is clearly superior, and thus the reason for this choice is only technical; since a number of measures of the internal division of labor rely on occupational ratios involving the total number of personnel, use of average daily patient census here is to maintain the conceptual independence between size measures involving the nature of the task on the one hand and the organizational labor force on the other.

46

Technological Complexity

The interaction between technology and social arrangements has been a topic of central concern to sociologists.[21] Most writers concerned with this issue share certain basic assumptions about the independent influence of inventions and technological change on social structure. However there is no agreement on the definition of the technological factor, nor on where to draw the line between technology and social structure. Consequently, there is a tendency to assign technology a fairly central, independent role and to define social structure in terms of the broadly conceived implications of technology.[22] Without entering into the discussion of the merits and validity of technological determinism, it should be noted that the present approach uses a somewhat more narrow conception of technology.[23] Here, technology is seen in terms of the uses and costs of machines, rather than as man-machine systems. It will be argued that such systems are socially defined structures. While they constitute a central aspect of the socio-technical organization of work and are closely related to the division of labor, both technology and division of labor are seen as dependent on the task and goal structure of an organization. Technological complexity, then, is defined in terms of the degree of mechanization and automation, the extent to which technical facilities and equipment are used in task performance.

Operationally, an indicator of technological complexity would be the number and kinds of special technical facilities, or alternatively, the proportion of technically trained personnel needed to operate the technical equipment. Obviously, similar measures could be obtained by computing the proportion of capital invested in equipment, the ratio of expenditures for capital and labor to gauge the capital intensity of production, the amount and cost of energy used, and the like. In hospitals, the corresponding variable is the complexity and extent of medical technology. Thus, the number of special technical facilities and services present, the percent of salaried physicians (radiologists, anesthesiologists, pathologists, etc.), and the per cent of technical personnel may all serve as operational definitions.

Significantly, all of these indicators of medico-technological complexity vary both with the complexity of the task structure and the type of ownership and external control. This observation, to be documented later, can be viewed as a partial confirmation of the claims of both technological and managerial determinists. I will return to this point in more detail.

Division of Labor

It is almost axiomatic that organizations are characterized by a division of labor. This is particularly true of modern work organizations. But the kind and degree of division of labor may vary among organizations, especially if they have different task structures. Of particular interest is the division of labor among specialized work functions and among specialized departments and subunits of an organization. In the following, I will discuss these concepts under the respective headings of "functional specialization" and "departmental specialization."

Functional Specialization

A central element in the notion of work division is the number of different functions which must be performed, sequentially or simultaneously, to accomplish a given task. For example, the number of different job titles in an organization provides a rough indication of the degree to which functions basic to the operations of the organization are specialized relative to each other and differentiated from each other. In other words utilizing such an indicator of overall functional specialization involves *inferring* activities from roles and job titles. Nevertheless, it can be assumed to measure the total amount or extent of division of labor within an organization.[24]

For hospitals, such a measure of the degree of functional specialization can be constructed on the basis of a list of 39 occupational categories. These categories, although not exhaustive of all job titles to be found in hospitals, can be assumed to constitute a reasonably comprehensive inventory of hospital-based occupations.[25]

The index of functional specialization uses the 39 distinct job titles as a standard baseline. Thus, in a given hospital, the degree of functional specialization is measured by the proportion of job titles actually occupied by personnel out of the maximum total of 39 titles. Since it is a proportion, this measure ranges theoretically from 0 to 1. For example, if in a given hospital, 20 out of the 39 occupational categories were actually filled, the value of this measure would be about .50. The greatest utility of this measure lies in its capacity as a comparative index; thus, an obvious advantage of its use as a baseline is the fact that it standardizes the range of categories for a given universe of organizations. All hospitals used this list of job titles to report the number of personnel in each category.[26]

In sum, the proportion of job titles actually occupied out of the maximum total of 39 yields an extremely sensitive measure of the degree of functional specialization in a given hospital. Let us now look at another way of conceptualizing the degree of internal differentiation and division of labor in a hospital, namely departmental specialization.

Departmental Specialization

The idea of departmental specialization involves the number and relative size of specialized and differentiated subunits of an organization. This concept is similar to that of functional specialization in that it refers to the internal differentiation of an organization, but it is different insofar as it is based on departments, subunits, and components (or blocks of functions) rather than the work functions themselves. Another difference is that departmental specialization can be defined in terms of both a priori as well as empirically grounded categories. It is thus theoretically relevant to basic structural characteristics of organizations, as well as to the characteristics of specific types of organizations such as hospitals. Furthermore, we can assume from the nature of work flow in hospitals that there is a high degree of interdependence between the various departments and components. While the actual number of such departments and components depends on how they are defined in a given hospital, the procedure adopted here is to use a fixed number of pre-defined departmental and personnel groups and to measure the relative distribution of the total hospital labor force among them. There are seven components which coincide with the major occupational groupings of the hospital-based labor force listed above; namely, the medical component (physicians), the professional nursing component (graduate professional nurses), the subprofessional nursing component (practical nurses, aides, and attendants), the technical component (technical personnel), the maintenance component (dietary, laundry, housekeeping, and maintenance personnel), and the administrative component (business and clerical personnel). In the following, each of these organizational components will be described and operationally defined.

The *medical component* includes salaried physicians, i.e., those members of the house staff who are employees of the hospital, as well as residents and interns. The total component is calculated as a percentage of the hospital labor force, i.e., the total full-time equivalent personnel. Salaried physicians listed as part-time were counted as one-third time.[27] Unfortunately, data on attending physicians were not available.

A separate measure, the percentage of *salaried physicians*, was calculated by excluding residents and interns from the medical component. In a study of "contractual" physicians in 757 general hospitals, Roemer had found that the proportion of salaried physicians in general hospitals is highly correlated with various measures of the technological complexity and quality of hospitals, holding size and type of control constant.[28] Furthermore, since only the teaching hospitals have residents and interns, it was desirable to have at least one measure of the medical contingent in terms of which all hospitals could be characterized and compared.

The proportion of graduate professional nurses, or the *professional nursing component*, was calculated by adding all full-time equivalent nursing personnel in each of eleven subcategories and taking the percentage of the total personnel. Part-time personnel in these categories was added at the rate of one-half time.[29]

The proportion of practical nurses and auxiliary nursing personnel, or the *subprofessional nursing component*, was calculated by adding the full-time equivalent personnel in all four subcategories, and taking the percentage of the total hospital personnel.[30]

The proportion of technical personnel, or the *technical component*, was calculated in a similar way, i.e., by combining 16 different occupational categories, adding the full-time equivalent personnel in these categories and taking the percentage of the total hospital personnel. (See Appendix D.)

The *maintenance component*, calculated by following the same procedure, includes laundry, housekeeping, maintenance, and nonprofessional dietary personnel. The proportion of business and clerical personnel, or the *administrative component*, was calculated directly from the number of full-time and part-time personnel given in this category. It includes, in principle, all personnel connected with the general administration of the hospital, such as controller, accountant, credit manager, admitting officer, bookkeeper, cashier, public relations director, personnel director, the hospital administrator and his assistants, secretaries, typists, stenographers, clerks, and telephone operators. A breakdown of the administrative staff in terms of these different categories was not available.

Finally, the residual proportion of all "other" personnel not included in the previous major categories was calculated. While the actual composition of this component is not known, there are indications that it contains mainly personnel in highly specialized or new technical categories.[31]

Gini's coefficient of concentration is used to measure the distribution of the hospital labor force among these major organizational components. First developed to describe income distribution, this coefficient measures the deviation from a theoretical distribution in which all categories are of equal size. In other words, this index measures the differentiation among the categories relative to each other, independent of an arbitrary origin.[32] For this reason it has also been called a coefficient of evenness of distribution.[33] The computation of this coefficient is based on the sum of cumulated proportions arranged by size. The formula adapted from Wright is as follows: $G = \frac{\Sigma c - P/2}{n P/2}$, where for a given population P with n classes or categories, c is the cumulated percentage in a given category and Σc is the sum of the cumulated proportions, summed over all n categories. If the categories are expressed in percentages, than $P = 1.0$ and the formula becomes $\frac{2 \Sigma c - 1}{n}$.

A perfectly even distribution corresponds to an area defined by the triangle $nP/2$, and the measure assumes the value of 1.0. Concentration of the population in only one or two out of several categories results in an area much smaller than that defined by $nP/2$. Consequently, the value of the coefficient decreases and ultimately approaches zero as the total population is concentrated in only one of the categories.[34]

The Gini index is similar to an index by Gibbs and Martin devised to measure the degree of division of labor based on the relative distribution of a country's labor force among its major industries.[35] Although the computation of the two differs, they measure essentially the same phenomenon. The correlation between the Gini index and an adaptation of the Gibbs-Martin index, both based on the seven major components of the hospital labor force, is relatively high (r = .95).

In sum, the measurement of the internal division of labor in hospitals is based on two concepts of work division and their operational definitions. The first one, functional specialization, deals with division of labor on the level of work functions and purports to measure the total *amount* of division of labor in an organization. The second one, departmental specialization, deals with division of labor on the level of departments and subunits, taking into account the *distribution* of the total hospital labor force among seven major organizational components. Departmental specialization, as measured by the Gini index, thus refers to the degree of internal structural differentiation of an organization, and by implication, to the degree of interdependence among the major organizational subunits. Since departmental specialization as measured by the Gini index is a truly *structural characteristic* of organizations, I will return to a more detailed discussion of the implications of this important measure in connection with its actual application below. The basic point here is the assumption that in hospitals the organizational components are themselves indicators of the phases or elements of the total work process which are interrelated and interdependent. On the basis of this assumption, the Gini index represents not only the structural complexity of the internal division of labor but also the degree of interrelatedness between the major components.

Professionalization

The role of professionalization as an organizational variable derives from the increasingly ubiquitous fact that certain work functions in organizations must be, or tend to be, performed by persons with special knowledge. We may speak of professional expertise and professional authority insofar as such special knowledge is based not just on experience or practical training, but on formal training in a body of theory and a "value-rational" orientation toward normative standards of service and conduct shared by a group of equals.[36]

Of central theoretical concern here is the idea that a professionalized labor force modifies the nature of organizational authority and control, and particularly bureaucratic authority. The core element of this idea is contained in Stinchcombe's suggestion that professionalization constitutes a nonbureaucratic mode of rational administration.[37]

It should be noted that professionalization as used here is conceived as a structural characteristic of the organization as a whole, not as an attribute of individuals, careers, or occupations. Moreover, it does not refer to the technical expertise of bureaucratic managers and officials, but to the skill level of the production component of the organizational labor force. Finally, the distinction between generalist and specialist professionals is relevant to a conception of professionalization as a basis of rational administration. Thus, both generalist and specialist professionalization are aspects of a rational division of work. But in contrast to the specialist form of professionalization, the generalist form as found in the traditional professions may in fact provide integration and coordination of specialized work functions and thus reduce procedural communications and supervisory enforcement of operative rules. Professional specialists, on the other hand, are themselves part of a system of division of labor, especially when they are employees of an organization. Rather than contributing to coordination, they are likely to require additional coordination and administrative regulation. It is noteworthy that in discussing the integrative functions of professions, Stinchcombe uses a generalist conception of crafts and of professional work, in explicit contradistinction to the more specialist concept of professionalization used by Nelson Foote.[38]

Professionalization of the organizational labor force contributes to coordination insofar as the work of generalist professionals is characterized by a high degree of "specification of function"[39] rather than specification of procedure. The work process is governed by the application of internalized norms and rules derived from a body of knowledge through formal training and practice. In hospitals, for example, decisions governing certain phases of the work process in general and operating procedures in particular can be made at the work level by those who have the requisite training and skill. Thus, the process of *patient care* (of which medical care is one aspect) is implemented predominantly by the professional nursing staff.

In general, the fact that members of a significant functional segment (e.g., the "production component") of the labor force have internalized the norms and rules relevant to their operations and task performance obviates the need for extended chains of procedural communication and hierarchically downward commands.

At the same time, professionals themselves provide coordination of major elements of the total work process, not only by articulating their own work with that of others but also by defining problems, by calling attention to potential or actual dysfunctions, and by taking corrective or even innovative action. This self-direction and discretion in decision-making constitutes in part what March and Simon have called "coordination by feedback," i.e., communication aiming toward adaptation in "contingency situations."[40] Professionalization may thus modify the structure of decision-making and of supervision, particularly the classical principle of "unity of command" and the degree of close supervision as reflected in a small span of control on a given organizational level.[41] It may also decrease the need for an elaborate administrative apparatus geared to centralized, routine communication and decision-making regarding procedures and operative rules.

In hospitals, professional nurses play a crucial role in the process of coordination by feedback on the level of the patient care unit. They do so by virtue of integrating professional and administrative functions more or less successfully in one role. It is commonplace that there are several structures of decision-making in the hospital which vary in their degree of centralization of the respective type of authority. The evidence indicates that physicians do not contribute significantly to the continuity and coordination of the work flow, i.e., total patient care, while the administrator does so mainly on the level of hospital departments. Thus, the joint professional and organizational status of nurses constrains them to assume coordinating functions which go far beyond formal work duties and role definitions. But whereas the administrative and supervisory nurse shares a measure of formal ("line") authority with the administrator, the lower-level staff nurse exercises a new kind of professional responsibility which derives from her multiple statuses and her pivotal work function at the "intersection of social circles."[42]

Thus, while the professional nurse may be supervised in her nursing function by higher-level nursing personnel and in her medical-auxiliary function by physicians, she exercises a considerable amount of discretion with respect to her coordinating functions. These functions are not formally part of a hierarchical structure above her level but constitute a relatively independent realm of decision-making and delegation of functions and of authority laterally or downward to practical nurses and aides. It is here that the internalization of work norms, the assumption of responsibility, and the exercise of discretion contribute to the coordination of specialized functions. Insofar as the total *amount* of coordination needed relative to a certain degree of functional specialization and of organizational units is assumed to be constant, the need for specific *kinds* of coordination, e.g., bureaucratic administration, may be reduced as nonbureaucratic and specifically professional forms of coordination are made available.

The degree of professionalization in hospitals is measured by the relative size of the professional nursing component, i.e., the proportion of graduate professional nurses of the total personnel.

There are, as we have seen, many other occupational groups in the hospital varying in the degree to which they possess the characteristics of professional status, such as formal training, discretion and self-regulation concerning work activity, a collectivity orientation, and a professional reference group orientation.

Some might argue that physicians and technical personnel should also be included in a measure of professionalization. But I have shown already that such a procedure would confound the functions of these different groups. One important aspect of what is to be measured here is that the nonmanagerial labor force is professionalized, i.e., the "production workers" of the organization.

There is abundant evidence in the literature that it is the nursing personnel who constitute the "production component" in hospitals, as against the medical and technical personnel, who constitute "staff" in the traditional terminology of industrial sociology. It is clear that "staff" and "line" are terms which are not unequivocally applicable to organizations like hospitals, since the physician-nurse axis constitutes a line of functional authority crucial to the work organization of the hospital. [43] But even here, as Hughes has pointed out, the nurse is not so much the physician's functional subordinate as his "right-hand man." [44] It is therefore not the physician's professional status and his ultimate responsibility which concern us in measuring the professionalization of the organizational labor force, but rather the nurse's continuous assumption of informal and unofficial (i.e., operative) responsibility, as over against the physician's episodic work pattern. [45] Even if we had complete data on the time attending physicians and house staff spend on the hospital floor, it would be misleading and theoretically indefensible to use the proportion of physicians as the crucial measure of professionalization, or to include physicians and other professionals together with nurses in such a measure.

Thus, attending physicians are responsible only for the medical care of their patients, not for comprehensive patient care. Physicians initiate and direct the crucial aspects of the work process, but nurses implement and coordinate it. From the point of view of patient care, then, the work of hospital physicians, like that of technical personnel and other specialists, is intermittent and episodic, while the nurses' work is continuous. [46]

Finally, it must be emphasized that from the viewpoint of the hospital organization as a whole the administrator-nurse axis is the administrative line of authority. Thus it is not incorrect to say that the therapeutic-clinical line runs parallel to the administrative line in the functional or informal organization of the hospital. But the expansion of the organizational and administrative aspects of hospitals becomes increasingly evident, rendering the view of the hospital in terms of the semi-charismatic doctor-nurse-patient relationship more and more inadequate.

Bureaucratization

The concepts of bureaucracy and bureaucratization have received their most important articulation through Weber's concern with the structural and historical implications of the nature of authority and "imperative coordination" in purposive corporate groups. For Weber, the crucial element of the monocratic, legal-bureaucratic form of rational administration is the exercise of control on the basis of special knowledge. Effective control is based on two structural elements: a specialized administrative staff, which is differentiated in terms of defined areas of competence and jurisdiction, and a hierarchy of offices occupied by experts whose decisions involve the application and implementation of formal rules and regulations on the basis of technical knowledge.[47]

The specialization of administrative functions assumes added importance if it is viewed as an instrument of communication and control at the disposal of the administrator for the purpose of routine decision-making with respect to procedures and operative rules, based on filed information and precedence. Hence, both the administrative staff and the hierarchy of authority are central aspects of the organizational control structure, and are referents of the more general term "bureaucratic structure." If the elements of bureaucratic structure, as conceived by Weber, are treated as variables, it becomes possible to generally characterize organizations or any of their subunits as more or less "bureaucratized" depending on the degree to which their bureaucratic structure approaches the monocratic form of rational administration.

Bureaucratic Hierarchy of Authority.

The direction of a specialized work process or a special organizational unit must frequently be provided by an expert. Professionals and technical specialists may therefore assume supervisory functions which are an integral aspect of their work function and not just something that is added to their otherwise "purely" technical area of competence and jurisdiction. Here, then, we encounter that well-known combination of technical and bureaucratic functions which Weber postulated as essential for the implementation of the functions of a legal-bureaucratic public authority. This combination of functions, i.e., authority based jointly on rank and expertise, provides a type of coordination referred to here as hierarchical coordination.

It should be noted that hierarchical forms of coordination and control may, of course, be independent of expertise and thus be based simply on formal, nonfunctional, "imperative" control or domination. Examples are the echelon authority of military officers in traditional army units, or the charismatic office authority of bishops in the Roman Catholic Church. Furthermore, hierarchical authority is frequently designed or maintained to legitimize and justify extra-organizational systems of status and power.[48]

In functionalist terms, bureaucratic authority represents an arrangement designed to regulate and coordinate operations. Thus, one would expect it to be dependent in large measure on the nature and complexity of the work process. However, charismatic and traditional types of authority exist prior to the assignment problem.[49] Hence, status considerations may enter into the determination of super- and subordination as well as work assignment, in the interest of maintaining given goals or a traditional status system. While there is no way of taking these extraneous influences into account in the present study, the possibility of their continuous operation should be kept in mind when interpreting the determinants and consequences of hierarchical authority.

Operationally, hierarchical coordination is measured here by the degree to which administrative-supervisory functions are exercised in a hospital. This measure involves the proportion of professional nurses in administrative-supervisory positions, calculated as a proportion of the professional nursing component. To the extent that nurses in administrative-supervisory positions constitute a significant proportion of the professional nursing component, we may speak of the "bureaucratization of professionals."[50]

The proportion of administrative-supervisory nurses yields an approximation to a measure of the total organizational hierarchy, since it represents the hierarchical structure of a key organizational component. The concept of bureaucratization of professionals may therefore be taken to refer to the degree of elaboration of administrative-supervisory authority. It suggests both a dynamic tendency of certain key occupations to become bureaucratized as well as the fact that professionals do exercise hierarchical authority. We have seen that this development is anchored in the role nurses play by virtue of their historically and functionally determined key position in the hospital. Nursing includes an extension of the administrative-managerial function, and this fact is formally manifest in the extent to which nurses provide supervision and hierarchical coordination not only to professional nurses and the total nursing department, including nonprofessional personnel, but also to housekeeping, dietary, and even technical functions.

In short, it is argued here that the proportion of professional nurses in administrative-supervisory positions measures the extent to which the organization has formally recognized and institutionalized this pattern of authority. We can therefore say that the larger the proportion of the administrative-supervisory subcomponent, the more have professionals been vested with administrative, bureaucratic authority. This is important as long as we focus on interplay between professional and bureaucratic modes of coordination, and if we want to know whether professionals obviate the need for bureaucratic coordination by virtue of having internalized the norms governing their work activity, or whether they simply take over some of these external, bureaucratic coordinating mechanisms themselves.[51]

Administrative-Clerical Staff

As an index of internal bureaucratization,[52] the administrative-clerical staff can be seen as an instrument of lateral and vertical communication, the filing and storage of information, and the diffusion of rules throughout the organization. As a process-specialized unit[53] attached to the office of the administrator, it is an example of an organizational component which is functionally centralized and serves the whole organization. Of course, administrative-clerical functions may or may not be dispersed throughout the organization, i.e., they may be attached to departmental subunits, or the executive office, or both.

While the administrative-clerical staff performs *regulative* functions from the point of view of the organization, it may itself be analyzed in terms of both regulative and operative functions which define subdivisions *within* the administrative-clerical unit.

Operationally, the relative size of the administrative-clerical staff can be defined in terms of the proportion of its personnel of the total personnel, excluding staff which performs maintenance and other "nonproductive" or "overhead" functions. Alternatively, and focusing more narrowly on the formalization of the communication structure, one may use the proportion of clerical personnel to the total administrative clerical staff, i.e., excluding personnel performing hierarchical-managerial functions.[54]

In this study, the degree of administrative coordination is measured by the relative size of the administrative component, or the proportion of personnel in business and clerical positions. Although the administrative component includes the hospital administrator and his assistants, the main dimension of this measure is not hierarchically differentiated authority, but lateral coordination and communication, especially since the role of the professional hospital administrator can be described as that of mediator.[55]

Administrative coordination also includes the management of relationships with the external environment, including other organizations. In governmental hospitals, particularly in federal hospitals, the relationships with the external environment include those with the superordinated agency (in our case, with the Veterans' Administration). This aspect of the administrative function parallels the degree of external control, i.e., the extent of "external bureaucratization."[56] For this reason alone, one would expect the V. A. hospitals to have a relatively larger administrative staff than hospitals operated under a different type of ownership and control.

Organizational Effectiveness

Effectiveness, more than any other of the variables discussed, must be understood in the light of the specific type of organization under consideration. At the same time, effectiveness of an organization is a question of inter-organizational and institutional analysis. In other words, it is almost meaningless to ask the question of effectiveness of one particular organization. Instead, it must be asked of a more or less homogeneous group of organizations (or a specific type), as well as of the institutional sector and the community that are served by these organizations.

As to the question of homogeneity, let us consider the teaching status of hospitals. For example, one of the obvious differences between teaching and nonteaching hospitals is illuminated by the distinction between medical care and patient care. Thus, teaching hospitals are often seen as providing high quality technical facilities and medical care, but not necessarily "good" bedside care.[57] But while the technical quality of the teaching hospitals can easily be demonstrated, this is not true of the quality of patient care. By the same token, one may use the proportion of the academic medical staff who are board diplomats as a measure of the quality of a teaching hospital; or, one may obtain an expert ranking of medical schools and then contextually infer the quality of affiliated hospitals. One may also use the number of first choices of teaching hospitals by interns and residents as a ranking device, or the ratio of accepted to offered internships and residencies as a measure of the desirability and attractiveness of a hospital as a teaching institution.

In all of these cases, however, the measure of effectiveness/quality is an indirect one and requires validation by means of more direct criteria. Moreover, the diversity or even incompatibility of hospital objectives is accentuated when one learns that a large public hospital with a great diversity among available patients may be preferable as a teaching institution to a small, private hospital in which the rights and privacy of patients are jealously protected. Similarly, the affiliation of a hospital with a nursing school and the consequent participation of student nurses in patient care is often seen as a quality factor. This is so not only because the nurse/patient ratio is higher but also because of the not-yet-routinized attention and care provided by student nurses.

Again, we can easily demonstrate the higher nurse/patient ratio, but not the actual time or quality of patient contact short of data based on a variety of intensive data-gathering techniques such as interviewing, participant observation, and expert judgment.

Finally, among psychiatric hospitals, small, private hospitals with a relatively high patient turnover (or low average length of stay) are usually found to be superior to the large state mental hospitals with a large chronic patient population:[58] But it is precisely the division of labor, or of types of patients, between these two kinds of institutions that makes them essentially incomparable unless one performs comparisons *within* these hospitals along the same lines as *between* them. These considerations concerning homogeneity and comparability have led to the adoption of the following specific indicators of quality and effectiveness: the net autopsy rate, accreditation, the personnel/patient ratio, average length of stay, the nurse/patient ratio, the proportion of technical personnel who are certified or registered, and the proportion of salaried physicians. In the following, these measures will briefly be defined and discussed.

Net Autopsy Rate

An autopsy is the post-mortem examination of a patient's body, often to evaluate the extent of a fatal illness or the cause of death. A scientific orientation among the medical staff would encourage post-mortem examinations in order to determine consistency between (prior) medical diagnosis and autopsy findings. A high autopsy rate would, therefore, indicate a high degree of professional-scientific orientation in a given hospital, where the medical staff *can afford to have their performance scrutinized.* Moreover, such an orientation can be expected to permeate the "therapeutic atmosphere" of the entire hospital and to influence attitudes and performance of all personnel toward higher quality. The net autopsy rate, in order to reflect such policies and orientations, is calculated as follows: the gross autopsy rate is the ratio of all autopsies to all deaths during a given period. The net autopsy rate is computed by deducting the number of coroner's cases, i.e., legally required autopsies, from the total number of deaths and autopsies.

The net autopsy rate is, of course, influenced by the composition of the patient population in terms of types of diseases. For example, a high proportion of cancer patients in a hospital will necessarily increase the autopsy rate. Another factor is the religious composition of the patient population. Autopsies require permission of the patient's family and may not be granted for religious reasons.[59]

Accreditation

Hospitals may be accredited as general hospitals by the Joint Commission on Accreditation of Hospitals, regardless of major type or types of medical service. (See also Appendix E.) Accreditation is a useful measure of quality in the sense that it implies compliance of the hospital with certain minimum standards. The minimum operational standards maintained by a given hospital also constitute, of course, an aspect of its goal structure, just as the accreditation of a hospital as a teaching institution implies that certain basic, additional requirements must be satisfied before the task structure is permitted to become diversified. Thus, teaching hospitals would almost by definition be "better" as long as medical-technical quality vs. patient care are not at issue.

Personnel/Patient Ratio

While this ratio can be used as a measure of the availability of personnel resources when comparisons across different types of hospitals are made, it is a rough measure of hospital quality *within* a given type. In both cases, the personnel/patient ratio depends on budget and policy considerations, as well as on the type of service. Obviously, teaching hospitals and general hospitals will tend to have a higher ratio, because of a higher level of technological and task complexity, than nonteaching, special hospitals.   -

Average Length of Stay

This measure is as much an indicator of "utilization" as it is one of "effectiveness." It is, therefore, practically useless for evaluative purposes in the absence of various controls, among which most important is the composition of the patient population and the distribution of diseases treated. This is only relatively less a problem in the case of psychiatric hospitals, since here, too, one has to evaluate separately the effect of the "total institution" [60] as against that of the actual composition of the patient population in terms of the initial diagnosis.

Finally, average length of stay may be influenced by budgetary and administrative considerations totally extraneous to the medical decisions involved. Thus, a study of V.A. tuberculosis hospitals shows that discharge rates did not exceed a certain limit so as to maintain a certain average daily patient census and to prevent budgetary cuts.[61]

Nurse/Patient Ratio

This is perhaps the only measure which comes close to gauging the quality of patient care in a hospital. Since the availability of nursing service is so closely tied to the type of medical service offered by a hospital, it would be desirable to define this ratio in terms of specific services, such as general medicine, surgery, obstetrics, pediatrics, and the like.

But even then there are a number of questions as to the validity of such a measure. First of all, the general shortage of graduate professional nurses often makes it necessary for hospitals to substitute lower-skilled personnel, or to remain understaffed. One might argue that the "better" hospitals are suffering less from this problem than others were it not for the many subtle organizational and labor market factors which influence the turnover and shortage among nursing personnel. Besides, the effectiveness measure might turn out to be one of "morale" or "atmosphere" which clearly introduces new dimensions and criteria.[62]

But even if we argue that high morale makes for "good" patient care, there are still other factors to be considered. Thus, there is the problem of the training of nurses in terms of quality, specialization, and certification, e.g., the differences between a three-year diploma and a four-year collegiate degree. Another question can be raised on the basis of findings that nurses do not necessarily spend more time with patients even if the nurse/patient ratio is increased. If there is more time, nurses may just spend it in the drug room, with the medical staff, with the charts, or with each other, rather than with patients.[63]

Finally, as a measure of effectiveness and quality, the nurse/patient ratio is somewhat vitiated by the fact that the percentage of graduate professional nurses is also used as a measure of professionalization. This problem exists, of course, for any occupational ratio which involves highly trained or "high quality" personnel. In short, the problem is that a position or job title, or generally, a structural element, is taken as an indicator of the function performed. While this assumption generally underlies the use of occupational ratios as indicators of organizational activities, the additional inference as to the "quality" of the activity or performance requires further validation by some independent criterion.

The Proportion of Qualified Technical Personnel

The presence of qualified technical personnel in a hospital can be taken as an indicator of the presence of the respective technical facilities, and vice versa. Thus, if psychiatric hospitals have a high proportion of qualified occupational therapists, we can assume the existence and operation of therapeutic programs.

The measure used in this study includes various categories of technical personnel and is, therefore, somewhat inferior to a function-specific measure such as, e.g., the proportion of occupational therapists in mental hospitals.

The Proportion of Salaried Physicians

This indicator is quite similar to the preceding one in that it measures the availability of qualified medical-technical personnel. Although the proportion includes such medical specialties as radiology, pathology, anesthesiology, medical education, and administration, it is nevertheless somewhat more homogeneous by virtue of the commonality of the medical degree. [64] However, here too one may raise questions similar to those in connection with nursing as to the type of training received and the "quality" of the medical degree, even though medicine is a more established profession than nursing.[65]

Of these seven indicators of effectiveness and quality, none would seem to satisfy the complexity of the issue. Yet, since it is precisely the complexity of a question which so often furnishes the excuse for not answering it or even defining it as problematic, I will disregard some of my own qualifications as to the validity of these measures, but will take their limitations into account in the application of them.

Summary

In this chapter I have attempted to define and discuss the concepts and variables in terms of which I propose to study hospitals as formal organizations. The main concepts have been operationalized as follows.

The degree of organizational autonomy is represented by the distinction between three types of ownership and control, viz. voluntary, nonprofit hospitals; local governmental hospitals; and federal (V. A.) hospitals. The complexity of the task structure is indicated by two sets of dichotomies: psychiatric vs. general hospitals, and teaching vs. nonteaching hospitals. Both autonomy and task complexity represent the major comparative dimensions of this study. Both of these variables, in other words, define the coordinate system or property space within which the 12 types of hospitals selected for intensive investigation are located. The complexity of the organizational environment is defined in terms of the size of the surrounding community and the number of af-filiations, accreditations, and approvals of the hospital. Some of these factors are related to the quality of the hospital.

The size of the organization is defined in terms of the total number of full-time equivalent personnel. The size of the task is defined in terms of volume of service, or average daily patient census. Both measures are used interchangeably for the purposes of this study.

The indicators of technological complexity are the proportion of technical personnel, regardless of qualification, and, for teaching hospitals, the number of technical facilities and services. The proportion of qualified technical personnel and the proportion of salaried physicians may serve as indicators both of technological complexity and of quality.

The internal division of labor is conceptualized on two levels. First, the degree of functional specialization measures the extent of the division of labor on the level of specific work functions, with 39 specific job titles serving as a baseline. Second, the degree of departmental specialization measures the evenness of distribution of the total personnel among seven major departments and organizational components, i.e., the size of all seven structural units relative to each other. The measure is based on an adaptation of the Gini coefficient of concentration.

The degree of professionalization is measured by the proportion of graduate professional nurses.

The extent of internal bureaucratization is conceptualized in terms of two elements of bureaucratic structure: hierarchical differentiation and administrative specialization. The first of these, the bureaucratic hierarchy of authority, is indicated by the proportion of nurses in administrative-supervisory positions. Administrative specialization is measured by the relative size of the administrative-clerical staff, i.e., the proportion of personnel in business and clerical positions.

Finally, organizational effectiveness is conceptualized in terms of seven indicators: the net autopsy rate, accreditation as a general hospital, the personnel/patient ratio, the average length of stay, the nurse/patient ratio, the proportion of qualified technical personnel, and the proportion of salaried physicians.

In the following chapter, these concepts will be integrated by relating them to their broader theoretical background, and by formulating specific hypotheses. These hypotheses are designed to cast the causal relationships outlined in the previous chapter into a form which is both more flexible and more specific. It is a form which emphasizes the probabilistic rather than the universal character of statements about relationships, which therefore permits their empirical exploration, testing, and evaluation.

Notes

1. A. A. Berle, Jr. and G. C. Means, *The Modern Corporation and Private Property* (New York: Macmillan, 1932); see also William R. Dill, "Environment As an Influence on Managerial Autonomy," *Administrative Science Quarterly*, 2 (1958), 409-443.
2. For an excellent study of this phenomenon, see Ray H. Elling and Sandor Halebsky, "Organizational Differentiation and Support: A Conceptual Framework," *Administrative Science Quarterly*, 6 (1961), 185-209; see also Joan Moore, "Patterns of Women's Participation in Voluntary Associations," *American Journal of Sociology*, 66 (1961), 592-603. On the theoretical implications of this phenomenon, see Peter H. Rossi, "Power and Community Structure," in Lewis A. Coser, ed., *Political Sociology* (New York: Harper Torch, 1966), pp. 132-145.

3. Eugene Litwak, "Models of Bureaucracy That Permit Conflict," *American Journal of Sociology*, 67 (1961), 177-184. See also, for a related concept of task structure, James Q. Wilson, "Innovation in Organization: Notes Toward a Theory," in James D. Thompson, ed., *Approaches to Organizational Design* (Pittsburgh, Pa.: University of Pittsburgh Press, 1966), pp. 196-204. Wilson's concept of task structure is different from the one discussed here, since it refers to the sum of individual rather than organizational tasks; he conceives of complexity as a function of the number of different tasks and the proportion of nonroutine tasks. Wilson sees diversity as a function of both the complexity of the task structure and the incentive system. In terms of the conceptual framework suggested here, diversity is an aspect of the complexity of the task structure, i.e., a consequence of the differentiation of organizational (as against individual) tasks. Given these differences, Wilson's task structure turns out to be more closely related to my concept of functional specialization.

4. James G. March and Herbert A. Simon, *Organizations* (New York: Wiley, 1958), pp. 154-158.

5. Anderson and Warkov, in their study of Veterans' Administration hospitals, also used the criterion of multiplicity of diseases treated for purposes of distinguishing between degrees of functional complexity. They write: "It is assumed . . . that the TB hospitals are less complex organizationally than are the GM&S hospitals in that fewer types of diseases are treated equal on a regular basis. . . . It is reasonable to consider the GM&S hospitals as more complex because, not only are all tasks performed in the TB hospitals also carried out in the GM&S hospitals, but many other services that are regularly rendered in the GM&S hospitals are not provided in the TB hospitals." Theodore R. Anderson and Seymour Warkov, "Organizational Size and Functional Complexity: A Study of Administration in Hospitals," *American Sociological Review*, 26 (1961), 25.

6. See the American Hospital Association, *Uniform Chart of Accounts and Definitions* (Chicago: American Hospital Association, 1959).

7. See, for example, the concept of "organization-set" as used by William M. Evan, "The Organization-Set: Toward a Theory of Interorganizational Relations," Thompson, ed., op. cit., pp. 173-191; see also Harold Guetzkow, "Relations Among Organizations," in Raymond V. Bowers, ed., *Studies on Behavior in Organizations* (Athens: University of Georgia Press, 1966), pp. 13-44; Eugene Litwak and Lydia F. Hylton, "Inter-Organizational Analysis," *Administrative Science Quarterly*, 6 (1962), 395-426; Richard L. Simpson and William H. Gulley, "Goals, Environmental Pressures, and Organizational Characteristics," *American Sociological Review*, 27 (1962), 344-351; Fred E. Emery and Eric L. Trist, "The Causal Texture of Organizational Environments," *Human Relations*, 18 (1965), 21-32; Burton R. Clark, "Interorganizational Patterns in Education," *Administrative Science Quarterly*, 10 (Sept. 1965), 224-237; James D. Thompson, *Organizations in Action* (New York: McGraw Hill, 1967); Sol Levine and Paul E. White, "Exchange as a Conceptual Framework for the Study of Interorganizational Relationships," *Administrative Science Quarterly*, 5

(1961), 583-601; William R. Dill, "The Impact of Environment on Organizational Development," in Sidney Mailick and E. H. Van Ness, eds., *Concepts and Issues in Administrative Behavior* (Englewood Cliffs, N.J.: Prentice Hall, 1962) pp. 29-48.

8. For an interesting attempt in this connection, see Christen T. Jonassen and Sherwood A. Peres, *Interrelationships of Dimensions of Community Systems: A Factor Analysis of 82 Variables* (Columbus: Ohio State University Press, 1960).

9. Erving Goffman, "On the Characteristics of Total Institutions," in his *Asylums* (Garden City, N. Y.: Doubleday Anchor, 1961), pp. 1-124.

10. See also James D. Thompson and William J. McEwen, "Organizational Goals and Environment: Goal-Setting as an Interaction Process," *American Sociological Review*, 23 (1958), 23-31, and Levine and White, op. cit.

11. Elling and Halebsky, op. cit.

12. See, for example, Mason Haire, "Biological Models and Empirical Histories of the Growth of Organizations," in Mason Haire, ed., *Modern Organization Theory* (New York: Wiley, 1959), pp. 272-306; see also William H. Starbuck, who distinguishes between size and age in terms of growth and development in his "Organizational Growth and Development," in James G. March, ed., *Handbook of Organizations* (Chicago: Rand McNally, 1965), pp. 451-533.

13. See Arthur L. Stinchcombe, "Social Structure and Organizations," in March, *Handbook*, pp. 142-193.

14. William G. Sumner, *Folkways* (Boston: Ginn, 1940), pp. 53-57.

15. Emile Durkheim, *The Division of Labor in Society* (Glencoe, Ill.: The Free Press, 1947), pp. 256-282; Hans H. Gerth and C. Wright Mills, eds. and trs., *From Max Weber: Essays in Sociology* (New York: Oxford University Press, 1946), pp. 181-195, 209-211, 261-262, 363-385 (hereafter referred to as Weber, *Essays*); Kurt H. Wolff, ed., *The Sociology of Georg Simmel* (Glencoe, Ill.: The Free Press, 1950), pp. 87-115.

16. Theodore Caplow, "Organizational Size," *Administrative Science Quarterly*, I (1957), 484-505.

17. Durkheim, op. cit., p. 262.

18. Weber, *Essays*, pp. 209-211, 261-262; Reinhard Bendix, *Work and Authority in Industry* (New York: Wiley, 1956), p. 222; Seymour Melman, "The Rise of Administrative Overhead in the Manufacturing Industries of the United States, 1899-1947," *Oxford Economic Papers*, 3 (1951), 69-102; Frederick W. Terrien and Donald L. Mills, "The Effect of Changing Size Upon the Internal Structure of Organizations," *American Sociological Review*, 20 (1955), 11-13; Amos H. Hawley et. al., "Population Size and Administration in Institutions of Higher Education," *American Sociological Review*, 30 (1965), 252-255.

19. Max Rheinstein, ed., *Max Weber on Law in Economy and Society*, Edward A. Shils and Max Rheinstein, trans. (Cambridge, Mass.: Harvard University Press, 1954), pp. 330-334; Robert Michels, *Political Parties* (Glencoe, Ill.: The Free Press, 1949), pp. 37-41.

20. A. W. Gouldner, "Reciprocity and Autonomy in Functional Theory," in

Llewellyn Gross, ed., *Symposium on Sociological Theory* (Evanston, Ill.: Row, Peterson, 1959), pp. 241-270; and A. W. Gouldner, "Metaphysical Pathos and Theory of Bureaucracy," *American Political Science Review*, 49 (1955), 506.

21. William F. Ogburn, *Social Change* (New York: Viking Press, 1922); Fred Cottrell, *Energy and Society* (New York: McGraw-Hill, 1955); Kenneth E. Boulding, *The Organizational Revolution* (New York: Harper, 1953).

22. James D. Thompson and Frederick L. Bates, "Technology, Organization, and Administration," *Administrative Science Quarterly*, 2 (1957), 325-343; Thompson, *Organizations In Action;* Charles Perrow, "Hospitals: Technology, Structure, and Goals," in March, *Handbook*, pp. 910-971; E. L. Trist et al., *Organizational Choice* (London: Tavistock, (1963).

23. See also Morris Janowitz, *The Professional Soldier* (Glencoe, Ill.: The Free Press, 1960); Stanley H. Udy, Jr., *Organization of Work* (New Haven, Conn.: Human Relations Area File Press, 1959), pp. 36-54; Joan Woodward, *Industrial Organization: Theory and Practice* (London: Oxford University Press, 1965); and Edward Harvey, "Technology and the Structure of Organizations," *American Sociological Review*, 33 (1968), 247-259.

24. Udy, op. cit., p. 41. It is interesting that functional specialization, as used here, corresponds roughly to March and Simon's "specialization among individual employees," except that my measure is based on job specialization rather than person specialization; departmental specialization, on the other hand, corresponds to "specialization among organizational units" (ibid., p. 158).

25. The major occupational groups covered by this list of categories are physicians, graduate professional nurses, practical nurses and aides, technical personnel, general maintenance personnel, and administrative (business and clerical) personnel. The detailed list of occupational categories was derived from the original questionnaire used by the American Hospital Association and is reproduced in Appendix D.

26. However, there are also certain limitations which should be pointed out. One is that the measure gives equal weight to occupational functions which vary according to the number of incumbents. Although it is independent of the size of the organization, it lumps together different kinds of specialized functions, some of which may be filled by one person, others by 10 or 100. Furthermore, it combines both functional and hierarchical role differentiation and thus measures the total amount of division of labor, horizontal and vertical.

Another minor limitation is due to the fact that the list of 39 occupational categories is to some degree arbitrary. A flexible list of all occupational titles present in a given hospital would provide a broader baseline against which variations in the degree of functional specialization could be measured. This would, moreover, permit one to use the ratio of the actual number of occupational titles to total personnel as a measure of the degree of division of labor in a given organization. Yet using a flexible list of job titles would also obscure changes in the general occupational structure of hospitals, and confound such changes with variations among individual hospitals.

An alternative measure of functional specialization would involve selecting only those occupational categories which are *minimally* necessary to operate a given type of organization and to measure the extent to which these are represented; or, one could rank organizations according to whether or not they perform certain specialized functions. The resulting scale would give an indication of which functions are basic or most important, and must be performed before others are added.

27. Milton Roemer, "Contractual Physicians in General Hospitals: A National Survey," *American Journal of Public Health,* 52 (1962), 1456.

28. Ibid., pp. 1458-1464.

29. See Appendix D for the specific occupational categories included in the professional nursing component. Although there is probably some variation in the exact proportion of time which part-time personnel other than physicians contribute, it can be assumed that the 50 per cent estimate is the best one available. This assumption is shared by the research department of the American Hospital Association.

30. The categories are listed in Appendix D.

31. This conclusion is based on personal interviews with hospital administrators, as well as on the correlation of this component with the technical component and the degree of functional specialization; see also note 34 below.

32. For a more detailed discussion, see Maurice G. Kendall, *The Advanced Theory of Statistics* (London: Griffin, 1943), I, pp. 43-47.

33. John K. Wright, "Some Measures of Distribution," *Annals of the Association of American Geographers,* XXVII (1937), 177-211. Generally, the Gini coefficient of concentration has been used to measure phenomena of distribution in economic, ecological, and geographic research. Gini himself used this index to study income distribution; see also the discussion of the Lorenz curve showing the degree of inequality in the distribution of income in W. Allen Wallis and Harry V. Roberts, *Statistics* (Glencoe, Ill.: The Free Press, 1957), pp. 257-258. For other uses of the Gini coefficient see Otis D. Duncan, "Urbanization and Retail Specialization," *Social Forces,* XXX (1952), 267-271; Philip M. Hauser et al., *Methods of Urban Analysis* (Montgomery, Ala.: Maxwell Air Force Base, Air Force Personnel and Training Research Center, 1957), pp. 31-56. As Duncan has shown, the Gini coefficient underlies most of the segregation indexes: Otis D. Duncan and Beverly Duncan, "A Methodological Analysis of Segregation Indexes," *American Sociological Review,* XX (1955), 210-217. In the present study, the Gini coefficient is used to measure the relative distribution of a given population among several categories rather than only two.

34. It will be noted that the Gini index includes the residual category of "other" personnel. The exploratory intercorrelations between all variables showed that the other component behaves much like the proportion of specialized functions, i.e., in the large, internally differentiated hospitals the proportion of additional occupational categories increases with the general

level of functional specialization. Thus, an increase of other personnel from a relatively low proportion does not detract from the capacity of the Gini index to measure the differentiation of organizational components relative to each other. On the contrary, since the proportion of other personnel will normally enhance the meaning of the Gini index in the intended direction, the other component was included in the total organizational labor force.

35. Jack P. Gibbs and Walter T. Martin, "Urbanization, Technology and the Division of Labor: International Patterns," *American Sociological Review*, XXVII (1962), 667-677.

36. See Everett C. Hughes, *Men and Their Work* (Glencoe, Ill.: The Free Press, 1958), pp. 78-87, 116-130; and his "Professions," *Daedalus*, 92 (1963), 655-668; Harold L. Wilensky, "The Professionalization of Everyone?" *American Journal of Sociology*, 70 (1964), 137-158; William J. Goode, "Community Within A Community: The Professions," American Sociological Review, 22 (1957), 194-200.

37. Arthur L. Stinchcombe, "Bureaucratic and Craft Administration of Production: A Comparative Study," *Administrative Science Quarterly*, IV (1959), 184-187. This idea is not to be confused with the alleged incompatibility or conflict between the authority of rank and of technical expertise in Weber's conception of bureaucracy, to which Parsons and Gouldner, among others, have called attention, and which will be discussed below. Talcott Parsons, "Introduction," in Max Weber, *The Theory of Social and Economic Organizations*, tr. A. M. Henderson and Talcott Parsons, ed. Talcott Parsons (New York: Oxford University Press, 1947), pp. 58-60, hereafter referred to as Weber, *Theory;* A. W. Gouldner, *Patterns of Industrial Bureaucracy* (Glencoe, Ill.: The Free Press, 1954), p. 22.

38. Cf. Stinchcombe, pp. 168-169; Nelson N. Foote, "The Professionalization of Labor in Detroit," *American Journal of Sociology*, 58 (1953), 371-380.

39. Weber, *Theory*, p. 226.

40. March and Simon, op. cit., pp. 160-161.

41. Morris Janowitz, *Sociology and the Military Establishment* (New York: Russell Sage, 1959), pp. 25-43; Luther Gulick and L. Urwick, eds., *Papers on the Science of Administration* (New York: Institute of Public Administration, 1937), pp. 3-45, 181-187.

42. Georg Simmel, *Conflict and the Web of Group Affiliations* (Glencoe, Ill.: The Free Press, 1955), p. 125; see also Merton's concepts of "role-set" and "status-set" in Robert K. Merton, *Social Theory and Social Structure* (rev. ed.; Glencoe, Ill.: The Free Press, 1957), pp. 368-384.

43. See, for example, Amitai Etzioni, "Authority Structure and Organizational Effectiveness," *Administrative Science Quarterly*, 4 (1959), pp. 43-67.

44. Hughes, *Men and Their Work*, p. 74.

45. Hans O. Mauksch, "The Organizational Context of Nursing Practice," in Fred Davis, ed., *The Nursing Profession* (New York: Wiley, 1966), pp. 109-137; Robert W. Habenstein and Edwin A. Christ, *Professionalizer, Traditionalizer, and Utilizer* (2nd ed.; Columbia: University of Missouri

Press), p. 48. In this context, it is significant that the Joint Commission on Accreditation of Hospitals requires an accredited hospital to have a professional nurse on duty at all times, but *not* a licensed physician; see *Hospital Accreditation References* (Chicago: American Hospital Association, 1961), pp. x-xi.

46. See also Lucile Petry, "Nursing Service in Hospitals," in United States Public Health Service, *The Chicago-Cook County Health Survey* (New York: Columbia University Press, 1949), pp. 1123-1161.

47. Weber, *Theory*, pp. 324-341.

48. Ibid., p. 325; Stanley H. Udy, Jr., "The Comparative Analysis of Organizations," in March, *Handbook*, pp. 692-699.

49. March and Simon, op. cit., pp. 23-25, 158-159.

50. Again, it may be argued that the proportion of physicians in administrative positions, or the proportion of all personnel in supervisory positions, would be an alternative measure of hierarchical coordination. Actually, it would be preferable to use a composite index of hierarchical authority which takes into account the hierarchical structure of different functional units in the organization, as over against a measure which assumes the existence of levels cutting across all departments and units (see my discussion of this point in Chapter 9). However, the proportion of physicians in administrative positions would yield a measure of centralization of *medical* decision-making parallel to the interdepartmental decision-making structure of the administrator and his managerial (non-clerical) staff. Such a proportion would not measure the *administrative* supervisory authority structure, which in hospitals reaches down to the work level of the organization only through the nursing department.

51. A more detailed discussion of this point and of a measure of delegation of authority in connection with the bureaucratization of professional nurses are presented in Chapter 9.

52. Bendix, op. cit., pp. 211-226.

53. Gulick and Urwick op. cit., p. 15.

54. See Stinchcombe, "Bureaucratic and Craft Administration."

55. Charles Perrow, "The Analysis of Goals in Complex Organizations," *American Sociological Review*, 26 (1961), 854-866; Paul J. Gordon, "The Top Management Triangle in Voluntary Hospitals," *Journal of the Academy of Management*, 4 (1961), 205-214; Harold L. Wilensky, "The Dynamics of Professionalism," *Hospital Administration*, 7 (1962), 6-24.

56. Bendix, op. cit. pp. 239-244.

57. Robert K. Merton, et al., eds., *The Student Physician* (Cambridge, Mass.: Harvard University Press, 1957); Renee Fox, *Experiment Perilous* (Glencoe, Ill.: The Free Press, 1959); Temple Burling et al., *The Give and Take in Hospitals* (New York: Putnam's Sons, 1956); Howard S. Becker et al., *Boys in White* (Chicago: University of Chicago Press, 1961). In non-teaching, small community hospitals, the opposite may be the case. See, e.g., Henry J. Southmayd and Geddes Smith, *Small Community Hospitals* (New York: Commonwealth Fund, 1944.)

58. Leonard P. Ullman, *Institution and Outcome: A Comparative Study of*

Psychiatric Hospitals (Long Island City, N.Y.: Pergamon Press, 1967); Kathleen Jones and Roy Sidebotham, *Mental Hospitals at Work* (London: Routledge & Kegan Paul, 1962); Ivan Belknap, *Human Problems of a State Mental Hospital* (New York: McGraw-Hill, 1956); S. Kirson Weinberg, "Organization, Personnel, and Functions of State and Private Mental Hospitals: A Comparative Analysis," in E. Gartley Jaco, ed., *Patients, Physicians, and Illness* (Glencoe, Ill.: The Free Press, 1958), pp. 478-491.

59. I am grateful to Dr. Seymour Glagov, Department of Pathology, University of Chicago, for drawing my attention to these limitations of the autopsy rate as a quality indicator, especially in the absence of appropriate statistical controls. He suggested, instead, the average number of the rate of medical (interphysician) consultations per patient as a measure of the quality of medical care. Although I have no data to construct such a measure, it stands to reason that teaching hospitals with a large house staff would rank comparatively high on this measure of quality.

60. Goffman, op. cit.

61. Seymour Warkov, "Irregular Discharge from Veterans' Administration Tuberculosis Hospitals: A Problem of Organizational Effectiveness" (unpublished Ph.D. dissertation, Department of Sociology, Yale University, 1959).

62. For an example of a study focusing on certain aspects of effectiveness in terms of coordination and morale, see Basil G. Georgopoulos and Floyd G. Mann, *The Community General Hospital* (New York: Macmillan, 1962).

63. This is based, in part, on field observation in a large teaching hospital; see Wolf V. Heydebrand, "Some Observations on the Problem of Teaching in Clinical Nursing: A Research Report" (Chicago: Presbyterian St. Luke's School of Nursing, 1961). (Mimeographed); see also Faye G. Abdellah and Eugene Levine, "Effect of Nurse Staffing on Satisfaction with Nursing Care," *Hospital Monograph Series, No. 4* (Chicago: American Hospital Association, 1958.)

64. See also Roemer, op. cit., who believes that the proportion of salaried physicians is definitely an indicator of quality in general hospitals.

65. Wilensky, op. cit.

4 Autonomy, Task Complexity, Division of Labor, and Coordination: Toward a Theoretical Synthesis

There are two fundamental questions in the study of organizations: how goals come to be defined and set in a society, particularly among organizations; and how goals are attained once they are defined and agreed upon. The first question is one of social innovation and change; the second, one of implementation of given objectives.[1]

Let us accept, for the moment, the definition of organizations as identifiable social structures formally established for the explicit purpose of achieving specific objectives and goals. This definition permits the treatment of organizational goals as both dependent and independent variables. Thus, on the one hand, goals obviously do not exist in a vacuum but must always be understood with reference to the socio-historical context in which they are formulated and realized. Such an analytical emphasis on goal-setting activities and their determinants tends to be concerned with the nature and complexity of problems and tasks and with the adequacy of task performance relative to the problems to be solved and the goals to be achieved. In the history of sociology, this emphasis has often led to a concern with the ad hoc valuational character of goal-setting activities (ideological or utilitarian), and to the well-known discussion focusing on the possibility and desirability of a value-free or value-neutral social science.[2]

In contrast, the analytical emphasis on goal-attainment activities tends to lead to a one-sided concern with internal structure. This approach tends to analyze structure and processes within the framework of given goals and is primarily concerned with the means-ends relationship between goals and subgoals, or goals and functions. An example of this conception is the hierarchically structured, analytical relationship postulated between system and subsystem, where in a complex, multilevelled system the goals of the lower level system, or subsystem, are the functions of the respective higher level system.[3]

"This relationship," says Parsons, "is the primary link between an organization and the larger system of which it is a part, and provides a basis for the classification of types of organizations."[4] By drawing from both theoretical traditions, it is possible to conceive a typology of organizational goals in terms of task complexity and conditions of problem-solving. This typology can then be transformed into a classification system that involves the different aspects of the division of labor, or kinds and degrees of technological and structural complexity.[5]

The theoretical framework necessary for such a transformation, and particularly for linking organizational goal structure and internal division of labor, requires the synthesis of certain elements of the historical and the structural-functional approaches to the study of social organization.[6]

It is not my purpose here to engage in the discussion of this broad theoretical problem. But from the point of view of a minimum theoretical synthesis, it is not difficult to view goal-setting and goal-attainment activities as different phases of a continuous process. It could, therefore, be argued that the goal-attainment phase always generates internal contradictions which can be resolved only by the redefinition of given goals or the formulation of new ones, assuming the organization is autonomous. Examples are the reconsideration of quality standards in the face of inadequate or insufficient goal-realization, the divergence and conflict among subgoals, or the emergence of new goals in response to the stagnating or harmful effects of established ones. But the new goal-setting phase must sooner or later provide for the establishment of mechanisms of goal-attainment, the mobilization of resources, and the coordination of activities. Classical formulations of this process are, of course,

Weber's discussion of the "routinization of Charisma" and Lenin's insistence on organization and high performance standards.[7]

It is in this sense that the definition of tasks, the division of labor, and the coordination of specialized task performance are phases of a larger process, insofar as the organization is a going concern, i.e., autonomous and viable. The conceptual framework outlined in the previous two chapters provides guidelines for the conceptualization of these two basic dimensions of organizations: goal-setting and goal-attainment. By including in this framework the ideas of task complexity and the various aspects of the division of labor, it is possible to avoid the conceptual limitations of an exclusive focus on the elements of control and their correlates in the study of organizations.[8]

Similarly, by reconceptualizing various aspects of authority, responsibility, and control in terms of coordination, it is possible to transcend the specific concern with the applicability of the model of legal-bureaucratic administration and to inquire into the non-bureaucratic and "post-bureaucratic" forms of organizational administration.[9]

In this chapter, then, I will discuss the theoretical context of these two major dimensions or phases: goal-setting and goal-attainment; or the definition of tasks, under different conditions of autonomy, the division of labor, and coordination. Of special interest here is Durkheim's theory of the division of labor, although it is usually applied to the societal level and not to the analysis of organizations. Next, I will examine Weber's ideas on the division of labor, as well as his better-known theory of authority and rational administration. I will then show the relevance of classical and neo-classical organizational theory to the approach taken here, particularly the work of Gulick and Urwick, Mary P. Follett, and the "neo-classicists" Barnard, Simon, and March. Finally, I will briefly discuss the systems-conception of organizations, particularly its somewhat one-sided concern with goal-attainment functions and internal structure.

The presentation and discussion of my approach to the study of organizations, which take up Part I of this book, will be concluded with the formulation of the major hypotheses that lead into the empirical work as presented in Part II.

Durkheim and the Idea of Organic Solidarity

Before Durkheim, the concept of social integration was understood essentially in relation to social contract [10] and economic exchange.[11] An exception is Marx, who conceives of social integration and conflict as based on the distribution of power and dependence as determined through property relations. In this context, division of labor and exchange are seen as alienated forms of human activity. [12] Consequently, Marx develops his views in opposition to the classical economists whom he discusses extensively regarding the concepts of division of labor and exchange.[13]

Like Marx, Durkheim credits Adam Smith with being the first political economist to "attempt a theory" of the division of labor.[14] "Occupations are infinitely separated and specialized, not only inside the factories, but each product is itself a specialty dependent upon others."[15] "But the division of labor," Durkheim continues, "is not peculiar to the economic world; we can observe its growing influence in the most varied fields of society. The political, administrative, and judicial functions are growing more and more specialized. It is the same with the aesthetic and scientific functions."[16]

Durkheim does not write about the division of labor in bureaucratic organizations as such.[17] His analysis of the joint effect of population volume and social density establishes a basic distinction between social integration as based on shared value orientations, in contrast to that based on cooperation and interdependence. "The first binds the individual directly to society without intermediary. In the second, he depends on society, because he depends upon the parts of which it is composed." [18] Durkheim is explicit about the causal relationship between density and division of labor when he says " . . . not that the growth and condensation of societies *permit*, but that they *necessitate* a greater division of labor."[19]

In contrast to Durkheim's collective type, the organic type is "a system of different special functions which definite relations unite."[20] It has been suggested that social density may lead not only to functional differentiation, but more generally to social differentiation, including the differentiation of status and power in the community which, in turn, influences the organization of production.[21] Thus, one could view the relationship between specialization and control in terms of two possible directions, namely, specialized functions leading to control functions and thereby to status differentiation, and vice versa, status and power differences leading to the ascription and allocation of specialized functions in the interest of maintaining a given status system.

For Durkheim, the normative element of reciprocity in contract relations is not possible without the relational element of cooperation which, in turn, is dependent on differentiation and specialization of function:

> To cooperate, in short, is to participate in a common task. If this is divided into tasks qualitatively similar, but mutually indispensable, there is a simple division of labor of the first degree. If the tasks are of a different character, there is a compound division of labor, specialization properly called.[22]

Durkheim recognizes the relationship between size of aggregate and structural differentiation when he says that "the division of labor varies in direct ratio with the volume and density of societies . . . for in order that functions may be more specialized, there must be more cooperators, and they must be related to cooperate."[23]

The "relatedness" of cooperators is dynamic in two principal ways. First, it emerges from the various forms of social interaction, such as competition and conflict,[24] spatial contiguity and temporal continuity of contact, and ease, frequency, and regularity of exchange. This is particularly true if

> instead of entering into or remaining in competition, two similar enterprises establish equilibrium by sharing their common task. Instead of one being subordinate to the other, they coordinate.[25]

Secondly, cooperative relations are dynamic because they lead to the development of regulative functions, such as federally organized administrative and governmental functions or administrative and constitutional law, as well as to self-regulation among the different parts of society by means of rules and legislation, e.g., industrial codes.[26]

These statements are complex. They sum up Durkheim's answer to Spencer's individualistic interpretation of the division of labor and to the theory of equilibrium of functions and harmony of interests of the classical economists, based on the assumption of unregulated, "free" competition and exchange. They also contain the elements of a rich conception of organization. The concept of organization emerging here includes, on the one hand, Sumner's idea of progressive institutionalization and formalization of initially habitual relationships.[27] On the other hand, it anticipates Weber's and other organization theorists' postulates that in a given organization functions must be specific, defined, determinate, and permanent in their relationship to each other, and regulated either through direct relations of interdependence or through rules, administrative regulation, planning, pre-coordination, self-regulation, and other explicit or implicit forms of coordination.[28]

Finally, it should be noted that Durkheim provides some of the theoretical relationships among the conceptions of "common" (agreed-upon) tasks, the pressure toward specialization and division of labor as a result of increasing numbers of actors and of transactions among them, and the emergence of *regulative* functions, i.e., rules of conduct as well as the regularization of conduct which builds up a "network of links." While the emergence of regulative rules leads to the proliferation of bureaucratic structures and administrative staffs, the regular interaction between functions engenders the consolidation of a network of links among status-roles and groups, a process which Simmel has called "sociation" or "societalization," the making of society.[29]

In other words, increased rates of interaction have consequences for both bureaucratic and nonbureaucratic modes of coordination, for the emergence of new goals and norms, as well as for the potential formalization of relations and the consolidation of structure. Thus, the consequences of the division of labor are potentially both integrative and innovative, but they are, at the same time, potentially divisive, oppressive, and destructive. The crucial condition, then, for one or the other consequence to be realized may well be related not only to the nature of the task, but, more importantly, to the degree of autonomy and control exercised in its implementation. It is this consideration which constitutes one of the major starting points for Weber's inquiry into the role of rationality, power, and legitimacy in social life.

Weber and the Idea of Rational Administration

Weber distinguishes much more explicitly than Durkheim between the sociological categories of economic action, notably the types of economic organization and division of labor on the one hand, and types of domination and "imperative coordination" and of regulative and legal-administrative order, etc., on the other.[30]

Weber on the Division of Labor

In his discussion and presentation of the technical division of labor, Weber follows Marx in distinguishing between economic-technical and social aspects of the division of labor. But substantively Weber is much closer to Durkheim. Weber's complicated classification procedure and the use of lengthy historical examples is cumbersome and therefore much less forceful than Durkheim's dynamic presentation. Nevertheless, both Weber and Durkheim come to essentially similar conclusions with respect to the development and the manifestations of the division of labor. For example, Weber distinguishes between the technically simple "primitive" household economies and those modes of "functional differentiation and combination . . . in which the services of a plurality of persons are combined to achieve a coordinated result."[31] Both accumulation and combination of functions constitute advanced, complex forms of division of labor, in contrast to the specification of functions. The latter involves a combination of different functions carried out by the same worker. Relative lack of specialization exists where, except for the differentiation of sex roles, "every individual performs every function as the occasion arises."[32] Weber's intermediate type, specification of functions, is

> typical of the occupational structure of the Middle Ages. Then there was a large number of crafts, each of which specialized in the production of a particular article, but with no reference to the technical heterogeneity of the functions involved.[33]

Obviously, modern professional activities involve this form of person-specialization, where one individual may carry out a combination of functions, such as a general medical practitioner's examination, diagnosis, and therapy of a patient. Both specification and interdependent specialization tend to occur in various combinations in modern organizations.

The social aspects of the division of labor correspond to its technical-economic forms. Leaving aside here Weber's treatment of the "unitary" economy, it is relevant to note the substantive similarity between his and Durkheim's formulations, if not terminology. Thus one type of division of labor may exist "between units which are heteronomous, but are autocephalous, which are thus oriented to an *order established by agreement or imposed*."[34] The other type is the "specialization of autocephalous and autonomous units in a market economy," which are oriented "to their own *self-interests* and to the order of a corporate group, such as the laissez-faire state, which enforces only *formal, rather than substantive rules*."[35] These distinctions clearly parallel those between "mechanical solidarity" and "organic solidarity," especially if one considers Durkheim's emphasis on the growth of administrative and restitutive law as accompanying the development of a complex division of labor.[36]

Weber's orientation toward exhaustive classification of the different types of division of labor prevents him from using the framework of a relatively simple but powerful dichotomy such as Durkheim's. Yet both the historical-morphological categories describing traditional and modern forms of socio-economic organization and the analytical categories of normative and structural integration are clearly present in Weber's work, although they are not easily isolated from the complex and often discontinuous presentation of socio-historical and analytical material. It is, therefore, of particular importance that Bendix, in his interpretation of Weber's work, has pointed to the conceptual distinction between interest and authority as basic to Weber's political sociology, if not to his whole work. Bendix writes:

> Though Weber nowhere discussed its significance for his work, it may be suggested that for him the conditions of solidarity on the basis of ideas or interests and the moral order of authority on the basis of a belief in legitimacy were the two perspectives through which a comprehensive view of society could be obtained.[37]

Weber on Bureaucracy

The definition of "legal authority with a bureaucratic administrative staff"[38] includes certain aspects of the division of labor such as a "continuous organization of official functions " and "a specified sphere of competence," the latter involving among other elements a "sphere of obligations to perform functions which has been marked off as part of a systematic division of labor." [39] Again, in his description of the "characteristics of bureaucracy," Weber refers to the "principle of fixed and official jurisdictional areas, which are generally ordered by rules, that is, by laws or administrative regulations" and to the "regular activities required for the purpose of the bureaucratically governed structure [which] are distributed in a fixed way as official duties." [40] In still another context, Weber states:

> Bureaucratization offers . . . the optimal possibility for carrying through the principle of specializing administrative functions according to purely objective considerations. Individual performances are allocated to functionaries who have specialized training and who by constant practice learn more and more. The 'objective' discharge

of business primarily means a discharge of business according to calculable rules and 'without regard for persons.' [41]

Since Weber includes the concept of formalized specialization of functions in his description of bureaucracy, the concept of division of labor in general has frequently been treated as bureaucratic in nature. However, the preceding discussion has shown that the concepts of the division of labor and specialization as such refer to any level of social organization. By contrast, a total organization may or may not be "imperatively coordinated" and, specifically, may or may not be governed by a monocratic-bureaucratic apparatus, i.e., by "legal authority . . . with employment of a bureaucratic administrative staff." That this staff may be highly differentiated in terms of formally specialized functions is thus a phenomenon of a different order, i.e., it is one that for Weber gives bureaucracy its special character as a particularly efficient and modern form of administration.[42] Weber shows that administrative functions multiply as a result of both quantitative and qualitative changes in the task structure, i.e., as a result of an increase in the size and complexity of the task.[43] Furthermore, Weber refers to the characteristic of hierarchical authority:

> The principles of office hierarchy and of levels of graded authority mean a firmly ordered system of super- and subordination in which there is a supervision of the lower offices by the higher ones.[44]

It is suggested here that the two principles of "fixed and official jurisdictional areas which are generally ordered by rules" and of "office hierarchy" are sufficient to describe and define the basic element of legal-bureaucratic authority of the monocratic variety. The widespread practice of sociologists to add characteristics of the position of officials to this definition is simply an elaboration of the consequences of the *systemic* or structural characteristics of bureaucracy for the *individual* (status and role) characteristics of the bureaucratic official.[45]

Based on the foregoing interpretation of Weber's conception of legal-bureaucratic administration, I choose to select the narrow meaning of this term. Thus the term "bureaucratic" will not be used to apply to the total organization or structure, including all aspects of functional specialization, nor to the characteristics of the position of officials, but only to the presence of a specialized administrative staff and to the organization of offices according to the principle of hierarchy. This use of the term "bureaucracy" assumes the variability of the structural characteristics of a bureaucratically administered organization. Therefore, in the course of analysis, the type of organizational structure always requires specification. Governmental organizations and agencies made up entirely of a specialized administrative staff are thus only special cases of organizations whose major functions and areas of jurisdiction are not particularly visible. It seems likely that this low visibility, partly a function of size and distance, is one of the reasons why government agencies have served as a prototype of "red tape," inefficient proliferation of administrative functions, and the negative attributes of bureaucracy in general.

There is considerable evidence that Weber originally did not describe business establishments or organizations in general, but governmental agencies and other administrative, official, public, etc. organizations.[46] The concept of bureaucracy is, of course, transferable so as to refer to the administrative staff of nongovernmental organizations. Thus, Weber speaks of the "development of modern capitalism [as] identical with the increasing bureaucratization of economic enterprise."[47] Consistent with the narrow interpretation of "bureaucratic," Bendix uses the proportion of salaried *administrative* employees in business organizations as an index of bureaucratization, excluding the proportion of salaried *technical* employees.[48]

From the perspective of establishing distinctions between different modes of coordination, it is of particular interest that Weber himself recognizes more than one form of rational administration and coordination of specialized functions. For example, he discusses a whole range of nontraditional organizational forms as well as types of coordination which differ in various ways from the case of bureaucratic administration. The role of contractual law in the development of organic solidarity has already been referred to in connection with Durkheim. Weber devotes a large section of his theory of social and economic organization to the discussion of the regulative functions of private law ("law of coordination"), especially the role of "purposive contracts" in creating a wide variety of organizational and administrative forms.[49] In addition, Weber's formulation of "pure" types of domination and authority is complemented by the presentation of a rich variety of mixed types. Some of these "combinations of the different types of authority" are discussed with respect to collegial authority, the separation of powers, various forms of representation, and political parties.[50] Of particular interest is Weber's concept of "democratic administration." Weber calls an administration democratic if it is based upon the assumption that everybody is equally qualified to conduct the public affairs . . . and that . . . the scope of power of command is kept at a minimum. . . . This type of administration can be found in many private associations, in certain political organizations, . . . or in universities (in so far as the administration lies in the hands of the rector and the deans), as well as in numerous other organizations of a similar kind. [51]

Weber also discusses the role of aptitude, skill, and incentives in connection with work organization and productivity. He even refers briefly to Taylor's scientific management system and to the role of various types of incentives as alternatives to direct or indirect coercion under free labor market conditions.[52]

Professional vs. Bureaucratic Authority

A crucial point in Weber's conception of bureaucracy is the fact that with a technically highly trained labor force it is possible to perform very complex tasks. At the same time, the organization has to expend only a minimum of the cost on "human relations," managerial control, and other forms of external coordination and control, such as close supervision. However, one condition must be assumed as given: that the goals and norms of the organization coincide with the goals and norms of the technical experts and their status group. Weber modeled his ideal type of rational, legal-bureaucratic administration in part after the governmental bureaucracy of his time. There is reason to believe that the institutionalization of the idea of a "civil service" provides a high degree of articulation between organizational and "professional" orientations in these organizational structures. [53] Weber is thus justified in treating technical knowledge and competence as an integral part of legal-bureaucratic authority, especially insofar as he defines bureaucracy as a system of control based on technical knowledge.[54]

Rather than criticizing Weber for confusing professional and bureaucratic authority, it may be more appropriate to recognize that the monocratic organizational model is of limited applicability, as Stinchcombe has suggested. Studies of staff-line conflict and of tensions between professional expertise and bureaucratic authority are not so much studies of governmental bureaucratic structures as of *professional organizations* (especially the voluntary hospital), of business concerns (especially under conditions of technological innovation), and of such organizations as unions, research foundations, social welfare agencies, and modern armies; again, especially under conditions of technological innovation.[55] In these types of organizations there is, indeed, much less coincidence between organizational and professional concerns, a situation which gives rise to Hughes' "itinerants vs. homeguard" and Merton's and Gouldner's "cosmopolitans vs. locals."

It is important in this context to attempt a clarification of the distinction between professional and bureaucratic authority. My use of the term "professionalization" corresponds to Weber's concept of "specification of function" as discussed above. It does *not* refer to the technical expertise of bureaucratic managers and officials, but to the skill level of the nonmanagerial production component of the organizational labor force. Similarly, my use of the term "bureaucratization," insofar as hierarchical differentiation is implied, corresponds to Weber's concept of bureaucratic authority as based on both rank and technical qualifications.

The widely noted problem of the potential incompatibility between professional and bureaucratic authority, then, is not to be confused with the question raised by Parsons concerning Weber's definition of bureaucratic officials as technical experts who occupy hierarchically differentiated positions.[55] The problem of the theoretical tension in Weber's conception of technically competent managers, as presented by Parsons, involves the incompatibility between legal or rank authority based on delegated "powers" on the one hand and functional authority based on technical competence and knowledge on the other. Unfortunately, however, in trying to clarify Weber's conception, Parsons introduces a new imprecision by identifying the competence of the technical specialist with the functional authority of the professional practitioner, particularly the physician. Parsons thus uses a conception of technical expertise that is more adequate to the description of the "general practitioner" whose work role is *specified* while the incumbent himself is *specialized*.[57]

Parsons correctly assumes that the role specification of "generalist" professional work may be in conflict with the specification of procedures and the enforcement of rules, the latter two being the responsibility of organizational rank authority.

It is interesting to note that Parsons continues to be quoted on this point as if the potential incompatibility between generalist professional practice and bureaucratic authority did, in fact, derive from tensions in Weber's conception of bureaucracy. In his critique, Parsons clearly uses a conception of the general practitioner operating in private practice, a conception spelled out in his famous essay on "The Professions and Social Structure."[58]

In short, the conflict between professional and bureaucratic decisions is of a jurisdictional nature and typically involves overlapping or conflicting areas of competence.

However, it is submitted here that Weber's conception of technical expertise is informed by the notion of specialization rather than specification of bureaucratic roles. Thus, the professionally trained and organizationally employed specialist may occupy a position of authority. In that position he performs administrative tasks, including the supervision of lower echelons and positions. Examples are professional civil servants in government or administrative-supervisory nurses in hospitals. But rather than being in jurisdictional conflict with rank superiors who may be less competent (empirically an ubiquitous phenomenon, often due to the inverse association of age and education) one of the specialist's typical problems is the predominance of administrative functions in his work role. The exercise of administrative-bureaucratic functions thus detracts from the full-time pursuit of a "purely" professional role.[59] While this latter problem is a form of *role conflict* experienced by the incumbent of a given status-role, the problem of overlapping areas of competence is a matter of potential *conflict among organizational roles*, subunits, and lines of authority.

The distinction between specialist and generalist professionals serves to articulate the difference between these two quite distinct problem areas. For example, in more complex organizational settings, the work of professionals tends to become part of the division and subdivision of labor itself, because it is here that professionalization assumes a more specialist character.[60]

Hughes has pointed out that an organizational setting provides both context and impetus for the increased specialization of professionals, and Rossi has described the same phenomenon in relation to research organizations.[61] In other words, rather than being the generalists whose insight into and control of the work process contributes to its coordination, professionals now perform more task-specific functions.

Moreover, although professionals in the more complex organizational context are more likely to be cosmopolitans rather than locals, it can be assumed that they increasingly acquire the trained capacity to reconcile their orientation toward specific task performance with a concern for organizational problems and priorities. Thus, the pervasive interpenetration of professional and organizational orientation, of functional and human-social job skills, and of specialist and administrative concerns has been noted by most students of organization.[62]

Of particular interest here is a recent elaboration of the local-cosmopolitan dichotomy which contrasts the organizational orientation of professionals with one of "professional self-gratification."[63] Goldberg and his associates call an orientation complex if it combines both organizational and personal-professional concerns. They do not, however, spell out the critical implication of the phenomenon of professional self-gratification for Parsons' conception of the professional role, which stresses collectivity orientation in the pattern variable of self vs. collectivity orientation. Moreover, collectivity orientation is characteristic of the generalist professional practitioner rather than the organizationally employed specialist.[64]

Two conclusions may be drawn from this discussion of Weber's contributions to a theory of organizations. First, both Weber and Durkheim distinguish between simple and complex forms of division of labor, and describe several forms of coordination of specialized or otherwise heterogeneous functions. This includes certain forms that are built into the division of labor itself, such as interdependent specialization of functions involving technically organized cooperation, the specification of functions in professionalized activities, the goal-setting functions of regulative groups, and the elements of democratic administration.

Second, it appears that a broadening of the analytical framework makes it possible to consider such ideas as functional interdependence, professional self-regulation, and hierarchical and regulative forms of administration on the basis of their relevance to organizational coordination.

I will now turn briefly to a third set of ideas which has been identified variously as "classical theory of organization," "administrative management theory," and "theory of departmentalization."[65] Its critique has led to what could be called a "neo-classical" version of the theory.

Classical and Neo-Classical Theory of Organization

For the classical theory of organization, the fundamental problems of the division of labor and of specialization are those of the assignment of tasks and the allocation of resources. The "optimal assignment problem" is then "the problem of allocating a given set of activities efficiently among a number of persons" and "organization units."[66] In contrast to the earlier human engineering approach of scientific management, the theory of departmentalization builds the chains of dependence and interdependence between specialized work functions into the work process itself. March and Simon have pointed out that if this view of the "assignment problem" is taken literally, "problems of coordination are eliminated." [67] The organization can be structured along four major dimensions based on the principle of homogeneity of work. According to this principle, the technical efficiency of a given organizational work unit is assumed to be directly proportional to the degree of homogeneity or similarity of specific tasks and work processes, including knowledge, skills, and machines. Corresponding to types of specialization, work elements as well as workers and organizational units can be grouped according to the major purpose they are serving or the major product they are putting out, the process they are using, the social or physical objects involved (e.g., the clientele served or the material utilized), and the place where services are performed. [68] This scheme of organizational division of labor seeks to describe on a structural level what earlier economic and sociological descriptions of the specialization of jobs and individuals have indicated for individuals, work groups, and workshops. [69] Thus, Weber's definition of interdependent specialization as a combination of functions involving "technically organized cooperation in the simultaneous performance of technically complementary functions" can now be applied to the whole organizational structure. Consequently, "technically complementary" departments and organizational units are "technically organized" so as to "cooperate in the simultaneous" (or successive, as the case may be) performance of functions. The conception of "organization as a technical problem" is basic to much of the literature on administrative science.[70]

Gulick postulates two primary ways in which the coordination of specialized function may be achieved. First, the coordination of work may be achieved

by organization, that is, by interrelating the subdivisions of work by allotting them to men who are placed in a structure of authority, so that the work may be coordinated by orders of superiors to subordinates reaching from the top to the botton of the entire enterprise.

Second, work coordination may be achieved

by the dominance of an idea, that is, the development of intelligent singleness of purpose in the minds and wills of those who are working together as a group, so that each worker will of his own accord fit his task into the whole with skill and enthusiasm.[71]

Since size, complexity, "time" (duration; permanence), and "habit" (routinization) are important "limiting factors in the development of coordination," the "question of coordination . . . must be approached with different emphasis in small and in large enterprises; in simple and in complex situations; in stable and in new or changing organizations." [72]

The concept or "structure of authority" refers to the well-known principle of the limited span of control and of unity of command providing an effective network of communication and control between the executive at the center and the subdivisions of work on the periphery. However, the relationship between structure and coordination is essentially seen in terms of the "interrelation of systems of departmentalization." [73] If a given organization is set up according to purpose specialization, the major task of coordination is the control of goal conflict and the maintenance of process consistency. If the major axis of organization is process specialization, "the work methods will be well standardized on professional lines" and the major coordinating task consists of timing and production control. But if an organization is built on two or more bases of departmentalization, the process departments may be used "as a routine means of coordinating the purpose departments." [74] Other means of interdepartmental coordination include the idea of the holding company, where the

> loose[st] type of coordinating authority . . . would give certain central services and require conformity to certain central plans and policies (while) each subsidiary, that is, each department would be given extensive freedom to carry on as it saw fit, and the [executive] at the center of the parent company would not pretend to do more than prevent conflict and competition. [75]

Finally, the coordination of work can be brought about by such organizational devices as planning boards and committees, interdepartmental committees, coordinators, and officially arranged meetings. Coordination of this type "greatly lessens the military stiffness and red tape of the strictly hierarchical structure. It greatly increases the consultative process in administration." [76]

The second major form of coordination is "by ideas," i.e., through a "dominant central idea as the foundation of action and self-coordination in the daily operation of all parts of the enterprise." [77] This formulation not only anticipates Barnard's concept of an organization as an "integrated aggregate of actions and interactions having a continuity in time" and as "a composition of cooperative acts;"[78] it also has important implications for the concept of the professionalization of the organizational labor force. Thus, Gulick lists seven "specific elements which bear directly upon the problem of coordination" and which focus on the proper selection and motivation of personnel, the building of "service morale" and conformity to the service ideal characteristic of professional work, the encouragement of the development of professional association, the encouragement of research, and the consideration of special aptitudes and skills.[79] The function of dominant ideals and of internalized work norms is thus clearly perceived as complementary to the structural, and as a possible alternative to the bureaucratic, form of coordination. Gulick thus concludes that

> the task of the administrator must be accomplished less and less by coercion and discipline and more and more by persuasion. . . . Management of the future must look more to leadership and less to authority as the primary means of coordination. . . . It may well be that the system of organization, the structure of authority is primarily important in coordination because it makes it easy to deal with the routine affairs, and thereby lessens the strain placed upon leadership, so that it can thus devote itself more fully to the supreme task of developing consent, participation, loyalty, enthusiasm, and creative devotion.[80]

Gulick's two primary ways of coordinating work, "by organization" and "by ideas," could be taken to correspond to Durkheim's organic and mechanical solidarity. However, for scientific management, the interdependence between specialized functions is not the end result of a process of growth and structural change, but of rational planning. Dominant ideals, moreover, serve less to provide mechanical solidarity than to instill a sense of professional commitment to work. In the ideal-type of the rational administrator, this commitment coincides, as it does for officials in Weber's legal-bureaucracy, with a commitment to the organization. Yet even Weber saw clearly that bureaucratic administration and the principle of hierarchical authority are only alternatives to other forms of coordination and control, notably in voluntary associations and in "private organizations," as over against those represented by public authority.

Despite the criticism to which it was subjected, the classical theory of organization permeates much of current thinking on organizational structure, and it is perhaps the critics who have contributed most significantly to its continuation in a modified and elaborated form.[81]

Most of the modifications of classical organization theory involve a conceptual move from a rigid, rationally planned structure to a flexible, adaptive, cooperative system. The emphasis shifts from structural arrangements to behavioral options, from command to communication, from legitimacy and loyalty to the motivational and cognitive limits of behavior, from internalized norms to morale, from sanctions, obedience, discipline, and coercion to incentives, compliance, rewards, and manipulation, from defined tasks and radical comprehensive planning to scanning, incremental decision-making, and "muddling through" in the face of uncertainty, from the "maximizing" pursuit of goals to "optimizing" and "satisfying" adaptation and survival.

A significant element in the neo-classical theory of organizations is the realization that motivation, participation, effort, and contributions cannot be taken for granted. Instead of relying on duty or the work obligations of a Protestant Ethic, or even on an understanding of the public-social good, "realistic" appeals to rational self-interest are backed by the exchange of rewards for compliance and contributions. The concrete, individual person, rather than an abstract social structure, becomes the salient element in organizational behavior, which is itself modeled after the goal-directed actor.[82]

But in spite of the differences between the classical tradition and the neo-classical reaction, the concern with motivation and the nature of incentives leads ultimately again to the question of the long-term stability of such exchange systems, and thus to the question of the internalization of norms. This issue provides a point of convergence for Weber's specification of functions and the idea of professionalization and craft administration, Durkheim's as well as Gulick and Urwick's coordination by shared ideas, Barnard's concern with communication, and March and Simon's coordination by feedback. The notion of incentive systems is, then, mainly an elaboration of the motivational assumptions grounded in these earlier organizational theories.

Clark and Wilson, for example, distinguish between material, status-related, and ideological-normative rewards. A typology corresponding to these different incentive systems distinguishes between utilitarian, solidary, and purposive organizations.[83] One is reminded of Etzioni's analytical typology which differentiates organizations on the basis of compliance relations, whereby the different kinds of involvement refer to the behavior of "lower participants."[84] In this scheme, the most frequent types of compliance relations are the congruent ones, i.e., coercive (alienative, remunerative-calculative, and normative-moral compliance).[85] Two of Etzioni's major organizational types, utilitarian and normative organizations, correspond quite closely to Clark and Wilson's utilitarian and purposive organizations. Etzioni, however, does not differentiate explicitly between moral and solidary involvement, except when he discusses solidary relations in normative and professional organizations.[86] On the whole, there are remarkable similarities between Etzioni's framework and Clark and Wilson's, especially if we consider the dynamic and conceptually close relationship between "involvement" and "incentives."

An important conclusion from this consideration of incentive systems is that we are dealing here with a continuum which describes different degrees of "tangibility" of rewards, i.e., different degrees of internalization of norms and constraints which induce men to participate and perform. The extent to which a high degree of professionalization may thus operate as a mechanism of coordination is strikingly illustrated by the fact that a company like Dupont may employ 150 Ph.D.'s in chemistry who do nothing but basic research in a giant laboratory with a minimum of supervision which is exercised, moreover, by another Ph.D. in chemistry.[87] While we may still be accustomed to think of this kind of work as lying outside the realm of incentives proper, agreeing, at best, to the notion of "symbolic rewards," the incentives here are clearly material and, to some extent, solidary and purposive, the involvement moral, and the commitment to perform according to independent professional standards high. In other words, the range of incentive systems encompasses a whole complex of orientations, which includes professional, organizational, and personal elements, in addition to material ones.

There is one final point which accentuates the continuity between the neo-classical theory, particularly Barnard and Simon, and Weber's work on bureaucracy. It concerns the definition of organizations as systems, regardless of whether they are rational or natural. Hopkins, for example, has shown the feasibility of a theoretical convergence of Weber's and Barnard's conceptions of bureaucratic authority.[88] While these two influential traditions have different philosophical and cultural roots and therefore have often been considered antithetical, they share a number of theoretical elements. Among these, perhaps the most important is a conception of organizations as unitary systems of collective action. Such systems are assumed to maintain continuity, integration, and identity, either in terms of the nature of legitimacy as a shared set of cognitive or normative symbols, or in terms of purposive cooperation and communication.

Both rational and natural system models are based on the functionalist logic of the goal-attainment process, i.e., the nexus between means and ends. A logical variant is the conception of organizations as social systems with goal-attainment primacy.[89]

In addition, Gouldner has commented on the affinity between Selznick and Parsons.[90] Parsons and Simon, in turn, share a system-conception of organizations, differentiated in terms of subgoals and levels and animated by the means-ends dynamic. For both, organizations are controlled by high-level programs. As to Simon, such plans or programs involve a series of linked choices and cognitive imperatives; for Parsons, they take the form of normative rules and value systems and, ultimately, culture patterns.[91]

Even Burns and Stalker's conception of an "organic" system of management, in contradistinction to the "mechanistic" type, represents an integrated although flexible, innovative, and open-ended system.[92] The formal similarity between the two types of system is greater than their substantive difference.

Conclusions and Hypotheses

The preceding review and analysis of certain theoretical perspectives on the problem of conceptualizing organizations has led to the further articulation of the basic dimensions of organizational structure considered here, notably autonomy, task complexity, division of labor, and coordination. We have seen that both Durkheim and Weber, as well as both classical and neo-classical organization theorists, find it necessary to take the variability of these factors into account, although with varying emphasis.

The relationship between these organizational dimensions can be expected to hold on the basis of three considerations: the theoretical frame of reference discussed in this chapter, the research findings relevant to organizational analysis in general, and the great number of studies specifically concerned with hospitals and various aspects of hospital organization.

The basic proposition here, common to these theoretical and empirical sources, is that the multiplicity and diversity of tasks and the internal division of labor require coordination if formal organizations are to achieve their objectives effectively. Although all hospitals are assumed to share the basic goals of patient care, they are expected to vary according to task complexity, according to different modes of dividing the work, and according to different modes of coordination.

More specifically, it is held that in hospitals the presence and operation of different modes of coordination varies with the kind and degree of task complexity and with type of ownership and control of the organization.

The greater the degree of task complexity, the greater the likelihood that *different* modes of coordination will be simultaneously present, i.e., that they are complementary rather than merely alternatives, that *structural* modes of coordination will be prevalent, and that *bureaucratic-hierarchical* modes of coordination are receding in importance.

Thus, the more complex general and teaching hospitals, in contrast to psychiatric and nonteaching hospitals, will have higher levels of functional specialization and medical technology, departmental specialization, and professionalization, as well as a larger administrative-clerical staff. But these complex hospitals will have a lower level of bureaucratic-hierarchical coordination.

These hypotheses, with the possible exception of the last one, follow directly from Durkheim's and Weber's general theories, and from the theory of departmentalization of Gulick and Urwick.

As to the expected inverse relationship between task complexity and bureaucratic-hierarchical coordination in hospitals, a significant intervening effect is that of departmental specialization and of professionalization, especially when these two factors are reconceptualized in terms of "coordination by plan" and "coordination by feedback", respectively. Thus, under conditions of comparatively low task complexity (psychiatric and nonteaching hospitals), departmental specialization and professionalization will tend to be on a relatively low level, implying homogeneity of the labor force and routinization of functions, and requiring external supervision and control. Bureaucratic-hierarchical coordination will therefore be highly developed. But under conditions of high task complexity, given a high level of division of labor and professionalization, work functions will be more differentiated and interdependent, but also more regulated by internalized professional work norms, and by lateral, inter-departmental coordination, both requiring comparatively less external supervision. Bureaucratic-hierarchical coordination will therefore be less prevalent under conditions of high complexity.

Variations in organizational autonomy are expected to affect these relationships both directly and indirectly, i.e., through task complexity and the division of labor. Thus, the relatively more autonomous private, voluntary nonprofit hospitals are expected to exhibit greater variations as to the internal division of labor and the modes of coordination than the less autonomous, public (local governmental, state, and federal) hospitals. The public hospitals are also expected to have a relatively larger administrative-clerical staff than the private hospitals, independently of task complexity and division of labor. In other words, we can expect the less autonomous organizations to be more bureaucratized in terms of administrative-clerical specialization.

Apart from task complexity and autonomy, organizational size is expected to have an effect on division of labor and the modes of coordination. Again following Durkheim, we expect the degree of functional specialization and departmental specialization to increase with size. Quantitative and qualitative changes in the task structure, e.g., increasing size and complexity of the tasks, should also have a direct, positive effect on the relative size of the administrative-clerical staff, according to Weber.

An assumption pervading the early literature on organizations is that size as such has a direct effect on coordination, especially on bureaucratization and hierarchical coordination.[93] Bendix's, Anderson's, and Warkov's qualifications as to the direct effect of organizational size on bureaucratization amount to the specification of task complexity and functional specialization as additional independent variables. Thus, Bendix shows that in business establishments size is directly related to technical specialization, but inversely to internal bureaucratization as measured by the relative size of the administrative component.[94] Discussing Dale's sequence of managerial problems, Bendix suggests that these problems increase as the task complexity of the organization increases. "Some small enterprises can be very complex, even if no large enterprises are simple."[95] Anderson and Warkov show that the administrative component is directly related to task complexity when size is controlled, and that it is inversely related to size.[96]

In Chapter 9, I will adduce further evidence from a 1935 Census of Hospitals bearing on the hypothesis that task complexity is directly, but size is inversely, related to administrative coordination as measured by the relative size of the administrative-clerical staff. The 1935 data also indicate that size is directly related to technical specialization, thus confirming Bendix's findings.

Turning now to the relationship between internal complexity and the operation of different modes of coordination, I will elaborate on the original hypotheses about the influence of task complexity and internal division of labor on coordination in terms of more specific aspects of this relationship. Thus, I would expect that a high degree of internal division of labor is associated with relatively high degrees of both bureaucratization and professionalization. But according to Stinchcombe, as well as March and Simon, I would also expect that professionalization ("coordination by feedback") is inversely related to bureaucratization in both of its major manifestations, i.e., as a specialized administrative-clerical staff, and as hierarchical control. It follows that internal division of labor should not be directly associated, or should even be inversely associated, with the relative size of the administrative staff and with hierarchical coordination, if professionalization is held constant; i.e., if it is treated as an intervening variable. In other words, the internal division of labor and professionalization interact in reducing the degree of bureaucratization in hospitals.

Furthermore, departmental specialization and the pre-coordination of functions (March and Simon's "coordination by plan") will reduce the need for supervision, i.e., for hierarchical coordination. Departmental specialization and the scheduling of activities will, moreover, counteract the specification of functions and thus be independent of, or even inversely related to, professionalization.

Where departmental specialization is, in fact, inversely related to professionalization, i.e., where both of these elements are impeding each other, one would predict an increase in the need for communication, and, therefore, an increase in the relative size of the administrative-clerical staff.

It can be expected, on the basis of Durkheim's "organic solidarity" as well as the assumptions of the classical and neo-classical theory of organization, that these relationships will obtain in complex, diversified types of organizations where the degree of internal division of labor is high. In other words, structural coordination based on departmental specialization will tend to be directly related to professionalization and administrative-clerical specialization only under conditions where the level of internal division of labor is relatively low, e.g., under conditions of incipient differentiation. But departmental specialization will always tend to be inversely related to hierarchical coordination, because the latter is functionally necessary only where the labor force is homogeneous or has a low skill level. Similarly, professionalization will tend to be inversely related to the relative size of the administrative-clerical staff only at a relatively low level of internal division of labor where neither structural nor professional coordination are prevalent and thus do not yet counteract each other. But professionalization will always tend to be inversely related to hierarchical coordination. We can expect this to be true partly because of the theoretical properties of these two modes of coordination as representing two potentially conflicting organizational roles, partly because of their differential association with the division of labor.

In sum, where the division of labor is on a low level, requiring external hierarchical control, professionals, insofar as they are present at all, will be most directly exposed to an alien, conflicting form of coordination which consists in specifying procedures rather than functions, goals, and results. But where the division of labor is highly developed, professional coordination will not only be more prevalent than hierarchical coordination, but it will also be more closely integrated with the division of labor itself. This absorption of professionals into the spectrum of specialized functions signifies the transformation of generalist into specialist types of professional work, or the demise of the general practitioner and the emergence of a wide variety of specialists. Although such specialists require, again, more coordination than their generalist archetypical predecessors, this coordination will more likely be provided by increasing administrative specialization and by new intra-specialty hierarchies, rather than by any single bureaucratic hierarchy.

Apart from the differential effect of size on these relationships, we may expect variations depending on the initial or absolute value of the variables referring to the internal division of labor. For example, psychiatric hospitals, although more specialized as units, can be expected to be internally less complex than general hospitals. If such specialized organizations have a smaller administrative staff, this may not only be due to the lower level of internal division of labor but could also be accounted for by the operation of alternative modes of coordination, namely, professional and bureaucratic-hierarchical forms of decision-making and control. Such a finding would be established through the demonstration of an inverse relationship between the relative size of the administrative staff and hierarchical coordination on the one hand and professionalization on the other.

Finally, it is hypothesized that organizations with low task complexity, a low degree of internal division of labor (i.e., a high degree of homogeneity), and a highly developed hierarchical structure will tend to be more impervious to external influences than organizations with a complex task structure and a high degree of internal division of labor. Thus, large psychiatric nonteaching hospitals will have fewer "external relations" and be less influenced by the size of the surrounding community than small or medium-sized general teaching hospitals. This hypothesis follows in part from the conception of the "total institution" developed by Goffman, and derives from the idea that simple, homogeneous social structures tend to have relatively rigid boundaries and may, in fact, operate much like "systems," while complex, heterogeneous structures are often more adequately described as amorphous, rapidly changing pluralistic clusters and coalitions. They are thus both more open *and* more responsive to external influences. We could also say that complex structures tend to be unstable from the point of view of the simple system, while the latter, in turn, appears insulated and defensively resisting change from the vantage point of the larger, more complex environment.

The major points of these hypotheses can be summarized as follows: There are structural differences between hospitals which can be conceptualized in terms of different aspects of task complexity and division of labor. Hospitals can therefore be seen as representing a variety of organizational forms and patterns of coordination.

The type of ownership and control, and hence the variations in organizational autonomy, will be related differentially to the task structure of hospitals, to the internal division of labor, and to the arrangements made 'to coordinate specialized functions and activities.

In addition to the external influences on the structure of the organization, there are certain systematic relationships between the various organizational dimensions. Thus different types and degrees of task complexity and different facets of the internal division of labor are major determinants, jointly with autonomy and size, of the various modes of organizational coordination. The different modes of coordination are, in turn, mutually dependent on or influenced by each other.

This concludes the first part of this book. Part II consists of three descriptive chapters dealing with hospitals as prototypes of complex work organizations. In Chapter 5, I will present the basic framework of the analysis in terms of organizational autonomy and the complexity of the task structure. The twelve types of hospitals resulting from the cross-classification of autonomy and task complexity will be compared with the total U.S. hospital population and with each other in terms of size of community, organizational size and age, accreditations and affiliations, average length of stay, and certain other criteria of effectiveness and quality. Chapter 6 deals with the complexity of medical technology in a comparative and historical perspective. Finally, the relationship between organizational size and the internal division of labor is discussed in Chapter 7.

Notes

1. One of the most lucid discussions of the alternatives of decision-making under given conditions of the means-ends-nexus is by James D. Thompson and Arthur Tuden, "Strategies, Structures, and Processes of Organizational Decision," in James D. Thompson et al., eds., *Comparative Studies in Administration*. (Pittsburgh, Pa.: University of Pittsburgh Press, 1959), pp. 195-216.
2. See, for example, Durkheim's critique of Spencer's utilitarianism, or Weber's critique of Marx's historical materialism.
3. Talcott Parsons, *Structure and Process in Modern Societies*. (Glencoe, Ill.: The Free Press, 1960), pp. 17-19; see also Herbert A. Simon, "On the Concept of Organizational Goal," *Administrative Science Quarterly*, 9 (1964), 1-22.
4. Parsons, op. cit., p. 19.
5. In this context, see especially Charles Perrow, "A Framework for the Comparative Analysis of Organizations," *American Sociological Review*, 32 (1967), 194-208.
6. See, for example, Pierre van den Berghe, "Dialectic and Functionalism: Toward a Theoretical Synthesis," *American Sociological Review*, 28 (1963), 695-705. Rather than approaching a synthesis, however, this attempt comes closer to a cooptation of the dialectic by functionalism. For a similar critique, see Andre Gunder Frank, "Functionalism, Dialectics, and Synthetics," *Science and Society*, 30 (1966), 136-148. See also Gouldner's distinction between natural and rational system models and the discussion of organizational tensions and of the functional autonomy of subunits; A. W. Gouldner, "Organizational Analysis," in Robert K. Merton et al., eds., *Sociology Today* (New York: Basic Books, 1959), pp. 413-428; and A. W. Gouldner, "Reciprocity and Autonomy in Functional Theory," in Llewllyn Gross, ed., *Symposium on Sociological Theory* (Evanston, Ill.: Row, Peterson, 1959), pp. 241-270.
7. Max Weber, *The Theory of Social and Economic Organization*, tr. A.M. Henderson and Talcott Parsons, ed. Talcott Parsons (New York: Oxford University Press, 1947), pp. 363-392 (hereafter referred to as Weber, *Theory*); V. I. Lenin, "What is to be Done?" and "State and Revolution," in Henry M. Christman, ed., *Essential Works of Lenin* (New York: Bantam Books, 1966).
8. See, for example, Amitai Etzioni, *A Comparative Analysis of Complex Organizations* (New York: The Free Press, 1961).

9. See, for example, Arthur L. Stinchcombe, "Formal Organizations," in Neil Smelser, ed., *Sociology* (New York: Wiley, 1967), pp. 169-172; Terence K. Hopkins, "Bureaucratic Authority: The Convergence of Weber and Barnard," in Amitai Etzioni, ed., *Complex Organizations* (New York: Holt, Rinehart, and Winston, 1961), pp. 82-98; Eugene Litwak, "Models of Bureaucracy Which Permit Conflict," *American Journal of Sociology*, 67 (1961) 177-184; E. Wight Bakke, *Bonds of Organization* (New York: Harper, 1950); see also Tom Burns and G. M. Stalker, *The Management of Innovation* (London: Tavistock, 1961); Michel Crozier, *The Bureaucratic Phenomenon* (London: Tavistock, 1964); Warren Bennis, *Changing Organizations* (New York: McGraw-Hill, 1966), pp. 3-15.

10. Thomas Hobbes, *Leviathan* (1651); Herbert Spencer, *Principles of Sociology*, Vols. II and III (1896).

11. Adam Smith, *The Wealth of Nations* (1776); James Mill, *Elements of Political Economy* (1821).

12. Karl Marx, *The Economic and Philosophic Manuscripts of 1844*, ed. D. J. Struik (New York: International Publishers, 1964), pp. 158-164; T. B. Bottomore and M. Rubel, eds., Karl Marx, *Selected Writings in Sociology and Social Philosophy* (London: Watts and Co., 1956), pp. 88-101 (hereafter cited as Marx, *Selected Writings*).

13. Marx, *Economic and Philosophic Manuscripts*, pp. 159-161. Unlike Durkheim, Marx distinguishes explicitly between division of labor on the societal level as against that of the workshop and factory, which amounts to a distinction between the economic and social aspects of the division of labor. Writing about modern society and industrial organization, Marx observes: "Society as a whole, like a workshop, has its division of labor. If the division of labor within a modern workshop were taken as a model to be applied to a whole society, the society best organized for the production of wealth would, without question, be that which had only a single entrepreneur in charge, apportioning the work to the various members of the community in accordance with a predetermined rule. But things are not at all like this. Whereas, in a modern workshop the division of labor is regulated in detail by the authority of the entrepreneur, modern society has no other rule, and no other authority for apportioning work, than free [sic] competition" (Marx, *Selected Writings*, p. 91).

It should be noted that Marx has generally a less "integrative" view of the division of labor in society than appears to be the case here; specifically, he tends to emphasize the divisive, conflict-producing aspects of capitalist division of labor. Nevertheless, Marx makes the interesting distinction between "heterogeneous" and "organic" manufacture, the latter corresponding to concepts used also by Durkheim (see below) and Weber. This distinction is made in *Das Kapital* (Berlin: Dietz, 1953), I, 352-387.

14. Emile Durkheim, *The Division of Labor in Society*, tr. George Simpson (Glencoe, Ill.: The Free Press, 1947), p. 39. Actually, it was Adam Ferguson who first gave a sociological description of the division of labor, in his *Essay on the History of Civil Society* (1767).

15. Durkheim, op. cit., p. 39.

16. Ibid., p. 40.
17. The only work in which Durkheim refers to the specific aspects of work organization on the level of the workshop or factory is his *Socialism*, ed. A. W. Gouldner (New York: Collier Books, 1962), pp. 167-211. As to the applicability of Durkheim's ideas to systems below the societal level, see Leo F. Schnore, "Social Morphology and Human Ecology," *American Journal of Sociology*, LXIII (1958), 620-634.
18. Durkheim, *Division*, p. 129.
19. Ibid., p. 262.
20. Ibid., p. 129.
21. Discussion of some aspects of this problem is contained in Stanley H. Udy, "Technical and Institutional Factors in Production Organization: A Preliminary Model," *American Journal of Sociology*, 68 (1961), 247-254; Arthur L. Stinchcombe, "Comment," *American Journal of Sociology*, 68 (1961) 255-259; and Stanley H. Udy, "The Comparative Analysis of Organizations," in James E. March, ed., *Handbook of Organizations* (Chicago: Rand McNally, 1965), pp. 692-699; see also Marx, *Selected Writings*, pp. 91, 92, and 95; and Weber, op. cit., pp. 246-250, 325-328.
22. Durkheim, *Division*, p. 24.
23. Ibid., p. 262.
24. Ibid., p. 266.
25. Ibid., p. 270.
26. Ibid., pp. 219-229, 364-371. Durkheim expresses these relationships as follows (all italics mine):

> For the same reason that *exchanges* take place among [solidary organs] easily, they take place *frequently*; being *regular*, they *regularize themselves* accordingly, and in time the work of *consolidation* is achieved (ibid., p. 368).
>
> Wherever organic solidarity is found, we come upon an adequately developed *regulation determining the mutual relations of functions*. For organic solidarity to exist, it is not enough that there be a system of organs necessary to one another, which in a general way feel solidary, but it is also necessary that the way in which they should come together. . . be *predetermined* (ibid., p. 365).
>
> What [regulative action] brings face to face are *functions*, that is to say, *ways of definite action*, which are identically *repeated* in given circumstances" (ibid., p. 366).
>
> The *fixity* and *regularity* . . . [of] the relations which are formed among these functions [is] transformed into *rules of conduct*. The rule does not . . . *create* the state of mutual dependence in which solitary organs find themselves, but only *expresses* in clear-cut fashion the result of a given situation . . . . Certain moralists have claimed that the division of labor does not produce true solidarity. They have seen in it only particular exchanges, ephemeral combinations, without past or future, in which the individual is thrown on his own resources. They have not perceived the slow work of *consolidation*, the *network of*

links which little by little have been woven and which makes something permanent of organic solidarity (ibid).

27. William G. Sumner, *Folkways* (Boston: Ginn and Co., 1940), pp. 53-57.

28. Hans H. Gerth and C. Wright Mills, trs. and eds., *From Max Weber: Essays in Sociology* (New York: Oxford University Press, 1946), pp. 196-244 (hereafter cited as Weber, *Essays*); Weber, *Theory*, pp. 145-153, 218-266, 324-423; Edward A. Shils and Max Rheinstein, trs., Max Rheinstein ed., *Max Weber on Law in Economy and Society*, (Cambridge, Mass.: Harvard University Press, 1954), pp. 98-197, 322-348 (hereafter cited as Weber, *Law*); Luther Gulick and L. Urwick, eds., *Papers on the Science of Administration* (New York: Institute of Public Administration, 1937). It should be noted that although it is necessary to formally distinguish markets from organizations, the latter may employ market and price mechanisms for purposes of coordination. See, e.g., Leon C. Marshall, *Industrial Society*, Part III, *The Coordination of Specialists Through the Market* (Chicago: University of Chicago Press, 1930); Robert E. Dahl and Charles Lindblom, *Politics, Economics, and Welfare* (New York: Harper and Row, 1953).

29. Kurt H. Wolff, tr. and ed., *The Sociology of Georg Simmel* (Glencoe, Ill.: The Free Press, 1950), pp. xiii, 3-11.

30. Weber, *Theory*, pp. 145-152, 229-233, 324-423; Weber, *Law*, pp. 322-348.

31. Weber, *Theory*, p. 226. According to Weber, there are two main possibilities: "First, the 'accumulation' of functions; that is, the employment of a number of persons all performing the same function to achieve a result. This may be organized in such a way that the functions are coordinated but technically independent of each other, are thus parallel; or they may be organized on a technical basis in relation to a single common purpose. [This is Durkheim's simple division of labor of the first degree.] The second type is the 'combination' of functions—that is, of functions which are qualitatively different, and thus specialized—in order to achieve a result. These functions may be technically independent and either simultaneous or successive; or they may involve technically organized cooperation in the simultaneous performance of technically complementary functions." (This is Durkheim's compound division of labor or interdependent specialization.)

32. Ibid., p. 225. This last type of division of labor is its simplest form and "may be due to the technical level of work which does not permit further dividing up, to seasonal variations, or to certain kinds of part-time work." This type obtains under the structurally undifferentiated conditions of homogeneous societies which Durkheim discusses in terms of integration on the basis of mechanical solidarity.

33. Ibid., p. 226.

34. Ibid., p. 229 (italics mine).

35. Ibid. (italics mine).

36. Durkheim, *Division*, pp. 63-69, 147-173, 200-229; Weber, *Law*, pp. 98-197. One may add here that Weber makes the corresponding distinction

between public law (law of subordination) and private law (law of coordination) (ibid, pp. 42-43).

37. Reinhard Bendix, *Max Weber: An Intellectual Portrait* (New York: Doubleday, 1960), p. 291.
38. Weber, *Theory*, pp. 329-341.
39. Ibid., p. 330.
40. Weber. *Essays*, p. 196.
41. Ibid., p. 215.
42. Ibid., p. 198. Closely tied to the "principle of fixed and official jurisdictional areas" is the fact that "the management of the office follows general rules," laws, and administrative regulations, which correspond to the jurisdictional areas (ibid., pp. 196, 198). Similarly, "the management of the modern office is based upon written documents ('the files')." (ibid., p. 197). Again, the system of filing corresponds to the official jurisdictional areas, while the files themselves have largely the function of documenting official decisions and action taken in accordance with the rules and regulations covering each jurisdictional area. Rules, files, and the formalization of information storage are thus integral parts of the specialization of administrative functions. It is clear that these elements also imply "the 'objective' discharge of business according to calculable rules and 'without regard for persons' " (ibid., p. 215); i.e., they imply the universalistic, impersonal nature of deciding "cases" according to the rules formally defined for a particular jurisdiction and implemented on the basis of precedent as documented in the files. The legal, court-like nature of these procedures is one of the reasons for calling this type of bureaucratic authority "legal," the other reason being its legitimation on the basis of laws.
43. Ibid., pp. 209-214.
44. Ibid., p. 197.
45. See, e.g., Robert K. Merton, "Bureaucratic Structure and Personality," Robert K. Merton et al., eds., *Reader in Bureaucracy* (Glencoe, Ill.: The Free Press, 1952), pp. 362-363; Peter M. Blau, *Bureaucracy in Modern Society* (New York: Random House, 1956), pp. 28-33; Stanley H. Udy, " 'Bureaucracy' and 'Rationality' in Weber's Theory," *American Sociological Review*, XXIV (1959), 791-795; Arthur L. Stinchcombe, "Bureaucratic and Craft Administration of Production: A Comparative Study," *Administrative Science Quarterly*, IV (1959), 168-187.
46. See Weber's reference to "officials" and "officialdom" in his *Essays*, pp. 196, 198; see also his definition of "public authority" (Behörde) as a "heteronomous and heterocephalous sub-unit" of a "governing body"; Max Weber, "Three Types of Legitimate Rules," tr. H. H. Gerth, in Etzioni, *Complex Organizations* pp. 5, 6-7; Weber, *Law*, p. 335; Max Weber, *Staatssoziologie*, ed. Johannes Winckelmann (Berlin: Duncker and Humblot, 1956).
47. Weber, "Legitimate Rule," p. 6.
48. Reinhard Bendix, *Work and Authority in Industry* (New York: Harper Torchbooks, 1963), p. 222.

49. Weber, *Law*, pp. 98-197.

50. Weber, *Theory*, pp. 382-386, 392-423; Weber, *Law*, pp. 322-348.

51. Weber, *Law*, p. 330. Weber writes further: "Normally this kind of administration occurs in organizations which fulfill the following conditions: first, the organization must be local or otherwise limited in the number of members; second, the social positions of the members must not greatly differ from each other; third, the administrative functions must be relatively simple and stable; fourth, however, there must be a certain minimum development of training in objectively determining ways and means" (p. 331).

52. Weber, *Theory*, pp. 261-266; see also his discussion of incentives.

53. One of the best studies of the formation of the Prussian professional bureaucracy is Hans Rosenberg, *Bureaucracy, Aristocracy, and Autocracy* (Boston: Beacon Press, 1958), especially pp. 88-108.

54. Weber, *Theory*, p. 339.

55. Harvey L. Smith, "Two Lines of Authority: The Hospital's Dilemma," in E. Gartley Jaco, ed., *Patients, Physicians, and Illness* (Glencoe, Ill.: The Free Press, 1958), pp. 468-478; A. W. Gouldner, *Patterns of Industrial Bureaucracy* (Glencoe, Ill.: The Free Press, 1954); Melville Dalton, *Men Who Manage* (New York: Wiley, 1959); Michel Crozier, *The Bureaucratic Phenomenon* (London: Tavistock, 1964); Harold L. Wilensky, *Intellectuals in Labor Unions* (Glencoe, Ill.: The Free Press, 1956); Simon Marcson, *The Scientist in American Industry* (Princeton, N. J.: Industrial Relations Section, Princeton University, 1960); William Kornhauser, *Scientists in Industry* (Berkeley: University of California Press, 1962); Harold L. Wilensky and Charles N. Lebeaux, *Industrial Society and Social Welfare* (New York: Russell Sage, 1958); Morris Janowitz, *The Professional Soldier* (Glencoe, Ill.: The Free Press, 1960).

56. See Talcott Parsons' introduction to Weber, *Theory*, pp. 58-60, note 4.

57. For the distinction between job specialization and person specialization, see Victor Thompson, *Modern Organization* (New York: Knopf, 1961), pp. 25-28; Georges Friedman, *The Anatomy of Work* (New York: The Free Press, 1961), pp. 2-19, 82-88.

58. Talcott Parsons, "The Professions and Social Structure," Chapter 2, in his *Essays in Sociological Theory* (rev. ed.; New York: Free Press Paperback, 1964), p. 22, where he too, invokes the role of the physician; and Peter M. Blau and Richard Scott, *Formal Organizations* (San Francisco: Chandler, 1962), p. 35; also Peter M. Blau, "The Hierarchy of Authority in Organizations," *American Journal of Sociology*, 73 (1968), 455.

59. Everett C. Hughes, *Men and Their Work* (Glencoe, Ill.: The Free Press, 1958), pp. 131-138.

60. These conclusions were presented in a paper based on a preliminary comparative study of general, special, and psychiatric hospitals; see Wolf Heydebrand, "Differential Modes of Coordination in Formal Organizations," read at the Annual Meetings of the American Sociological Association, Los Angeles, 1963; see also Wolf Heydebrand, "Bureaucracy in

Hospitals: An Analysis of Complexity and Coordination in Organizations" (unpublished Ph.D. dissertation, Department of Sociology, University of Chicago, 1965). Some supporting evidence was found in a study of Civil Service Commissions; cf. Peter M. Blau et al., "The Structure of Small Bureaucracies," *American Sociological Review*, 31 (1966), 189. The relevant hospital literature indicates that the more complex hospitals do not only attract a larger proportion of professional nurses who have graduated from cc1legiate nursing programs, but also have more specialized nursing personnel on their staff, in addition to other professional-technical specialists. Cf. Milton Greenblatt et al. *From Custodial to Therapeutic Patient Care in Mental Hospitals* (New York: Russell Sage Foundation, 1955), p. 13; Esther Lucile Brown, *Newer Dimensions of Patient Care, Part II* (New York: Russell Sage Foundation, 1962); Everett C. Hughes et al. *Twenty Thousand Nurses Tell Their Story* (Philadelphia: Lippincott, 1958); George W. Albee, *Mental Health Manpower Trends* (New York: Basic Books, 1959), and National Commission on Community Health Services, *Health Manpower* (Washington, D.C.: Public Affairs Press, 1967), pp. 64-65, 128-131.

61. Cf. Everett C. Hughes, "Professions," *Daedalus*, 92 (1963), 663; Peter H. Rossi, "Researchers, Scholars, and Policy-Makers: The Politics of Large-Scale Research," *Daedalus*, 93 (1964), 1151-1153.

62. See, for example, Bendix, *Work and Authority*, pp. 198-253, 287-340; Litwak, op. cit., Harold L. Wilensky, "The Professionalization of Everyone?" *American Journal of Sociology*, 70 (1964), 137-158; Warren Bennis et al., "Reference Groups and Loyalties in the Outpatient Department," *Administrative Science Quarterly*, II (1958), pp. 481-500.

63. Louis C. Goldberg et al., "Local-Cosmopolitan: Unidimensional or Multidimensional?" *American Journal of Sociology*, 70 (1965), 704-710.

64. Parsons, "Professions."

65. James G. March and Herbert A. Simon, *Organizations* (New York: Wiley, 1958), p. 22.

66. Ibid., pp. 23, 26.

67. Ibid., pp. 25-26.

68. Gulick, "Notes on the Theory of Organization," in Gulick and Urwick, op. cit. p. 15.

69. For a modern economic description of specialization, see Harvey Leibenstein, *Economic Theory and Organizational Analysis* (New York: Harper, 1960), pp. 89-115.

70. Urwick, "Organization as a Technical Problem," in Gulick and Urwick, op. cit. pp. 47-88.

71. Ibid., p. 6.

72. Ibid.

73. Ibid., pp. 7, 9, 31-37.

74. Ibid., p. 34. These and the subsequently described modes of coordination anticipate the idea of decentralization which grew out of the realization that structural factors may influence human relations and morale. See, e.g., James C. Worthy, "Organizational Structure and Employee Morale," *American Sociological Review*, XV (1950), 169-179; see also

H. Baker and R. R. France, *Centralization and Decentralization in Industrial Realtions* (Princeton, N.J.: Princeton University Press, 1954). Baker and France define administrative decentralization as "... the minimization of decision-making at the highest, central point of authority, and maximization of the delegation of responsibility and authority in decision-making to lower levels of management" (ibid., p. 14). Structurally, this can be achieved by planning work groups in such a way that coordination and cooperation between frequently interacting workers and work groups is facilitated. The careful grouping of interrelated functions gives maximum autonomy to the first-line supervisor, thus encouraging leadership behavior and further delegation of authority. See also Ernest Dale, *Planning and Developing the Company Organization Structure* (New York: American Management Association, 1952), pp. 38-67, 98-119.

75. Gulick, "Notes," in Gulick and Urwick, op. cit. p. 34.

76. Ibid.

77. Ibid., p. 37.

78. Chester I. Barnard, *Organization and Management* (Cambridge, Mass.: Harvard University Press, 1948), pp. 112, 118; see also his *Functions of the Executive* (Cambridge, Mass.: Harvard University Press, 1968), pp. 96-113.

79. Gulick, "Notes," in Gulick and Urwick, op. cit. pp. 37-38.

80. Ibid., p. 39. See also the broad concept of coordination used by Mary Parker Follett, "The Process of Control," in Gulick and Urwick, op. cit. pp. 161-169: Henry C. Metcalf and L. Urwick, eds., *Dynamic Administration: The Collected Papers of Mary Parker Follett* (New York: Harper, 1940), pp. 30-49, 71-117.

81. Herbert A. Simon, *Administrative Behavior* (2nd ed.; New York: Macmillan, 1957); James G. March and Herbert A. Simon, op. cit.; Schuyler C. Wallace, *Federal Departmentalization: A Critique of Theories of Organization* (New York: Columbia University Press, 1941); Barnard, *The Functions of the Executive.*

82. It seems that these elements of a neo-classical theory constitute a conservative reaction against the more rational and progressive, socially conscious earlier scientific management theorists. On the elements of a conservative style such as "concreteness," "individuality," the "organismic" model, etc., see Karl Mannheim, "Conservative Thought," in his *Essays on Sociology and Social Psychology*, (London: Routledge & Kegan Paul, 1953), pp. 102-119; see also Gouldner's view of the "natural-system model" as "infused with a conservative and anti-liberal metaphysical pathos" in his "Organizational Analysis." p. 410.

83. Peter B. Clark and James Q. Wilson, "Incentive Systems: A Theory of Organization," *Administrative Science Quarterly*, 6 (1961), 129-166; see also James Q. Wilson, "Innovation in Organization: Notes Toward a Theory," in James D. Thompson, ed., *Approaches to Organizational Design* (Pittsburgh, Pa.: University of Pittsburgh Press), pp. 193-218.

84. Etzioni, *Complex Organizations*, pp. 16-20.

85. Ibid., p. 12.

86. Ibid., pp. 168-171.

87. From personal communication with Harris Hartzler, Ph.D., Dupont Company, Wilmington, Delaware.

88. Terence K. Hopkins, "Bureaucratic Authority: The Convergence of Weber and Barnard" in Etzioni, *Complex Organizations.*

89. Parsons, *Structure and Process,* pp. 16-96.

90. Gouldner, "Organizational Analysis," p. 404.

91. Parsons, *Structure and Process*; Simon, *Administrative Behavior,* pp. 110-153. Also Herbert A. Simon, *Models of Man* (New York: Wiley, 1957), pp. 170-175, 261-273; and his "On the Concept of Organizational Goal," p. 20; also Nicolas Rashevsky, "Is the Concept of an Organism as a Machine a Useful One?" in Philipp G. Frank, ed., *The Validation of Scientific Theories* (New York: Collier, 1961), pp. 142-148.

92. Burns and Stalker, op. cit., pp. 96-125.

93. See Frederick W. Terrien and Donald L. Mills, "The Effect of Changing Size Upon the Internal Structure of Organizations," *American Sociological Review,* XX (1955), 11-13; Theodore Caplow, "Organizational Size," *Administrative Science Quarterly,* I (1957), 484-505.

94. Bendix, *Work and Authority,* p. 222, Table 7.

95. Ibid., p. 227, note 38.

96. Theodore R. Anderson and Seymour Warkov, "Organizational Size and Functional Complexity," *American Sociological Review,* XXVI (1961), 26.

Part II: Modern Hospitals: Prototypes of Complex Work Organizations

5   Organizational Autonomy and Task Structure

For the comparative organizational analysis carried out in this study, hospitals are classified along three dimensions: ownership and control, teaching status, and type of medical service. The classification of hospitals according to these criteria constitutes, at the same time, their systematic ordering along the three major dimensions of autonomy, diversification, and multiplicity of objectives. Both diversification and the number of objectives have, in turn, been defined as integral aspects of an organization's task structure. After an overview of this classification which is both theoretically and empirically grounded, I will describe the nature of the differences between federal, local governmental, and voluntary control, i.e., low, medium, and high autonomy, between teaching and nonteaching hospitals, i.e., high and low task diversification, and psychiatric and general hospitals, i.e., low and high task complexity in terms of number of objectives.

Finally, I want to provide a somewhat broader perspective on these distinctions by showing their implications for a number of contextual and structural characteristics of hospitals. These characteristics should serve to define each of the twelve hospital types in more detail. Methodologically, most of these characteristics are correlates of autonomy and task structure and can be considered "controlled" for the purposes of this study.

The Twelve Hospital Types: A Systematic Framework

The general idea of a systematic research design is to classify the data into homogeneous subgroups, to compare the subgroups according to certain significant dimensions and variables, and to study the relationships among the variables within each of the subgroups. Such a procedure is justified if it can be assumed that there are significant differences between the groups. For example, if there was no reason to assume that federal and local governmental hospitals or general and psychiatric hospitals are in any way different from each other, one could analyze these institutions as belonging to only one category: hospitals. But empirical observation as well as theoretical reasoning suggest that type of external control and of medical service should have a significant effect on the structure of the hospital.

Classification by Service, Teaching Status, and Control

The classification of hospitals according to service, teaching status, and ownership and control results in the distribution of 3,544 hospitals among twelve subgroups. Table 1 shows the number of hospitals in each of the categories. The 3,544 hospitals that are divided into these twelve groups constitute 51.9 per cent of the 6,825 hospitals included in this study.[1]

Table 1 shows, first of all, the prevalence of nonteaching over teaching hospitals and of general over psychiatric hospitals. This distribution corresponds to that in the total hospital population. Of all U.S. hospitals listed by the American Hospital Association in 1960 (N=6,845), 22.1 per cent are teaching hospitals; in this study (N=3,544), teaching hospitals constitute 23.5 per cent. Similarly, psychiatric hospitals make up 6.3 per cent of the national total; the corresponding figure from this study is 8.8 per cent. As Table 1 shows, over two-thirds of the psychiatric institutions included are controlled by state and local governmental authorities. Among these, state-controlled institutions constitute over 90 per cent. If we add the forty psychiatric V.A. hospitals to the other "public" hospitals, we see that 270 out of 313 or almost nine-tenths of the psychiatric hospitals are under some form of governmental control.

Table 1
Number of Hospitals by Type of Service, Teaching Status, and Control

Control and Teaching Status	Type of Service		Total
	Psychiatric	General	
Voluntary	43	1,974	2,017
Teaching	13	467	480
Nonteaching	30	1,507	1,537
State and Local Governmental	230	1,141	1,371
Teaching	91	185	276
Nonteaching	139	956	1,095
Federal (V.A.)	40	116	156
Teaching	17	60	77
Nonteaching	23	56	79
Total	313	3,231	3,544

Among the voluntary hospitals, the largest group (1,507 hospitals) is represented by the general nonteaching "community" hospitals. Among the voluntary hospitals we also find the largest group of general teaching hospitals, as well as the smallest group of psychiatric teaching hospitals.

The V.A. system has the most balanced distribution of psychiatric and general hospitals in the teaching and nonteaching categories. More than one-half of the V.A. general hospitals are teaching institutions, a fact which is not only related to the characteristics of the V.A. patient population, but also to the generally favorable orientation of the Veterans' Administration to teaching and research and to the relatively high quality of V.A. hospitals. In short, Table 1 shows the distribution of hospitals among the twelve types that result from the classification of the data in terms of service, teaching status, and control. This arrangement should become more meaningful once the nature of the three basic dimensions has been described; at the same time, their description and discussion (which follows) includes references to the various categories and hospital types as presented in Table 1.

Autonomy vs. External Control

In order to study the possible effect of the type of controlling organization on the hospital structure, three types of ownership and control were selected. These are (1) voluntary, nonprofit hospitals without religious affiliation, (2) state and local governmental hospitals, and (3) federal hospitals, specifically those of the Veterans' Administration system. The subgroups selected on this basis include 2,017 voluntary nonprofit hospitals, 1,371 state and local governmental hospitals, and 156 federal hospitals (see Table 1). Let us briefly look at the nature of the difference between voluntary, state and local governmental, and federal hospitals.

Voluntary or community hospitals are governed by voluntary, nonprofit associations or corporations. Members tend to be interested and influential citizens in the community who elect a board of trustees or directors from among themselves. The board has the primary responsibility for the operation of the hospital, a function which is usually delegated to an executive committee. The majority of community hospitals are managed by nonmedical professional or lay administrators. There is a tendency, however, for voluntary psychiatric hospitals, in contrast to general hospitals, to have a physician as their chief administrative officer.

112

In general hospitals, the medical staff is divided into major clinical services. Each service is headed by a chief, who is usually elected by the service itself, but occasionally he is appointed by the board of trustees. A joint board-staff committee is usually maintained to set policy and to act on both medical and administrative matters.

In voluntary, nonprofit hospitals, the payroll component of total expenses was over 60 per cent in 1956, about 6 per cent below the average of all hospitals combined. For all teaching hospitals, the mean payroll component rose from 42 per cent in 1951 to 75 per cent in 1960.[2] It can, therefore, be assumed that the average payroll component of total expenses in the nonteaching community hospitals was considerably below 60 per cent in 1956.

The second major group in this study consists of state and local governmental hospitals. The local or "public" hospitals tend to be controlled by specific departments, boards, or administrative agencies of respective government. State hospitals are usually controlled by state departments of health and welfare; but in some cases, they are controlled by special boards or commissions appointed by the governor. These groups, while usually submitting a budget to the legislature or some department of the state government, are relatively autonomous. The local governmental, or "public" hospital includes county hospitals, city-county, and city hospitals, as well as district hospitals.

City-county hospitals are under the joint control of municipal and county governments. Such a hybrid organization is established mainly for the purpose of distributing the costs of hospital operation. The boards, therefore, represent both city and county governments.

Although the governing authority of city hospitals varies considerably, the most common form is still the hospital board or commission composed of certain citizens of the community. The board members are usually appointed by the mayor or the city council, and they tend to be relatively autonomous within the limits of the budget.

Among the various types that constitute the local governmental hospitals, the district hospital is perhaps most similar to the voluntary, nonprofit or "community" hospital, since its board, elected by the residents of the district, is also responsible for operating the hospital, as is the board of trustees of the voluntary hospital.

Hospital districts are political subdivisions created for the purpose of establishing and maintaining a hospital. They have the advantage of meeting the need for suburban and rural hospital facilities on a local level without external government controls, and, at the same time, they contain a taxable population which is large enough to insure adequate financing for the construction and maintenance of a hospital.[3]

In state hospitals, the medical staff is usually composed of physicians who are full-time salaried employees of the hospital; but in county and city hospitals, only part of the medical staff is made up of salaried physicians. The others are usually private practitioners who donate their services. They are not, as a rule, permitted to admit their own private patients. However, to what extent such regulations are enforced in smaller local hospitals is difficult to assess.

In district hospitals, medical staff membership is usually open to all qualified physicians. In these, as well as in the state teaching hospitals, part-pay and full-pay patients, who are frequently private patients of staff members, are admitted in addition to "free" patients who are unable to afford private hospital and medical care.

In the teaching institutions, patients who qualify in terms of "medical suitability" for teaching purposes tend to be admitted as "free" patients.[4]

Payroll expenses in state hospitals are estimated to constitute about 64 per cent of the total expense; in county hospitals, this figure is 69 per cent, as against 67 per cent in city hospitals and 62 per cent in both city-county and district hospitals. These figures were estimated for 1956.[5] The estimates reflect variations in the relative expenditures for personnel which, in turn, are related to differences in the personnel/patient ratio and the composition of the hospital labor force. Again, teaching hospitals can be expected to have much higher payroll/expense ratios.

Generally, the differences between public and voluntary, non-profit hospitals are mainly in the nature of the financial limitations and control which tend to be imposed on the state and local governmental hospitals, and in the characteristics of the patient population. These factors, in turn, have an important effect on the size of the organization, and, generally, on the resources available to the hospital.

The third major group of hospitals selected for comparative purposes are those federal hospitals which are under the jurisdiction of the Veterans' Administration. In many studies and descriptions of hospitals, federal hospitals are excluded because they are thought to be too "different" from other types of controlling organizations. V.A. and other federal hospitals do perform the same range of functions as other nonfederal hospitals, although they are probably more specialized with respect to a client population.

The Veterans' Administration is an independant agency of the executive branch of the federal government. One of its three basic operating departments is the department of Medicine and Surgery, headed by a chief medical director, who is responsible to the Administrator of Veterans' Affairs, appointed by the President of the United States. This director is aided by a deputy and four assistant chief medical directors, a controller, and seven area medical officers. The area medical officers have limited supervisory authority and serve primarily in an advisory capacity.[6]

Managers of V.A. hospitals are appointed by the Administrator of Veterans' Affairs and tend to be physicians.[7] Hospital managers are responsible for the operation of the individual V.A. hospital, and report to the chief medical director. Physicians are appointed to full-time positions and are salaried employees of the Veterans' Administration. In addition to physicians, the V.A. Department of Medicine and Surgery also appoints dentists and nurses to positions in V.A. hospitals. All other employees, including the administrative staffs, pharmacists, dieticians, and nonprofessional personnel are appointed under the rules and regulations of the U.S. Civil Service Commission.

It is generally recognized that the quality of medical and hospital care in V.A. hospitals is comparatively high. This is, in part, indicated by the fact that the payroll component of total expenses is about 80 per cent, much higher than the 66 per cent national average for all hospitals in 1956, even though V.A. hospital payroll expenses include salaries paid to physicians and dentists that are normally not included in the personnel expenditures of nongovernmental hospitals.[8] Finally, V.A. hospitals, unlike most other types, provide complete rehabilitation services, i.e., vocational rehabilitation or re-training, and physical and occupational therapy.[9]

Persons eligible for care in V.A. hospitals consist of four groups. First are those persons requiring care and treatment for service-connected disabilities. According to a 1956 census, about 35 per cent of the total number of patients receiving care in V.A. hospitals were in this category. Second are those persons requiring treatment for conditions not service-connected who were either discharged from military service for a disability incurred or aggravated in line of duty or who have a compensable service-connected disability. In 1956, 8.6 per cent of all V.A. patients were in this group. In the third category are other veterans with wartime service who require treatment for nonservice conditions (55.4 per cent in 1956). The fourth group consists of nonveterans with specific entitlement, who in 1956 constituted less than 1 per cent of all V.A. patients.[10] We will now turn to the discussion of the complexity of the task structure, i.e., to the distinction between types and degrees of task complexity in terms of medical service and medical education.

Complexity of Task Structure: Multiple Services

In Chapter 3, I have already indicated the possibility of conceptualizing the number of medical specialties represented in a hospital in terms of a continuum of task complexity, ranging from one to as many as 30 specialties.[11]

The multispecialty hospital is usually referred to as a general hospital, regardless of the number of different medical and surgical specialties present. There are only a few one-specialty hospital types, such as psychiatric or tuberculosis hospitals. "Chronic disease" hospitals are often referred to as "long-term," both designations referring to a generic disease category which is considered overriding from the point of view of patient care. The proper distinction is therefore between long-term general and long-term special hospitals. Average length of stay is, indeed, frequently considered a more important criterion for distinguishing types of hospitals than the degree of specialization of the hospital as a whole. For example, the American Hospital Association often groups short-term general and short-term special hospitals together for certain purposes of statistical reporting.[12] However, because of the comparatively small number of special hospitals as well as of tuberculosis and other long-term hospitals, this intermediate category has been excluded from the present study. Moreover, a listing of medical specialties is available only for teaching hospitals.[13] Thus, short of using the actual number of medical specialties represented in the hospital as a quantitative indicator of task complexity, I am simply using the dichotomy between general and psychiatric hospitals instead.

The numerical breakdown between psychiatric and general hospitals within the three types of ownership and control represents the actual number of hospitals in these categories. Thus, of the 2,017 voluntary, nonprofit hospitals, only 43, or about 2 per cent are psychiatric institutions. The percentage is somewhat higher (with 230, or 17 per cent) among state and local governmental hospitals, and 40, or 26 per cent for the federal V.A. hospitals.

General hospitals have multiple services and are "multifunctional" in the sense that potentially all patients and diseases are treated. Among the 1,031 general hospitals with approved residency programs in 1960, the mean number of medical specialities per hospital was 3.4, including, typically, internal medicine and surgery. Two hundred and five (or about 20 per cent) of these general hospitals had seven or more different specialities.

If, by contrast, psychiatric hospitals are defined here as "unifunctional" organizations, i.e., as having only one medical specialty, the question may be raised as to what extent mental illness may be seen as a "specific" diesease so as to justify this definition. For example, one could consider mental illness as representing a whole range of mental and emotional disturbances, from organic disorders of the brain and central nervous system to disturbances and disorders associated with the mental apparatus to the different psychoses and psycho-neurotic syndromes. In other words, it could be argued that mental hospitals treat as great a variety of different diseases as the general medical-surgical hospital.

At least two points can be made in response to this argument. First, it is clearly a matter of diagnostic differentiation and sophistication to what extent "mental illness" is treated as just one kind of illness, or as a residual category of nonphysical illnesses. Insofar as this is not the case, we could say that, given a variety of mental illnesses, the greater the adequate differentiation of diagnosis and treatment of these illnesses, the greater the technological complexity of the mental hospital, and the higher its quality.

In other words, the range of variation would correspond to the difference in treatment goals, often referred to by the terms "custodial" and "therapeutic" (control vs. treatment orientation), a difference that also relates to the quality of the institutions involved. Similar differences have also been observed in prisons and correctional institutions,[14] and they serve as a frame of reference for Goffman's concept and description of the "total institution," viz. one where custodial functions are carried out to the point of coercion.

The second point is that even if mental hospitals treat a variety of mental disorders and thus have not only multiple objectives but also a high level of technological complexity, general hospitals have comparatively more objectives because they treat a potentially much larger variety of different diseases, including psychiatric disorders. Consequently, the general medical-surgical hospital is a non-specialized, multifunctional organization, even if not all functions are carried out all the time. In the absence of data on the finer diagnostic distinctions between subcategories of diseases and in view of the problems concerning distinctions between dominant treatment orientations (such as custodial and therapeutic) and their empirical assessment, it seems appropriate for our purposes to treat mental hospitals as unifunctional, specialized organizations limited to a specific medical specialty, and general medical-surgical hospitals as multifunctional, nonspecialized organizations, which are characterized by a multiplicity of major objectives and services.

Complexity of Task Structure: Diversification

Assuming that the institutionalization of medical education and research in a hospital profoundly alters its goal and task structure, the general and psychiatric hospitals within the three types of control are further subdivided into teaching and nonteaching hospitals.

A hospital is defined as a teaching hospital if it has a residency and/or internship program approved by the American Medical Association; it is defined as a nonteaching hospital if it does not engage in the education of medical practitioners or students. The definition of a hospital as a teaching hospital does not necessarily imply that it is affiliated with a specific medical school or university. Although, on occasion, I will distinguish between those teaching hospitals affiliated with a medical school or university and those that are not, the present definition of "teaching hospital" combines both types. The reason for this inclusive definition is the need for a sufficiently large case base for meaningful comparisons in terms of the objectives of this study.

The technical definition of diversification in terms of heterogeneity of products for a variety of markets applies only in the sense that medical education and research are hospital "products" which are different from medical service and patient care. The widely held assumption that business organizations diversify as a precautionary or adaptive economic measure does not, of course, apply to hospitals. Nevertheless, the fundamental difference between teaching and nonteaching hospitals points to a divergence of objectives which has many elements of the economic phenomenon of diversification.[15] For example, if a psychiatric or general hospital adds a certain medical specialty, e.g., obstetrics, to those already present, this would mean an increase in the number of major functions or objectives and thus in the level of both technological and overall task complexity. One could also assume that the impact of an additional similar function would be greater on the "unifunctional" as compared to the "multifunctional" organization, since it would *introduce* functional differentiation in the first case, but merely *increase* it in the second. If a hospital, however, adds a new function which is dissimilar to those already present, we would assume that the impact is equally great, if not greater, than that assumed to derive from adding a new similar function. Although degree of similarity depends necessarily on the criteria of comparison used, the reference here is to similarity in terms of different medical service categories.

Organizational diversification, conceived as a process, represents a form of innovation and change. While it is not possible within the framework of the present study to investigate the effect over time of adding functions as such, it can be assumed that the teaching hospital is an organization that has undergone considerable innovation and change in the direction of increased diversity and complexity. In other words, the presence of different medical specialties, represented by board-certified medical specialists and diplomates, as well as presence of medical interns and residents can be assumed to change the task structure and the content of the division of labor in that they introduce new, specific demands and contributions which have ramifications throughout the organizational structure.

The following statement illustrates the difference between teaching and nonteaching hospitals from the perspective of the medical administrator:

> While recognizing the fact that the care of a patient accepted by an institution is of paramount importance, the point of view is maintained that teaching institutions differ in several important ways from hospitals and clinics which have been designed primarily for the medical care of the community. Perhaps the most striking difference lies in their desire, universally felt, occasionally realized, to select their patients on the basis of their suitability for teaching or investigation. . . . The costly facilities for teaching and research are an extravagance when used for patients who are not suitable medically for the work at hand. The facilities include trained teachers and

investigators as well as laboratories, special-diet kitchens and other provisions not usual in non-teaching hospitals.[16]

The eligibility of hospitals as teaching institutions is based on certain criteria stated in the *Directory of Approved Internships and Residencies.* The following is a summary of the most important criteria for eligibility determined by the Council on Medical Education and Hospitals of the American Medical Association.

While scope and diversity of clinical services, rather than size of the hospital, are a major requirement for residency programs, internship programs are approved only in hospitals with a minimum of 150 beds, excluding bassinets. For internship programs, moreover, three of the four major divisions, i.e., internal medicine, general surgery, obstetrics, and pediatrics, must be present. In addition, adequate training facilities in pathology, psychiatry, and radiology, as well as an active and well organized out-patient department, should be present. It is also required that the hospital maintain a minimum autopsy rate of 25 per cent of all inpatient deaths. Obviously, the hospital should be properly organized, staffed, and equipped: "Equipment, appliances, and apparatus such as are commonly employed in the practice of modern scientific medicine should be available."[17] Finally, not only does the eligibility of a hospital presuppose a certain level of quality; the teaching program itself will tend to affect the hospital's quality: "A well-organized, effective, educational program inevitably results in the improvement of the quality of patient care in a hospital."[18]

I will now turn to a comparison of the twelve hospital types in terms of a number of basic hospital characteristics. The comparison will serve to articulate the differences between the twelve types, but it will also underline the pervasive effects of organizational autonomy and the complexity of the goal and task structure on the hospital's internal organization.

Some Correlates of Autonomy and Task Structure

So far, the twelve hospital types have been described "as such," i.e., on the basis of the dimensions used for the construction of the typology. In addition, a variety of illustrative, historical, and descriptive material was introduced, hopefully to render this classification of hospitals meaningful and plausible, even commonsensical.

But before a systematic comparison of the twelve types is possible, two additional criteria have to be met: (1) all twelve types must be comparable in a meaningful sense, independent of the actual analysis, and (2) each type must be sufficiently self-contained and homogeneous so that the likelihood of spurious relations is reduced.

In order to approximate these requirements,[19] the twelve types will now be described and compared on the basis of the following selected variables. The first description is in terms of size, an important general variable relating to both organizational task structure and resources. The second is in terms of a number of environmental characteristics, among them age (only for teaching hospitals), size of community, and the number of "external relations." Finally is a comparison of the twelve types in terms of a number of criteria of effectiveness and quality, notably accreditations and approvals, average length of patient stay, net atuopsy rate, personnel/patient ratio, and nurse/patient ratio.[20]

Size and Age of Hospitals

The size of hospitals, measured here in terms of the average daily patient census, constitutes an important dimension of differentiation among the twelve hospital types, as shown in Table 2.

Table 2 shows that the largest types are public psychiatric hospitals. The voluntary psychiatric hospitals, in contrast, are relatively small. All teaching hospitals are larger than their non-teaching counterparts. This is, in part, due to the fact that there is a positive correlation between size, complexity and (as we shall see later) quality, a combination of relationships which results from the fact that the larger, more complex, higher quality hospitals are more likely accredited as teaching institutions by the American Medical Association. Thus hospitals tend to be large when they are psychiatric hospitals and when they are teaching hospitals. Ownership and control are related to size as follows. Generally, voluntary hospitals are small. V.A. general hospitals tend to be large compared to other general hospitals. Finally, while V.A. psychiatric hospitals are relatively large, the (nonfederal) public psychiatric hospitals are, on the average, considerably larger. Table 2a summarizes the main effects of control, teaching, and service on size, based on an analysis of variance.

It shows, for example, that the F-ratio for the teaching effect on size, i.e. the difference between all teaching and nonteaching hospitals with respect to size, is largest (F=2,149.85), while the

Table 2
Means and Standard Errors of Hospital Size, by Service, Teaching Status, and Control

	U.S. Hosp.	All 12 Groups	Voluntary				State and Local Governmental				Federal (V.A.)			
			Nonteaching		Teaching		Nonteaching		Teaching		Nonteaching		Teaching	
			Psy	Gen	Psy	Gen	Psy	Gen	Psy	Gen	Psy	Gen	Psy	Gen
(N)	6,825	3,544	30	1,507	13	467	139	956	91	185	23	56	17	60
$\bar{x}$	193	253	80	58	195	249	1,812	49	2,326	385	1,161	281	1,595	611
$s_{\bar{x}}$	6.1	10.7	28.1	1.2	43.7	7.8	115.6	2.2	161.5	34.1	97.6	26.3	108.3	46.1

[a] Standard errors are given in order to facilitate cell-by-cell comparisons. A formula useful for this purpose is $t = \dfrac{\bar{x}_1 - \bar{x}_2}{s_{\bar{x}_1} + s_{\bar{x}_2}}$ where t with N $>$ 30 can be referred to a table of normal probability.

Table 2a gives the results of the 3-way analysis of variance.

Table 2a
Effects of Control, Teaching Status and Service on Size

Dependent Variable:		Main Effects			Interactions			
					First Order			Second Order
		Control	Teaching	Service	Control X Teaching	Control X Service	Teaching X Service	
		F-Ratios[a]						
Size		404.00	2,149.85	1,834.87	14.15	215.37	153.12	15.29
	$df_1 =$	2	1	1	2	2	1	2

[a]F-Ratios needed for significance at the .01 level:
4.60 ($df_1 = 2$) and 6.64 ($df_1 = 1$); $df_2 = 3,532$ (for all effects).

123

difference between the three types of ownership and control is comparatively much smaller (F=404.00). The effect of service, i.e., the difference between psychiatric and general hospitals, is intermediate, but closer to the teaching effect (F=1,834.87).

Although the main effects of control, teaching, and service on size are statistically significant, we cannot conclude that they are independent of each other, since there is significant first and second order interaction among the main effects.[21] Substantively, the overriding effect of teaching and service on size means that there is a strong relationship between task complexity and organizational size. While I would favor the general interpretation of size as a function of the nature and complexity of the task structure, it must be recognized, at least in the case of teaching hospitals, i.e., diversification, that the relationship is one of mutual dependence. As to the effect of control on size, we can tentatively conclude that size is inversely related to the degree of organizational autonomy. In other words, the less autonomous public hospitals tend to be larger, due in part to the nature of the patient population and the assumption of certain kinds of tasks, while the more autonomous private hospitals tend to be of limited size. This would include church-affiliated as well as proprietary hospitals, where the average sizes are 135 and 50, respectively, for general hospitals, and 130 and 80, respectively, for psychiatric hospitals.

As to organizational age, information is available at this point only for teaching hospitals as a whole. The average age of teaching hospitals in 1960 was about 45 years, with a standard deviation of about 30. Of the 877 teaching hospitals for which the information was obtained, 222 (or about 25 per cent) were less than 38 years old, while 200 (or about 23 per cent) were 74 years and older. It is noteworthy that there is no relationship between "growth" and "development," as indicated by the absence of any correlation between size and age among teaching hospitals. Older hospitals tend to have a larger number of accreditations and A.M.A.-approved programs, while hospitals with a history of gaining, losing, and regaining their teaching accreditation tend to be younger. Thus, the only generalizations from these relationships worth entertaining would be that high-quality hospitals tend to be older, and that older hospitals are more stable. However, this is not saying very much, considering the fact that drastically unstable or ineffective hospitals are likely to have dropped out of the picture, and are therefore not available for analysis.

Size of Community

The size of the community in which the hospital is located, or the degree of urbanization of the organizational environment is, strictly speaking, an independent variable, at least with respect to teaching status and type of service. We can therefore consider the results of the analysis of variance only in terms of association rather than "main effects."

This analysis shows that teaching hospitals tend to be located in metropolitan communities, specifically, in SMSA's in which the central city has a population of one million or more. The state and local governmental teaching hospitals tend to be located in SMSA's where the central city has a population of between 800,000 and one million. The concentration of teaching hospitals in metropolitan areas accentuates their character as multifunctional, diversified organizations with a high degree of dependence on and interdependence with other organizations as well as with specialized markets and populations.

As to the relationship between type of service and community size, it is interesting to note that psychiatric hospitals tend to be located in larger communities than general hospitals. The relationship is not as strong by far as it is in the case of teaching hospitals. However, it is statistically significant, and will prove to be of considerable importance in the specific comparisons between the less complex, nonteaching psychiatric hospitals and the highly complex, teaching general hospitals, both of these types representing opposite poles on a continuum of task complexity.

With respect to the factor of ownership and control, we could assume that size of community is a dependent variable insofar as state legislatures and the Veterans' Administration exercise some control over the location of hospitals under their jurisdiction.

Extent of Accreditations, Affiliations, Approvals, and Memberships

Accreditation. In my discussion of organizational effectiveness, I have suggested that the minimum operational standards maintained by a given hospital, documented by presence or absence of accreditation, indicate a certain aspect of the hospital's goal and task structure. Accreditation, as reflecting higher quality, is thus also closely related to the dimension of control and ownership. In order to get an overall impression of the quality differentials for the twelve group s in quantitative terms, the percentage of accredited

Table 3
Means and Standard Errors of Size of Community, by Service, Teaching Status, and Control

	U.S. Hosp.	All 12 Groups	Voluntary				State and Local Governmental				Federal (V.A.)			
			Nonteaching		Teaching		Nonteaching		Teaching		Nonteaching		Teaching	
			Psy	Gen	Psy	Gen	Psy	Gen	Psy	Gen	Psy	Gen	Psy	Gen
(N)	6,825	3,544	30	1,507	13	467	139	956	91	185	23	56	17	60
Size of Community[a] $\bar{x}$	25	23	45	19	71	58	13	5	38	36	14	6	50	54
$s_{\bar{x}}$	.5	.7	8.5	1.1	16.7	2.6	2.5	.6	5.3	3.5	7.7	1.1	15.0	6.4

[a]See Appendix C for explanation.

Table 3a
Association of Control, Teaching Status, and Service With Size of Community

| Dependent Variable: | Main Effects | | | Interactions | | | |
| | | | | First Order | | | Second |
	Control	Teaching	Service	Control X Teaching	Control X Service	Teaching X Service	Order
			F-Ratios[a]				
Size of Community	101.87	906.08	29.99	1.55	12.33	21.94	.71
$df_1 =$	2	1	1	2	2	1	2

[a]F-Ratios needed for significance at the .01 level: 4.60 ($df_1 = 2$) and 6.64 ($df_1 = 1$); $df_2 = 3,532$ (for all effects).

127

hospitals was calculated within each of the twelve groups.[22] Table 4 shows the accreditation rates for both general and psychiatric hospitals.[23]

Table 4 shows the significantly higher rates of accreditation of teaching hospitals. Moreover, it is interesting to note that all psychiatric hospitals are more likely to be accredited as general hospitals than as psychiatric ones, the V.A. psychiatric hospitals, teaching and nonteaching, ranking highest here with 91 per cent and 88 per cent respectively. With the exception of general teaching hospitals, there are obvious differences in the accreditation rates among the ownership and control categories. For example, a comparison of the three nonteaching general hospital types shows the V.A. hospitals highest, with 98 per cent, the state and local governmental hospitals lowest, with 32 per cent and the voluntary hospitals, with 52 per cent, close to the average for all U.S. hospitals.

In sum, accreditation emerges as a significant correlate of both medical education and federal control. Thus the medical profession and the federal government, unlikely partners, perform the crucial role of guardians of quality and high standards in health care. It appears that the potential conflict between the overlapping areas of professional competence and administrative regulation is repeated here on the extra-organizational, institutional level. The fact that the concern for quality standards is shared by both parties (while their relationship is potentially one of competition) reduces the possibility that standards become fixed arbitrarily; each "side" is watched closely by its "opponent," not only for possible violation of existing standards and practices, but also for the effort made toward "helping the people"—the raison d'etre for the medical profession and a powerful government.

Affiliations. Accreditation is an indicator of compliance with *minimum* standards. In order to get at the problem of quality in more depth, we may look at two contextual variables, the affiliation of hospitals with a medical school or university, and affiliation with a professional nursing school. Hospitals so affiliated are assumed to rank higher in quality because of the greater availability of medical and nursing manpower and the generally high standards maintained for purposes of training. Table 5 shows the differential affiliation of hospitals.

Obviously, the voluntary and public (state and local governmental) teaching hospitals almost monopolize both types of affiliation. However, as we shall see below, hospitals with a high proportion of affiliations tend to rank high on other indicators of quality as well.

Table 4

Percentages of Hospitals Accredited As General and As Psychiatric Hospitals, by Type of Service, Teaching Status, and Control

Accreditation	U.S. Hosp.	All Groups	Voluntary				State and Local Governmental				Federal (V.A.)			
			Nonteaching		Teaching		Nonteaching		Teaching		Nonteaching		Teaching	
			Psy	Gen	Psy	Gen	Psy	Gen	Psy	Gen	Psy	Gen	Psy	Gen
(N)	6,825	3,544	30	1,507	13	467	139	956	91	185	23	56	17	60
As General Hospital	53	56	37	52	85	99	10	32	67	99	91	98	88	98
As Psychiatric Hospital	4	4	23	0	31	9	9	0	54	16	13	2	18	0

Table 5
Percentage of Hospitals Affiliated with Medical Schools and Nursing Schools, by Type of Service, Teaching Status, and Control

Affiliation with (N)	U.S. Hosp.	All 12 Groups	Voluntary				State and Local Governmental				Federal (V.A.)			
			Nonteaching		Teaching		Nonteaching		Teaching		Nonteaching		Teaching	
			Psy	Gen	Psy	Gen	Psy	Gen	Psy	Gen	Psy	Gen	Psy	Gen
	6,825	3,544	30	1,507	13	467	139	956	91	185	23	56	17	60
Medical School	5	6	0	0	8	27	0	0	6	50	0	0	0	0
Nursing School	16	17	0	9	8	68	0	3	20	64	0	0	0	0

130

Moreover, affiliation is a contextual, indirect measure of quality: there is little question that affiliation as such increases the complexity of the task structure; yet it does not—by itself—assure an adequate response to that increased complexity.

Extent of External Relations. In order to gauge a hospital's viability in still another way, let us briefly look at the whole range of possible affiliations, accreditations, approvals, and memberships.[24]

Unfortunately, data for this particular test are available for teaching hospitals only. For the 1,262 teaching hospitals included, the mean number of such "approval codes" in 1960 is 5.6, with a standard deviation of 2.0. The distribution of hospitals along this dimension is surprisingly even, with 19 per cent having three or fewer "relationships," and 18 per cent having eight or more.

In shifting the interpretation of the approval codes from a qualitative-substantive to a more quantitative-formal meaning, i.e. from quality to number of "external relations" or extent of interaction between organization and environment, we are gaining a new perspective on the question of organizational activity across boundaries.

Thus, the greater the extent of inter-organizational relationships, the larger the number of medical specialties present and the higher the degree of technological complexity as measured by the number of technical facilities and services.[25] Extensive external relationships are presumably also encouraged by a large, diversified staff.[26] but inhibited by the size of the task (average daily patient census) and an extended average length of stay.[27]

The extent of external relations thus becomes a determinant of the organization's ability to procure resources and to organize in such a way as to respond effectively to the size of the task. Thus, the positive relationship between the number of external ties and organizational resources gives an extended meaning to the term "resources" including the complexity of the organizational response to a given task. To the extent, then, that the ability of an organization to procure and organize its resources is a measure of its effectiveness,[28] we can conclude that extensive external relations will increase its effectiveness. Moreover, insofar as federal hospitals have fewer external relations than others, the extent of external relationships is inversely related to external control, or stated differently, it is directly related to the degree of organizational autonomy. However, it is important to be aware of the limitations of this generalization within the present context for two reasons. One is that these external relationships are by definition "positive" relationships, and therefore reflect only more or less favorable interaction between organization and environment. The second point is that federal hospitals operate on the basis of "independent" resources, too, except that they can do so as a matter of expectation or guarantee, while the voluntary hospitals are more autonomous only in the sense that they have a right to operate on a deficit budget. Autonomy thus boils down to the right to be poor.

Finally, it is interesting to note that the extent of external relations is greater when the hospital is more stable as a teaching institution, when it is older, and when the turnover or succession rate among administrators is lower, i.e., when the top administrative structure is more stable.[29]

Again, viewed in terms of effectiveness, the latter relationship would seem to confirm the obvious stereotype, namely that administrative stability contributes to organizational effectiveness, since the administrator can build up external relations if his tenure of office is longer. By the same token, however, long tenure may imply lower flexibility and innovative capacity, thus ultimately decreasing effectiveness. It is conceivable, therefore, that the relationship between administrative stability and effectiveness is curvilinear; i.e., that very high and very low turnover rates are both detrimental to effectiveness, and that there is an optimal period of office tenure.[30]

Average Length of Patient Stay

The variation in length of stay is, of course, first and foremost a function of type of service (Tables 6 and 6a). Thus, there is a big difference between general and psychiatric hospitals, with the large psychiatric hospitals representing the characteristic long-term "custodial" institution. Of course, we cannot say on the basis of this table which type of psychiatric hospital is more custodial in character and which might be more therapeutic. However, it is obvious that the voluntary psychiatric hospitals have a lower average length of stay. The V.A. hospitals, as a whole, have the highest averages, reflecting in part the influence of a different general and psychiatric patient population. We can conclude from these differences that length of stay is influenced jointly by type of service and type of control. The analysis of variance presented in Table 6a bears this out, since there is significant interaction between these two factors (F=93.34).

The effect of teaching status, although significant, is relatively

Table 6
Means and Standard Errors of Average Length of Stay, by Service, Teaching Status, and Control

| | U.S. Hosp. | All 12 Groups | Voluntary | | | | State and Local Governmental | | | | Federal (V.A.) | | | |
| | | | Nonteaching | | Teaching | | Nonteaching | | Teaching | | Nonteaching | | Teaching | |
			Psy	Gen	Psy	Gen	Psy	Gen	Psy	Gen	Psy	Gen	Psy	Gen
(N)	6,825	3,544	30	1,507	13	467	139	956	91	185	23	56	17	60
Average Length of Stay x̄	67.0	52.5	153.1	6.3	462.4	8.1	511.7	7.0	524.4	10.4	847.0	43.4	609.4	39.5
s x̄	8.1	4.4	25.9	.1	242.8	.3	44.7	.4	106.6	.9	198.2	3.0	103.5	2.1

Table 6a
Effects of Control, Teaching Status, and Service on Average Length of Stay

Dependent Variable:	Main Effects			Interactions			
				First Order			Second Order
	Control	Teaching	Service	Control X Teaching	Control X Service	Teaching X Service	
	F-Ratios[a]						
Average Length of Stay	1,204.62	255.09	8,453.23	3.67	93.34	31.85	29.17
$df_1 =$	2	1	1	2	2	1	2

[a]F-Ratios needed for significance at the .01 level: 4.60 ($df_1 = 2$) and 6.64 ($df_1 = 1$); $df_2 = 3,532$ (for all effects).

smaller compared to the factors of service and control. We note that average length of stay is slightly higher in the teaching hospitals, with the exception of the V.A. teaching hospitals. The slightly higher length of stay in teaching hospitals is probably due to the composition of the patient population, i.e., a somewhat higher proportion of "rare cases," as well as the greater medical interest in retaining patients for purposes of teaching and observation.

In general, it appears that average length of stay can be considered "controlled" by the type of ownership and control and to an even greater degree, by the complexity of the task structure, especially type of service. For the purposes of this study, therefore, we can consider average length of stay as an integral aspect of a hospital's task structure, even though it is true that accreditations, approvals, and other quality elements favor short-term hospitals.

Net Autopsy Rate

As I have explained earlier, in the present study it is held that the net autopsy rate is an indicator of the scientific orientation of the medical staff, and thus of the general quality of the hospital. If we examine the variation of the mean net autopsy rate among the different hospital types (Table 7), we can see the strong association between autopsy rate and teaching status, confirmed by the high F-ratio for this factor (Table 7a).

However, the influence of control is also quite obvious in that the V.A. hospitals rank highest in terms of this measure of quality, with voluntary hospitals taking an intermediate position between V.A. and state and local governmental hospitals. These differences were already apparent in Table 4, which showed the percentage of accredited hospitals by service, teaching status, and control. The autopsy rate, although a factor in the approval of a hospital for teaching status, is likely to increase *after* a hospital has become a teaching institution, i.e., it is both a dependent and an independent indicator of quality. Incidentally, as to the influence of hospital inpatient mortality on the frequency of autopsies, it should be noted that there is no correlation between the two rates. The correlation between gross mortality rate and autopsy rate is $r=-.013$ for all 6,825 hospitals, and $r=-.005$ for the 3,544 hospitals (all 12 groups combined), with only minor variations around zero within each of the 12 groups. While teaching hospitals, again, rank high on this indicator of quality, there is also considerable variation *among* teaching hospitals with respect to the autopsy rate.

Table 7
Means and Standard Errors of Net Autopsy Rate, by Service, Teaching Status, and Control

	U.S. Hosp.	All 12 Groups	Voluntary				State and Local Governmental				Federal (V.A.)			
			Nonteaching		Teaching		Nonteaching		Teaching		Nonteaching		Teaching	
			Psy	Gen	Psy	Gen	Psy	Gen	Psy	Gen	Psy	Gen	Psy	Gen
	6,825	3,544	30	1,507	13	467	139	956	91	185	23	56	17	60
Net Autopsy Rate $\bar{x}$	.32	.30	.49	.23	.57	.48	.24	.19	.39	.49	.74	.68	.76	.73
$\bar{x}$	.003	.003	.016	.004	.073	.007	.015	.004	.022	.015	.017	.020	.036	.014

Table 7a
Effects of Control, Teaching Status, and Service on the Net Autopsy Rate

	Main Effects			Interactions			
				First Order			Second Order
	Control	Teaching	Service	Control X Teaching	Control X Service	Teaching X Service	

F-Ratios[a]

Dependent Variable:							
Net Autopsy Rate	559.14	1,366.78	20.34	30.08	28.08	30.59	1.53
$df_1 =$	2	1	1	2	2	1	2

[a]F-Ratios needed for significance at .01 level: 4.60 ($df_1 = 2$) and 6.64 ($df_1 = 1$); $df_2 = 3{,}532$ (for all effects).

137

For example, the role of autopsies in advanced medical education is suggested by the fact that the autopsy rate increases with the number of medical specialties present (r=.23) and with the number of resident positions offered by the hospital (r=.24), but *not* with the number of internships offered (r=.07). The university and medical school affiliation of hospitals is, of course, also a factor in the frequency of autopsies (r=.28). This is particularly noteworthy in view of the fact that there is no relationship between the autopsy rate and the number of "external relations" (r=—=.07), indicating that the nonevaluative external relationships of the hospital, such as memberships and nonmedical affiliations, must have a negative effect on the net autopsy rate. This interpretation is consistent with the frequent observation that the teaching functions of the hospital have radically different implications for structure than the service and patient care functions. For example, there is no relationship between the net autopsy rate and the nurse/patient ratio (r=—.01), or the ratio of student nurses to graduate professional nurses (r=—.06).

There is a slight association between the autopsy rate and the proportion of certified technical personnel (r=.15) as well as the proportion of salaried physicians (r=.14), but not with the sheer number of medical technical facilities present in the hospital (r=.08).

Assuming that the net autopsy rate says something about medical-technical quality, one may wonder about the effect of the relative size of the administrative staff on this aspect of quality. Among teaching hospitals, the effect is surprisingly strong (r=.30), indicating a positive contribution of administrative functions to quality. However, the relationship is probably not unidirectional, since a high autopsy rate may imply additional legal-clerical work, independent of medical records.

Personnel/Patient Ratio

Another factor which helps to define the profile of differences between the twelve hospital types is the personnel/patient ratio. With the exception of the voluntary hospitals, the psychiatric hospitals have a very low level of resources in terms of personnel, ranging from 40 (per 100 patients) in the public, nonteaching psychiatric institutions to 79 in the teaching counterpart. The voluntary psychiatric hospitals have a significantly higher personnel/patient ratio, which in the case of the psychiatric teaching hospitals exceeds even that of the voluntary nonteaching general hospitals (208 vs. 203 personnel per 100 patients).

As can be seen from an inspection of the differences between the means in Table 8, there is a sizeable joint effect of service and control which is borne out in the significant first-order interaction among these two factors (Table 8a). Although significant, too, the main effect of teaching on the personnel/patient ratio is surprisingly low.

In general, one can conclude that the great difference between psychiatric and general hospitals with respect to the number of personnel per 100 patients reflects their difference in task complexity and technology. Psychiatric and other long-term patients require a less intensive and less differentiated work force. However, this is only part of the picture; two additional points are relevant here. First, a psychiatric hospital need not be a long-term hospital. Both voluntary (teaching and nonteaching) psychiatric hospital types have a somewhat lower average of stay (see Table 6). They have correspondingly higher personnel/patient ratios (Table 8). In other words, average length of stay and personnel/patient ratio are inversely related, with a correlation coefficient of $r=-.54$ for all U.S. hospitals and $r=-.66$ for the 12 groups combined.

The second point is that type of ownership and control should not have an influence on the personnel/patient ratio if it were only a function of task complexity and technology. However, there are considerable differences between types of ownership and control in this respect. Thus, the personnel/patient ratio for voluntary and nonfederal governmental *general* hospitals is similar and relatively high compared to the V.A. general hospitals. But among *psychiatric* hospitals, the situation is reversed. Both types of "public" psychiatric hospitals have relatively low ratios, compared to the "private" voluntary psychiatric hospitals.

It can be concluded that among general hospitals the effect of technology is greater, but that among psychiatric hospitals, the effect of "low autonomy" and of limited resources becomes more visible.

The Nurse/Patient Ratio

The variation of the nurse/patient ratio among the twelve hospital types follows essentially similar patterns as those of the personnel/patient ratio.

Table 8
Means and Standard Errors of the Personnel/Patient Ratio, by Service, Teaching Status, and Control

	U.S. Hosp.	All 12 Groups	Voluntary				State and Local Governmental				Federal (V.A.)			
			Nonteaching		Teaching		Nonteaching		Teaching		Nonteaching		Teaching	
			Psy	Gen	Psy	Gen	Psy	Gen	Psy	Gen	Psy	Gen	Psy	Gen
	6,825	3,544	30	1,507	13	467	139	956	91	185	23	56	17	60
Personnel/Patient Ratio $\bar{x}$	2.08[a]	2.02	1.30	2.03	2.08	2.34	.40	2.27	.79	2.36	.75	1.49	.77	1.52
$s_{\bar{x}}$	.08	.06	.07	.04	.19	.02	.03	.20	.12	.08	.03	.04	.04	.03

[a]The figures presented in this table are the means of the *ratio* of personnel to patients. The ratio 2.08, for example, expressed as a *rate*, would read: 208 personnel per 100 patients.

Table 8a
Effects of Control, Teaching Status, and Service on the Personnel/Patient Ratio

Dependent Variable:	Main Effects			Interactions			
				First Order			Second Order
	Control	Teaching	Service	Control X Teaching	Control X Service	Control X Service	
	F-Ratios[a]						
Personnel/Patient Ratio	391.17	25.71	4,393.08	8.33	340.97	24.21	1.76
$df_1 =$	2	1	1	2	2	1	2

[a] F-Ratios needed for significance at .01 level: 4.60 ($df_1 = 2$) and 6.64 ($df_1 = 1$); $df_2 = 3,532$ (for all effects).

The influence of task complexity is even stronger here, with general hospitals having ratios several times higher than psychiatric hospitals. Presumably, this pattern reflects to some extent the scarcity of professional nurses and the possibility of substituting lower-skilled personnel in psychiatric hospitals. At the same time, nurses assume a larger share of supervisory and administrative functions in psychiatric hospitals.

While the influence of task complexity is accentuated, that of ownership and control is more graduated. The number of nurses per 100 patients is highest in voluntary general hospitals, hovers about the average for all U.S. hospitals in state and local governmental hospitals, and is lowest among V.A. hospitals. I will show later that nurses in voluntary hospitals assume a greater burden of administrative-clerical functions. Consequently, the effective utilization of nursing manpower may not be too different in voluntary and federal hospitals, although one could argue that the use of nurses for administrative-clerical functions is inefficient.

I have already noted that among teaching hospitals, the nurse/patient ratio is strongly influenced by the extent of external relations ($r=.48$). Of course, "external relations" includes the qualitative element of affiliation with a nursing school, which explains part of this relationship. Nevertheless, it can be assumed that the "effective" hospital tends to have a higher nurse/patient ratio, provided professional nurses are permitted by organizational arrangements to perform task-specific nursing functions rather than delegated medical and administrative functions.

Summary and Conclusions

In this chapter, I have described the major dimensions of the comparative framework of this study: autonomy and the complexity of the task structure. The classification of hospitals in terms of ownership and control, teaching status, and service results in twelve hospital types which, as a whole, constitute about half of the U.S. hospital population.

In order to describe the twelve types and to show the similarities and differences between them, we have looked at a number of basic hospital characteristics and their variation as a result of the influence of autonomy and task complexity.

The following conclusions can be drawn from this comparison. In contrast to psychiatric hospitals, the more complex general hospitals are smaller, are located in smaller communities, have a short

Table 9
Means and Standard Errors of the Nurse/Patient Ratio, by Service, Teaching Status, and Control

| | U.S. Hosp. | All 12 Groups | Voluntary | | | | State and Local Governmental | | | | Federal (V.A.) | | | |
| | | | Nonteaching | | Teaching | | Nonteaching | | Teaching | | Nonteaching | | Teaching | |
			Psy	Gen	Psy	Gen	Psy	Gen	Psy	Gen	Psy	Gen	Psy	Gen
N=	6,825	3,544	30	1,507	13	467	139	956	91	185	23	56	17	60
Nurse-Patient Ratio $\bar{x}$	.44*	.46	.17	.54	.25	.54	.02	.46	.08	.43	.06	.21	.07	.22
$s_{\bar{x}}$	.01	.01	.07	.01	.11	.01	.003	.02	.02	.02	.03	.005	.04	.01

*The nurse/patient *ratio* of .44, if expressed as a *rate*, reads: 44 graduate professional nurses per 100 patients.

143

average length of stay, a high personnel/patient ratio, and a high nurse/patient ratio.

Teaching hospitals, in contrast to nonteaching institutions, are somewhat larger, are located in larger communities, have a slightly longer average length of stay, and have a higher proportion of accreditations, approvals, and affiliations, as well as a higher net autopsy rate. Older teaching hospitals are likely to be more stable and have a larger number of "external relations," a factor which in turn is positively associated with the top administrator's tenure of office.

Finally, public hospitals, in contrast to private ones, are larger, have a somewhat longer average length of stay, and lower personnel/patient and nurse/patient ratios. The pervasive influence of ownership and control on these characteristics supports my original assumption that autonomy is a kind of higher-order independent variable. Even though it is treated as if it were on one level together with task complexity, it co-determines important aspects of the organizational task structure, a phenomenon which parallels the differential effect of public vs. private ownership and control of certain industries.

Federal hospitals are different in many respects from both state and local governmental institutions as well as voluntary hospitals, especially general hospitals. They rank highest in terms of accreditations and net autopsy rate, although not in terms of personnel/patient and nurse/patient ratios. These differences, however, seem to indicate that there can be no clear-cut distinction between "public" and "private" medical and hospital care. Autonomy with respect to legal status and goal-setting does not necessarily imply autonomy with respect to resources, or the ability to maintain high standards of quality. In the next chapter, these structural differences will be further explored in terms of medical technology.

Notes

1. The residual 48.1 per cent of these 6,825 hospitals are not included in the systematic comparison because of an insufficient number of cases relative to the total required for each category. Put differently, the case base in any category or group has to be large enough to permit analysis in terms of ten major variables. For example, while there is a total of about 1,200 church-affiliated voluntary hospitals, it cannot be used here, because there are only three hospitals within this group that can be classified as both teaching and psychiatric. The problem is similar in regard to the more than 1,000 proprietary hospitals (these are 1959 figures). The remaining hospitals,

outside of 20 cases with insufficient data, represent a variety of categories, each of them too small for systematic comparative analysis. For purposes of comparing the twelve hospital types used here to the ungrouped total, i.e., all twelve groups combined (N=3,544), as well as to the total U.S. hospital population (N=6,825), the analysis always includes these two additional categories. Each data table has, therefore, fourteen columns.

2. See James A. Hamilton, *Patterns of Hospital Ownership and Control* (Minneapolis: University of Minnesota Press, 1961), pp. 8, 121. The figures for teaching hospitals were calculated on the basis of data derived from the 1952 and 1961 A.H.A. Guide Issues.

3. Hamilton, op. cit., p. 72; see also Franz Goldman, *Public Medical Care* (New York: Columbia University Press, 1945).

4. It can be assumed that these patterns have changed drastically since the establishment of Medicare and Medicaid programs in 1966.

5. Hamilton, op. cit. pp. 67-85.

6. Ibid., pp. 47-49.

7. Ibid., p. 55; see also Louis Block, "Hospital Trends, A Ready Reference of Hospital Facts and Figures," *Hospital Topics*, 1956, p. 178.

8. Hamilton, op. cit., p. 52.

9. Laura G. Jackson, *Hospital and Community* (New York: Macmillan, 1964), p. 374.

10. Hamilton, op. cit. p. 52.

11. I am grateful to Professor Jack Feldman, formerly of the National Opinion Research Center, University of Chicago, for first suggesting to me the idea of using the number of residency programs as well as the types of internships available at a given teaching hospital as indicators of the complexity of the organizational task structure. For a listing of the medical specialties, see the "Directory of Approved Internships and Residencies," *Journal of the American Medical Association*, 174 (1960), 675.

12. *Hospitals*, Guide Issue, Part 2 (1960), p. 365. Short-term hospitals are those with an average length of stay of 30 days or less.

13. This information on the number of medical specialties per hospital is taken from the "Directory of Approved Internships and Residencies," op. cit., and will be used mainly for a separate analysis, "in depth," of U.S. teaching hospitals. When relevant, however, results of this analysis are included here.

14. David P. Street et al. *Organization for Treatment* (New York: The Free Press, 1966).

15. See, for example, Michael Gort, *Diversification and Integration in American Industry* (Princeton, N.J.: Princeton University Press, 1962); also William W. Alberts and Joel E. Segall, eds., *The Corporate Merger* (Chicago: The University of Chicago Press, 1966).

16. Emmet B. Bay, *Medical Administration of Teaching Hospitals* (Chicago: The University of Chicago Press, 1931), pp. 15, 16.

17. "Directory of Approved Internships and Residencies," op. cit., p. 352.

18. Ibid., p. 663.

19. Satisfaction of these conditions may be considered a ritual by some;

purists, on the other hand, would argue that as long as a given investigation has not evaluated all of the possible variables for their effects, the findings are necessarily of limited value. In my judgment, it is possible and useful, from an "optimizing" perspective, to consider certain variables that help define the twelve hospital types as both comparable and distinct.

20. All variables used in this study, except accreditations and approvals, as well as variables on teaching hospitals as a whole, were transformed into different scales before the statistical analysis was performed. (See the more detailed discussion in Appendix F.)

21. For example, the first-order interaction between teaching and service $(F= 153.12)$ means that if the effect of teaching status and service on size is considered simultaneously, the two factors have a differential effect on size: the difference between psychiatric and general hospitals with respect to size is in general smaller than the difference between teaching and nonteaching hospitals with respect to size. Second-order interaction may occur if we consider the simultaneous effect of all three main dimensions of the comparative framework with respect to size. In Table 2a, the second-order interaction $(F =15.29)$ is significant, indicating that all three dimensions are different from each other in their effect on size, in addition to the first-order differences between any two of the three dimensions. In general, statistical interaction means that the simultaneous effects of two factors (e.g., teaching and service) in relation to a third one (e.g., size) may be different, depending on how they are related to each other and to the third one. (For technical discussions of statistical interaction and the analysis of variance, see the references in Appendix F.)

22. Hospitals are accredited as "general" hospitals by the Joint Commission on Accreditation of Hospitals. The American Psychiatric Association also publishes minimum standards for psychiatric hospitals used for purposes of accreditation as psychiatric institutions. See Appendix E for the principles and criteria of accreditation as a general and as a psychiatric hospital.

23. The rates of psychiatric accreditation for general hospitals must be interpreted with caution, since there is the possibility that some general hospitals do not have psychiatric facilities. As it appears from Table 4, public and voluntary nonteaching general hospitals, as well as V.A. teaching general hospitals, do not have any psychiatric accreditation. Only 2 per cent of the 56 V.A. nonteaching general hospitals have such an accreditation, while the public teaching general hospitals have the highest rate, with 16 per cent.

24. *Hospitals*, Guide Issue, Part 2, (1960), p. 14. For the variable of "extent of external relations" a maximum of 12 so-called "approval codes" was used, including State Hospital Association and Blue Cross membership, and combining the two codes for nursing school affiliation (i.e., affiliation with vs. control of nursing school) and the two psychiatric approvals (actual vs. conditional). For a discussion of a hospital's "external relations," e.g., membership and participation in various hospital associations, see: American Hospital Association, "Study to Delineate Proper Relationships

between the A.H.A. and Allied Hospital Associations" (Chicago: American Hospital Association, 1965).

25. The correlation coefficients are .41 and .42, respectively, based on 1,260 teaching hospitals. Data were missing on two hospitals.

26. The correlation with size (personnel) is r=.21; with the proportion of different job titles occupied, r=.47.

27. The correlation with number of patients is r=—.23; with average length of stay, r=—.28. It is interesting to note the fine, but consistent and significant differentiation between different size measures in relation to the extent of external relations. Thus, the correlation with another task size measure, the number of beds, is also negative, with r=—.21, while the correlation with total expenses for 1960 is r=.13. Both expenses and personnel can be interpreted as size of resources, in contrast to size of task. See also Chapter 7, especially the section on "Organizational Size: Task vs. Resources."

28. See Ephraim Yuchtman and Stanley E. Seashore, "System Resource Approach to Organizational Effectiveness," *American Sociological Review*, 32 (1967), 891-903; and Stanley E. Seashore and Ephraim Yuchtman, "Factorial Analysis of Organizational Performance," *Administrative Science Quarterly*, 12 (1967), 377-395. I am grateful to Dennis Magill for alerting me to the implications of this approach.

29. The correlations here are as follows for "external relations": with frequency of changes in teaching status, r=—.19, with age, r=.33, and with administrator's turnover rate. r=—.14, the latter coefficient being based on only 1,130 teaching hospitals due to missing data.

30. Based on 1,141 teaching hospitals, the mean turnover rate for hospital administrators between 1951 and 1960 is 1.3. In other words, for this ten-year period, teaching hospitals had between 1 and 2 different administrators, on the average, and more likely only one. The average tenure period was therefore between 6 and 7 years. There is no evidence in these data that this average represents an "optimum" tenure period for hospital administrators.

I am grateful to Harry Perlstadt and Charles Rosen for their assistance in the coding and preparation of some of the special data on teaching hospitals.

6   Structure and Change in Medical Technology

In this chapter, I will consider both developmental and structural aspects of medical technology. Specifically, I will describe the changes in the technical facilities and services of hospitals since 1946, as well as certain changes in technical manpower since 1935. In the comparison between hospitals in 1935 and 1959, I will show the development of medical technology in terms of the personnel/bed ratio, the proportion of salaried physicians, and the proportion of technical personnel. Finally, I will describe the variation among the twelve hospital types of the proportion of salaried physicians,[1] the proportion of technical personnel, and of all those the proportion of qualified technicians and their distribution among eight technical specialties.

Technological Development in Hospitals

The range and availability of medico-technological services and facilities have increased to an unprecedented degree in the last twenty to thirty years, and have been major factors both in the quality and the cost of hospital-based medical care. Let us first look at the change in facilities as such, and then analyze the corresponding changes in technical manpower.

Technical Facilities and Services

In 1961, eleven out of twenty technical services and facilities were available to at least 50 per cent of all nonfederal, short-term general and other special hospitals, with operating rooms, diagnostic X-ray, and clinical laboratories being available in virtually all of these hospitals. Most of these special facilities represent, in structurally differentiated form, the diffuse, rudimentary "technical functions" performed by the physician and the nurse of the early hospital of over a century ago. However, in recent years, the greatest proportional increase has occurred in those specialized facilities characterized by a high degree of technological complexity and sophistication, such as electroencephalography, electrocardiography, blood banks, and the like, as well as in the recent developments of radiation therapy, such as the use of radioactive isotope facilities. It is clear that just as new technical facilities are developed from year to year and adopted by the leading hospitals, hospitals, in general, are under pressure to acquire those facilities which have come to be defined as standard equipment. Thus, hospitals have to respond to these pressures even in the face of financial limitations if they do not want to be known as second-rate institutions that have to refer their complicated cases to technically more advanced hospitals. The rapid increase and diffusion of technical facilities is further illustrated by the fact that in the six years between 1961 and 1966, the proportional increase in hospitals having certain facilities is equal to that between 1946 and and 1961. For example, in 1966 the proportion of nonfederal, short-term general and other special hospitals (N=5,374) with physical therapy departments had increased to 52.4 per cent, those with pharmacies to 61.7 per cent.[2] At the same time, while hospitals with radioactive isotope facilities had increased to 29.2 per cent in 1966, other developments in radiation therapy had been adopted, quite possibly often in the same hospitals. Thus, in 1966, 31.3 per cent of short-term general hospitals reported having radium radiation therapy facilities, and 10.6 per cent had cobalt facilities. Typically among the largest of these hospitals (those with 500 beds and over), 95 per cent had adopted radium and radio-isotope facilities, and about 70 per cent had cobalt facilities. As expected, the overall relationship between hospital size and the number of facilities is, of course, also positive. Thus, among teaching hospitals in 1960, the correlation of the number of facilities with the number of residency positions offered is $r=.38$, with number of internships offered, .44, with total expenses, .49, and with full-time equivalent personnel, .53.

Table 10

Percent of Nonfederal, Short-Term General and Special Hospitals (N 5,309) with Selected Technical Facilities in 1961)

Technical Facility	Percent Hospitals
Operating Room	97.5
X-Ray, Diagnostic	97.4
Clinical Laboratory	96.3
Electrocardiography	93.8
Emergency Room	93.1
Obstetrical Delivery Room	90.0
Post-operative Recovery Room	56.6
Premature Nursery	56.5
Blood Bank	56.2
Pathology Laboratory	51.1
Pharmacy	50.7
Physical Therapy Department	42.8
Outpatient Department	41.3
X-Ray, Therapeutic	36.7
Dental Clinic	28.7
Radioactive Isotope Facility	24.6
Electroencephalography	15.8
Intensive Care Unit	12.7
Occupational Therapy Department	9.4

Source: *Hospitals*, Guide Issue, Part II (1962), p. 404.

Apart from the fact that for larger hospitals it is relatively more efficient to acquire expensive technical equipment simply in terms of economies of scale, the most obvious explanation for any correlation between size and technology is that the use of facilities requires the services of specialized technical personnel. Yet there is no automatic increase in the *number* of specialized personnel with technical facilities. Thus, the correlation between technical facilities and per

Table 11

Percent of Nonfederal, Short-Term General and Special Hospitals with Selected Technical Facilities in 1946 (N = 4,444) and 1961 (N = 5,309)

Technical Facility	Percent 1946	Hospitals 1961
Radioactive Isotope Facility	0.0	24.6
Electroencephalography	6.2	15.8
Dental Clinic	17.0	28.7
Blood Bank	24.7	56.2
Physical Therapy	32.3	42.8
X-Ray, Therapeutic	35.7	36.7
Pharmacy	38.2	50.7
Electrocardiography	56.3	93.8
Clinical Laboratory	79.4	96.3
X-Ray, Diagnostic	88.0	97.4

Source: *Hospitals,* Guide Issue, Part II (1962), p. 406.

---

cent of salaried physicians is r=-.03, and between facilities and percent of qualified technicians r=.04. But when using a measure of *differentiation* among eight separate technical specialties,[3] the correlation between technical differentiation thus defined and the number of facilities is r=.25, and between facilities and functional specialization (based on the 39 job titles) is r=.55. Thus, the growth of technical facilities is related to the overall size and amount of division of labor within the hospital, and only secondarily and indirectly to the more specific factor of specialized technical personnel.

Before discussing the role of technicians in the present-day hospital structure, let us first look at some historical changes in the employment of technical personnel in hospitals.

A Historical Comparison: 1935 and 1959

We have already seen that among indicators of medical-technological complexity, the proportion of physicians and of technical personnel is particularly useful. Of these two, the proportion of salaried physicians has also been suggested as an indicator of quality of medical care in hospitals.[4]

In addition, the number of personnel per beds, almost identical with the personnel/patient ratio, has been discussed as a function of task complexity and technology, and as an indicator of the differential allocation of personnel resources in terms of the overall goal of "good patient care." A comparison between hospitals in 1935 and 1959 in terms of these three indicators reveals both historical change as well as structural stability.

Let us first look at the net change that has taken place in these 25 years. While general and special hospitals increased both in number and size, the "long-term" TB and mental hospitals decreased in numbers but became much larger on the average. The growth in the number of personnel per 100 beds is probably, in part, due to this general growth in size, with mental hospitals having the largest increase in both respects.

But, more importantly, the larger personnel/bed ratio for all service types suggests an increasing differentiation of personnel in terms of specialized functions. Thus, the most interesting indicator of the changing organization of medical technology is the simultaneous increase of technicians and decrease of physicians between 1935 and 1959. This double change suggests not only the development of a more complex division of labor, but the delegation of medical-technical functions from physicians to other technicians. While less highly trained, i.e., less person-specialized than physicians, technicians are more job-specialized. By the same token, however, they have become part of a hierarchial structure in which salaried physicians have come to occupy the top level. This development of a hierarchy of medical-technical functions and responsibilities explains the observation that there are proportionately fewer salaried physicians and more technicians.[5]

The decrease in the proportion of physicians requires perhaps an additional comment. For both 1935 and 1959, this category includes physicians in all medical specialties employed by the hospital, as well as residents and interns. However, the recent history of the medical profession, particularly the increasing number of medical specialties, suggest that hospitals have come to employ fewer general

Table 12
Change in Structure of Medical Technology: 1935 and 1959, by Type of Service

Year Type of Service	Number of Hospitals		Average Size		Personnel/100 beds		% Physicians		% Technicians	
	1935	1959	1935	1959	1935	1959	1935	1959	1935	1959
General and Special	4,733	5,777	91	147	77	127	4.8	2.2[a]	5.4	9.4[a]
Tuberculosis	506	272	140	235	45	76	4.1	2.5[b]	4.4	7.3[a]
Mental	597	441	892	1,484	18	68	2.7	3.2	5.3	6.3[b]
All Hospitals	5,836	6,490	177	241	45	120	4.3	2.3[a]	5.3	9.1[a]

Source for 1935: Adapted from E. H. Pennel et. al., "Business Census of Hospitals, 1935," *Public Health Reports* (Washington, D. C.: U.S. Government Printing Office, 1939), Supplement No. 154, p. 32, Table 27.

Source for 1959: Adapted from American Hospital Association, Annual Survey of Hospitals, 1959.

a=Significant at .01 level.
b=Significant at .05 level.

(These figures established according to Vernon Davies, "Rapid Method for Determining Significance of the Difference Between Two Percentages," Circular 151, Agricultural Experiment Stations: Washington State University, July 1962.)

154

Table 13
Change in Structure of Medical Technology: 1935 and 1959, by Type of Service and Size of Hospital.

Service Type and Size (No. of beds)	Number of Hospitals		Personnel/ 100 beds		% Physicians		% Technicians	
Year	1935	1959	1935	1959	1935	1959	1935	1959
General and Special	4,733	5,777	77	127	4.8	2.2	5.4	9.4
Under 25 beds	1,282	423	56	98	3.5	2.3	3.8	13.2
25 - 49 beds	1,150	1,391	58	99	3.4	1.2	4.4	10.9
50 - 149 beds	1,540	2,246	72	127	4.3	1.4	5.1	9.0
150 and over	761	1,717	85	156	5.3	4.0	5.8	7.8
Tuberculosis	506	272	45	76	4.1	2.5	4.4	7.3
Under 50 beds	135	24	38	86	5.4	1.9	3.7	8.2
50 to 149 beds	231	117	43	71	4.5	2.5	3.9	8.1
150 and over	140	131	47	79	3.8	2.5	4.6	6.5
Mental	597	441	18	68	2.7	3.2	5.3	6.3
Under 50 beds	144	48	67	104	4.3	5.1	6.2	9.8
50 - 499 beds	189	144	35	107	4.1	3.8	6.3	7.9
500 and over	284	249	17	38	2.3	2.6	5.2	4.7
All hospitals	5,836	6,490	45	120	4.3	2.3	5.3	9.1

Sources: Same as Table 12.

practitioners and more specialists. Thus, while the proportion of salaried physicians has decreased, the proportion of specialists among them has probably increased. There is some supporting evidence for this interpretation in the fact that among mental hospitals, there is a small *increase* in the proportion of physicians, especially among the very small and the very large, as Table 13 shows.

Thus, although psychiatrists are differentiated in terms of training and orientation,[6] they tend to belong to one major medical specialty, viz., psychiatry. Psychiatric hospitals have therefore not seen the dramatic shift from general practice to a variety of specialties experienced by many general hospitals.[7]

The increase in the proportion of psychiatric specialists was therefore a more or less continuous development and, for psychiatric hospitals, visible from the beginning. Thus, mental hospitals had the lowest percentage of physicians of all service types in 1935, general and special hospitals the highest proportion. In 1959, the situation is exactly reversed, with mental hospitals having the highest proportion.

By the same token, in 1959 the proportion of technicians was lower in mental than in general hospitals, although both started at about the same level in 1935, viz., at 5.3 and 5.4 per cent respectively.

The personnel bed ratio is, as expected, much lower in mental than in general hospitals, with TB hospitals in an intermediate position. This holds for both 1935 and 1959.

In general, the gain in technological complexity is relatively greater for the short-term general and special hospitals than for TB or mental hospitals and, among all service types, for smaller than for larger hospitals (Table 13).

Thus, the personnel bed ratio increases with size in the general and special hospitals both in 1935 and 1959, and in the TB hospitals in 1935. However, it decreases with size in TB hospitals in 1959, and in mental hospitals both in 1935 and 1959.

Thus, while the smallest category of general hospitals (under 25 beds) had an increase in technicians of almost 10 percentage points, the largest mental hospitals had a net loss of half a percentage point. Size, however, does not affect the loss in the percentage of physicians to the same extent as it does the gain in the percentage of technicians. In addition, ownership and control influences the loss in the percentage of physicians and the gain in the proportion of technicians most in the "autonomous" (voluntary nonprofit as well as proprietary) hospitals, and least in the "externally controlled" (federal, state, and local governmental) hospitals. The main reason for this pattern is that of all service types, public hospitals, especially federal ones, had a higher proportion of technicians to begin with, while the private hospitals, especially the proprietary ones, started from a very low level in 1935, and thus had gained comparatively more by 1959.

In sum, the most important aspect of the technological development of hospitals since 1935 is the significant increase in the proportion of technicians and in the personnel/bed ratio, with a corresponding general decrease in the proportion of salaried physicians. I have interpreted these complementary changes as indicating the delegation of medical-technical functions from physicians to an increasing number and variety of technical specialists. This process of delegation of functions in medical technology is most pronounced in small general and special hospitals (under 150 beds), and least in large mental hospitals (over 500 beds).

It is conceivable that this delegation of functions has, in part, been prompted by the increasing relative scarcity of medical professional manpower, and the increasing specialization within the medical profession. However, the major factor has probably been the growing technological complexity of diagnostic and therapeutic medical functions, requiring a corresponding variety of technically trained personnel able to assume many of the former responsibilities of physicians.

A Hierarchy of Experts

The development of medical technology in hospitals since 1935 has led to an increasing horizontal and vertical differentiation among technical functions. We have seen the results of this development for salaried physicians as well as technical personnel in general. Let us now look at the structure of medical technology in terms of an additional distinct level, namely, the proportion of those technicians who are certified, registered, or in any other way qualified on the basis of formal, specialized training.[8]

The variation among the 12 hospital types of these three levels of employed specialists is shown in Table 14.

The variation of the proportion of salaried physicians among the twelve hospital types shows clearly that type of control is a major factor. Nevertheless, the absolute size of the proportions, as well as their differences, are small.

It is interesting to note that the effect of type of service, although significant, is less important than that of teaching and control. We also note again that state and local governmental and voluntary psychiatric hospitals have higher proportions of salaried physicians than general hospitals. However, in the V.A. hospitals the opposite is the case.

When we look at the distribution of the proportion of technical personnel among the hospital types, we find that service has the most powerful effect (Table 14). Just as average length of stay, the personnel/patient ratio, and other characteristics were shown to be influenced most significantly by the differences between psychiatric and general hospitals, so is the technical component influenced by task complexity. Thus, the relative size of the technical component indicates the degree to which the hospital is performing basic medical-technological functions. This component is also affected by type of control, indicating that the performance of these basic functions is in part dependent on such factors as budget, resources, and other policy considerations.

Since the technical component is made up of a variety of different occupational specialties, variations in its exact composition may be confounded by variations likely to be dependent on service, control, and teaching. For example, an interesting reversal occurs among the voluntary hospitals, where the psychiatric types have a larger technical component than the general hospitals. But although it is larger, it is somewhat less differentiated in terms of the various technical specialities. This is. probably due to the fact that, in contrast to general hospitals, the psychiatric hospitals have a higher proportion of occupational therapists and psychiatric social workers within the technical component, but fewer or no personnel in some of the other technical specialties.

Finally, let us examine the variation in the proportion of qualified technicians across the twelve hospital types (Table 14). The main effect derives not from type of service but from the teaching status of the hospital. Thus, teaching hospitals have a significantly larger proportion of qualified personnel among technicians. The second main influence is type of ownership and control, with the V.A. hospitals having consistently the highest proportions of qualified technical personnel. If we conceive of technicians, qualified technical personnel, and physicians as levels in a hierarchy of experts, the question arises as to how these categories of technical

Table 14

Means and Standard Errors of Salaried Physicians, %Technicians, % Qualified Technicians, and Degree of Technical Differentiation, by Service, Teaching Status, and Control

Medical and Technical Components		U.S. Hosp. 6,825	All 12 Groups 3,544	Voluntary				State and Local Governmental				Federal (V.A.)			
				Nonteaching		Teaching		Nonteaching		Teaching		Nonteaching		Teaching	
				Psy 30	Gen 1,507	Psy 13	Gen 467	Psy 139	Gen 956	Psy 91	Gen 185	Psy 23	Gen 56	Psy 17	Gen 60
% Salaried Physicians	$\bar{x}$	.01	.01	.03	.01	.04	.01	.01	.01	.02	.01	.02	.04	.02	.04
	$s\bar{x}$	.000	.000	.010	.000	.008	.001	.001	.001	.002	.001	.001	.002	.001	.003
% Technicians	$\bar{x}$	.09	.09	.10	.09	.10	.08	.05	.09	.06	.08	.04	.07	.04	.07
	$s\bar{x}$	.001	.001	.011	.001	.013	.001	.002	.001	.003	.002	.003	.004	.004	.003
% Qualified Technicians (of all technicians)	$\bar{x}$	.34	.34	.34	.33	.44	.41	.24	.29	.37	.41	.59	.52	.66	.57
	$s\bar{x}$	.003	.004	.059	.007	.061	.008	.017	.009	.020	.015	.043	.029	.043	.020
Degree of Differentiation among 8 technical specialties (Gini coefficient for technical differentiation)	$\bar{x}$	.41	.41	.35	.39	.46	.47	.46	.37	.49	.51	.61	.57	.62	.58
	$s\bar{x}$	.002	.002	.028	.003	.028	.004	.01	.004	.009	.008	.016	.011	.017	.011

Table 15

Correlations Between Proportion of Salaried Physicians and % Qualified Technicians, Degree of Technical Differentiation and % Qualified Technicians, and Between All Four of These Measures and Size, by Service, Teaching Status, and Control

	U.S. Hosp.	All 12 Groups	Voluntary				State and Local Governmental				Federal (V.A.)			
			Nonteaching		Teaching		Nonteaching		Teaching		Nonteaching		Teaching	
	6,825	3,544	Psy 30	Gen 1,507	Psy 13	Gen 467	Psy 139	Gen 936	Psy 91	Gen 185	Psy 23	Gen 56	Psy 17	Gen 60
A. Correlations Between % Salaried Physicians and:														
% Qualified Technicians	.16	.23	.60	.18	.10	.17	.15	.09	.33	.08	.61	.62	-.36	.37
Degree of Technical Differentiation	.17	.29	-.15	.15	-.22	.13	.11	.17	.01	.06	.02	.06	-.26	-.06
% Technicians	.09	.09	-.10	.09	-.29	.02	.12	-.04	-.002	-.10	-.16	-.08	-.52	-.13
B. Correlations Between % Qualified Technicians and Technical Differentiation	.22	.25	-.25	.23	.51	.17	.16	.09	.00	.28	.25	.36	.01	.18
C. Correlations Between Size (Average Daily Census) and:														
% Salaried Physicians	.19	.36	-.15	.18	-.17	.10	.04	.23	-.02	.14	.07	-.16	-.26	-.24
% Qualified Technicians	.28	.27	-.32	.32	.55	.20	.06	.28	-.12	.19	-.04	-.12	-.33	.20
% Technicians	-.42	-.37	.17	-.25	-.38	-.20	-.28	-.24	-.60	-.26	-.05	-.32	-.16	-.28
Degree of Technical Differentiation	.52	.54	-.01	.45	.22	.40	.19	.47	.35	.51	-.06	.11	.18	.37

manpower are related to each other. According to the generalization advanced earlier that physicians have delegated medical-technical functions to technicians, we should find these two categories to be *inversely* related to each other. Similarly, insofar as qualified technical personnel perform an intermediate, supervisory role, their proportion should change *directly* with the proportion of salaried physicians.

Both of these relationships are, in fact, borne out by the data, as Table 15 shows. While these correlations are not particularly strong, they show consistently the increase of qualified technical personnel with the proportion of salaried physicians.[9]

At the same time there is a slight negative relationship between the per cent of salaried physicians and the technical component as a whole for the majority of the twelve hospital types, and most pronounced among voluntary and federal psychiatric teaching hospitals. This finding parallels the earlier observation made on the basis of the historical comparison, namely that the hospital-employed medical specialist tends to delegate medical-technical functions to a technical staff which becomes in itself more or less hierarchically differentiated.

But the relationships discussed here reflect an ongoing process, rather than the net result of a 25-year development. The correlations, therefore, reflect the fact that there are other influences at work, as well as more exceptions. Thus, in the voluntary general nonteaching hospitals, the largest single group of all, the proportion of technicians, varies directly with that of salaried physicians, suggesting that medical-technical functions as a whole are internally less differentiated or hierarchically less elaborated.

Table 14 shows that these relatively small community hospitals rank below the U.S. average in terms of technical differentiation. Among the nonteaching state mental hospitals, the positive relationship between the proportion of physicians and of technicians appears to be due to the fact that there are simply not enough qualified technicians (state mental hospitals rank lowest, with 24 per cent qualified technicians, as shown on Table 14). Thus, it is likely that the more experienced subprofessional technicians take over some of the supervisory functions ordinarily performed by qualified technicians.

Let us carry the analysis of the structure of medical technology one step further. We had already noted that the number of technical facilities in a hospital is to some extent a function of its size. The question arises, therefore, as to the effect of size on the per cent of salaried physicians and on the per cent of technical personnel, both professional (qualified) and subprofessional. In the literature, there is some evidence that the proportion of salaried technicians increases with the size of the establishment, as Bendix has shown for businesses. [0]

In hospitals, this relationship appears to hold for qualified technicians, but not for the technical component as a whole. On the contrary, the technical component varies inversely with organizational size, especially in the more complex general and psychiatric teaching hospitals (see Table 15). By contrast, the proportion of qualified technicians and the degree of technical differentiation tend to increase with size, especially in general hospitals. There is some further support for the hypothesis of the transfer and delegation of functions from physicians to technicians and for the coordinating role of the professionalized technicians in the fact that the effect of size on the proportion of salaried physicians tends to parallel the effect of size on the proportion of qualified technicians, and that the latter are directly associated with technical differentiation (Table 15). In other words, the top levels of the technological decision-making structure as a whole become relatively larger with increasing organizational size. But assuming that the number of intermediate levels also increases with size, our finding suggests that medical technology takes on a pyramidal character in the larger hospitals, that there is an increasing amount of delegation of technical functions from the higher to the lower levels and that the growing differentiation of technical activities and the addition of the new technical facilities leads to the development of a hierarchy of technical experts within the larger organization. From the point of view of the larger organization, this process can itself be interpreted as a form of delegation and decentralization.

In sum, the differential effect of hospital size on medical-technical manpower shows that size tends to favor horizontal and hierarchical differentiation of technical functions rather than their mere quantitative expansion.

Let us now briefly examine the variation of the proportion of qualified technicians in the light of autonomy and task complexity, but with size and the proportion of salaried physicians controlled (Table 16). [11]

The first three rows of Table 16 summarize the effects of ownership and control, teaching, and service on the three compositional measures of medical-technical manpower which we have already observed in Table 14. Thus, the variation in the proportion of salaried physicians derives mainly from the differences in ownership and control (federal vs. nonfederal, in this case), although the influence of teaching status and service are also strong.

Similarly, the technical component varies mainly as a result of differences in the number of major objectives and services, but there is also an influence of ownership and control in that the governmental (local, state, and federal) hospitals have a somewhat smaller component than the voluntary hospitals. Finally, the per cent of qualified technicians varies mainly as a result of the teaching status of the hospital, with federal hospitals in general having a larger proportion, corresponding to the larger proportion of salaried physicians in this group as compared to the other types. The extent to which organizational size influences structural factors is demonstrated by the fact that the effect of the teaching status of the hospital on the per cent of qualified technicians is completely eliminated when size is controlled. Thus, the teaching effect is really due to the larger size of teaching hospitals. At the same time, the effect of service is increased significantly when size is controlled, since psychiatric hospitals are larger than general hospitals (Table 16, row 4). This seems to indicate that due to the direct effect of size and of the per cent of salaried physicians on the per cent of qualified technical personnel (Table 15), such factors as a larger hospital or more physicians in a given hospital should have essentially the same positive effect on the professionalization of technicians. This is not quite the case, however. When we control for the per cent of salaried physicians, the effects of ownership and control as well as teaching on the per cent of qualified technicians are considerably reduced, while the effect of service is not significant, just as if we had not controlled for the per cent of salaried physicians (Table 16, row 5).

Only when the joint influence of both size and the per cent of salaried physicians is controlled (Table 16, row 6) do we see that the crucial relationship beween salaried and qualified technicians pertains to their *service*-related functions. The difference between teaching and nonteaching hospitals with respect to this relationship has disappeared.

This finding suggests, again, that professional technicians in addition to their medical-technical function, also perform administrative and supervisory functions with respect to the nonprofessional technicians, i.e., with respect to the rest of the technical component.

In sum, there are more qualified technicians in hospitals with a larger medical staff. But the hospital's size, too, tends to be associated with a higher degree of medical-technological complexity. It is quite plausible, then, to infer that qualified technicians play a

Table 16
Effects of Control, Teaching Status, and Service on Three Measures of Medical-Technical Personnel, and Effects on % Qualified Technicians, with Size and % Salaried Physicians Controlled

	Main Effects			Interactions			Second Order
				First Order			
	Control	Teaching	Service	Control X Teaching	Control X Service	Teaching X Service	
				F-Ratios[a]			
Dependent Variables Alone:							
1. % Sal. Physicians	279.69	156.94	109.06	2.98	37.43	1.11	2.73
2. % Technicians	77.52	20.33	236.06	1.46	28.09	8.08	1.20
3. % Qualified Technicians	63.66	110.83	.01	2.82	1.87	.00	.07
With Controls:							
4. % Qualified Technicians, with Size Controlled	33.43	.59	77.27	1.11	22.43	9.37	.87
5. % Qualified Technicians, with % Sal. Physicians Controlled	30.16	71.68	2.40	2.02	4.56	.02	.13
6. % Qualified Technicians, with both Size and % Sal. Physicians Controlled	26.10	1.74	85.53	.84	23.04	8.86	1.16
$df_1=$	2	1	1	2	2	1	2

[a] F-Ratios needed for significance at the .01 level: 4.60 ($df_1=2$), 6.64 ($df_1=1$); $df_2=3,532$ (for all effects).

mediating and vertically coordinating role between physicians and subprofessional technical personnel. The effects observed in these data suggest that professional technicians constitute an important organizational-functional link in the diagnostic and therapeutic processes initiated by the physician. The structure of medical technology plays a crucial role in these processes in the sense that the hierarchical organization of technical experts, supposedly a contradiction in itself, nevertheless appears to be an effective response to the increasing "mechanization" of medical care.

Summary and Conclusions

In this chapter, I have examined the growth of medical technology from the point of view of technical facilities and of specialized technical manpower. The rapid increase in the percentage of hospitals having certain technical facilities testifies to the central role of technology in medical di gnosis and therapy. Changes in manpower, taken as indicators of technological development, reveal a pattern of delegation of technical functions from physicians to technicians.

An explicit comparision between a 1935 business census of hospitals and the 1959 data shows that the proportion of salaried physicians has decreased, while that of technicians has increased. The interpretation of this change as a process of delegation of functions is supported by the data on the proportion of qualified technicians and the differentiation among technical specialities. The proportion of formally trained technicians is assumed to constitute the top stratum among technicians and forms a hierarchical link between the technical component as a whole and the medical-professional component of salaried physicians. It is likely that this stratum of qualified technicians is itself further stratified into organizational levels, depending on its size relative to the technical component as a whole.

On the basis of this assumption, one can generalize the findings to the effect that medical technology assumes a more hierarchical structure with increasing task complexity and division of labor. The net effect of these changes in the structure of medical technology is a successive delegation of functions to both new technical specialities and new organizational levels. The process of horizontal-functional differentiation is thus paralleled by vertical-hierarchical differentiation.

It is an interesting paradox, however, to find that technicians become administrators at the very point where they become more professionalized. The proportion of salaried physicians and of qualified technical personnel were used mainly as structural indicators rather than as quality measures. An interpretation of the changes described in this chapter in terms of quality of hospital care would require additional information.

But as salaried physicians have decreased over the years, it stands to reason that the increase in qualified technicians has largely served to compensate for that loss. Besides, there is reason to believe that in the future both the proportion of salaried physicians and of qualified technicians will increase as hospitals continue to change in medical technology and seek to maximize the "mechanization of medical care" by improving its administrative and professional coordination.

Notes

1. In discussing the proportion of salaried physicians as an important measure of medical-technological complexity, it will not be necessary (nor particularly relevant) to touch on the controversial issue of the physician who works in an organization rather than as a private practitioner, and who is paid by an organization rather than by the patient. For lack of the appropriate data, it will also not be possible to compare the "open-staff system" prevailing in American community hospitals, and emerging to some extent in American public nonfederal and federal hospitals as well as in university-affiliated, teaching, and research institutions, with the organization of medical care in England and continental Europe. For useful information on this question, see William A. Glaser, "American and Foreign Hospitals: Some Sociological Comparisons," Eliot Freidson, ed., *The Hospital in Modern Society* (Glencoe, Ill. The Free Press, 1963), pp. 37-72; also Joseph K. Owen, *Modern Concepts of Hospital Administration* (Philadelphia; Saunders, 1962).
2. *Hospitals*, Guide Issue, Part 2 (1967), 470-471.
3. The measure used is the Gini coefficient of concentration, based on eight technical specialties listed in Appendix D. The logic and calculation of this measure are discussed in chapter 3 in connection with "departmental specialization."
4. See Milton Roemer, "Contractual Physicians in General Hospitals: A National Survey," *American Journal of Public Health*, 52, (1962), 1457.
5. In preparing the 1959 data for this comparision, I have made the category of technicians as similar in composition as possible to that of 1935. Since for 1935 Pennel and his associates had included such job titles as dentists and psychologists, which are not included in the 1959 data under technicians, the bias would tend to operate in the direction of *underestimating* the percentage increase in technicians between 1935 and 1959. However, it can be assumed that these extra job categories constitute

only a very small percentage of the technical component in 1935. Salaried physicians, as well as residents and interns, reflect about the same specialties in 1935 and 1959; i.e., radiology, pathology, anesthesiology, psychiatry, medical education, research, and administration.

6. See, for example, Anselm L. Strauss et al., *Psychiatric Ideologies and Institutions* (New York; The Free Press, 1964).

7. On the increasing specialization within medicine, see Herman M. Somers and Anna R. Somers *Doctors, Patients, and Health Insurance* (Washington D.C.: Brookings Institution, 1961), pp. 28-33.

8. See Appendix D for the list of technical functions with special qualifications. These categories represent *actual* qualifications rather than *required* ones.

9. The one exception, i.e., the negative correlation among V.A. psychiatric hospitals, is conceivably due to the already very high proportion of qualified technical personnel. In other words, it can be assumed that there are several hierarchical levels among qualified technicians here, so that only the top echelon of qualified technicians would be directly related to the proportion of salaried physicians while the lower levels assume delegated functions. They should, therefore, be inversely related to the proportion of physicians, a point which could be demonstrated only if we could distinguish operationally between *levels* of qualified technicians. In absence of such a distinction, however, the above interpretation can be seen as supported by the relatively high negative correlation between salaried physicians and the technical component as a whole (r=—.52), the highest coefficient among all twelve types.

10. Reinhard Bendix, *Work and Authority in Industry* (New York: Harper Torchbooks, 1963), pp. 221-222.

11. The last three rows of Table 16 show the results of an analysis of covariance, with service, teaching status, and control as the "main effects," % salaried physicians, % technicians, and % qualified technicians as the dependent variables, and with size and the % salaried physicians "controlled", i.e. used as covariates. This means that the *relationship* between covariates and the dependent variables is being analyzed in the light of the three main variables or "effects".—Other examples of covariance analysis used in this book appear in connection with Tables 22, 32, and 40. For a clear exposition of covariance analysis, and the terminology associated with it, see Karl Schuessler, "Covariance Analysis in Socoiological Research", in Edgar Borgatta et al., eds. *Sociological Methodology 1969* (San Francisco: Jossey-Bass, 1969), pp. 219-244.

7 Division of Labor, Size, and Task Complexity

The division of labor among specialized functions and units raises one of the central questions of organizational analysis: why and how is work subdivided, and what are the consequences of this subdivision? This chapter deals with the first part of the question, i.e., with the determinants of the internal division of labor in hospitals. But it is clear since Marx, Durkheim, and Weber that the crucial role of the division of labor derives from its dual status among organizational phenomena: it is an integral element of the complexity of the organizational task structure and technology, and it is a way of dealing with that complexity.

Accordingly, I will first examine the variation in the degree of functional and departmental specialization among the twelve hospital types. Then I will analyze the effect of organizational size on these two kinds of specialization. In this analysis, I will use different indicators of size, distinguishing particularly between size of task and size of resources.

Finally, I will examine the two different aspects of the division of labor from a comparative perspective, with special emphasis on the effects of teaching status and type of medical service on internal differentiation while controlling for the effect of size.

Specialization: Functional and Departmental

In an attempt to specify some of the more immediate determinants of hospital bureaucracy, I have distinguished between two aspects of the division of labor in organizations. The first, functional specialization, refers to the amount of division of labor between specific work functions. Operationally, it is defined as the proportion of specialized functions filled in a given hospital. A value of 1.0 would mean that all 39 specific occupational categories are filled. A value of .51, for example, indicates that slightly over one-half—i.e., about 20—of the categories are filled, the average for all U.S. hospitals. The second aspect of division of labor, departmental specialization, refers to the differentiation among organizational components, assuming, of course, that they represent groups of specialized, interdependent activities such as those designated by separate departments or categories of personnel. Operationally, departmental specialization is defined by the Gini coefficient of concentration, based on seven major departments or personnel categories.[1]

On the basis of previous empirical research as well as theoretical considerations, I had hypothesized that the more complex general and teaching hospitals, in contrast to the psychiatric and non-teaching hospitals, are not only more advanced in terms of medical technology, but have a more complex internal division of labor, i.e., higher levels of functional and departmental specialization.

The variation of these two forms of specialization across the twelve hospital types strongly confirms these expectations (Table 17).

The mean values of functional specialization and departmental specialization are consistently higher for teaching as compared to nonteaching hospitals, and they tend to be higher for general hospitals in contrast to psychiatric hospitals.[2]

The strong effect of the complexity of the task structure on internal specialization and differentiation raises the question as to what extent organizational size adds to, or detracts from, this effect.

The Effect of Size on Specialization

Theoretically, increasing size should lead to increasing functional specialization and differentiation. We have seen already that this is the case with respect to technical facilities and services and the differentiation of technical functions in general. As expected, the influence of size on functional specialization is strong (Table 18).

Table 17
Means and Standard Errors of Functional Specialization and Departmental Specialization, by Service, Teaching Status, and Control

Type of Specialization		U.S. Hosp.	All 12 Groups	Voluntary				State and Local Governmental				Federal (V.A.)			
				Nonteaching		Teaching		Nonteaching		Teaching		Nonteaching		Teaching	
				Psy	Gen	Psy	Gen	Psy	Gen	Psy	Gen	Psy	Gen	Psy	Gen
		6,825	3,544	30	1,507	13	467	139	956	91	185	23	56	17	60
Functional Specialization	$\bar{x}$	.51	.54	.37	.49	.58	.75	.53	.43	.67	.72	.67	.65	.74	.75
	$s\bar{x}$	.002	.003	.017	.004	.029	.006	.010	.004	.010	.011	.012	.010	.017	.009
Departmental Specialization	$\bar{x}$	.53	.54	.52	.52	.61	.63	.43	.50	.51	.63	.56	.65	.58	.72
	$s\bar{x}$	.001	.002	.020	.002	.034	.003	.007	.002	.011	.006	.007	.006	.009	.009

Table 18

Intercorrelations Between Size, Functional Specialization, and Departmental Specialization, by Service, Teaching Status, and Control

	U.S. Hosp.	All 12 Groups	Voluntary				State and Local Governmental				Federal (V.A.)				Within Group Homogeneity[a]
			Nonteaching		Teaching		Nonteaching		Teaching		Nonteaching		Teaching		
			Psy	Gen	Psy	Gen	Psy	Gen	Psy	Gen	Psy	Gen	Psy	Gen	
(N)	6,825	3,544	30	1,507	13	467	139	956	91	185	23	56	17	60	
Size & Functional Specialization	.75	.74	.61	.79	.83	.82	.51	.17	.67	.83	.39	.79	.01	.54	7
Size & Departmental Specialization	.29	.30	-.17	.35	-.32	.53	-.17	.18	-.79	.52	-.41	.17	-.53	-.13	5
Functional & Departmental Specialization	.59	.62	-.03	.54	-.02	.51	.50	.43	-.44	.61	.10	.20	.54	.14	12

[a]Number of groups (hospital types) with a correlation coefficient lower (in absolute numbers) than that of all 12 groups combined; see Note 3.

172

The values shown in Table 18 are Pearsonian coefficients of correlation, based on the number of cases given at the top of each column. The values in the last column represent the number of groups, out of the total of twelve, in which the coefficients are smaller, regardless of sign, than the coefficient observed in the ungrouped total of all 12 groups combined. This number will be used as an index of the degree to which the 12 groups are more homogeneous with respect to a given relationship or set of variables.[3]

A brief comparison between columns 1 and 2 in Table 18 shows that the correlations in the 12 groups combined approximate those in the universe of U.S. hospitals. This parallels the earlier observation that the means of the respective variables in the 12 groups combined are similar to those in the total aggregate of U.S. hospitals.

The correlations between size and functional specialization tend to be fairly high, especially among teaching hospitals. The V.A. psychiatric teaching hospitals are an exception here insofar as functional specialization does not vary with size.[4]

The correlations between size and departmental specialization are generally lower than those between size and functional specialization. An examination of the correlations across the twelve types shows that in psychiatric hospitals departmental specialization tends to decrease with increasing size. This relationship is even more pronounced among psychiatric teaching hospitals.

As to the relationship between functional and departmental specialization, we note first of all that there is a high degree of within-group homogeneity. This is to be expected on the basis of the classification of hospitals in terms of task complexity.

More important from a theoretical perspective is the fact that functional specialization is not uniformly nor very highly correlated with departmental specialization. Moreover, in the case of the public psychiatric teaching hospitals, the relationship is clearly inverse.[5]

Assuming that the *amount* of division of labor among specialized functions has some empirical, temporal priority over their *structural pattern*, it is to be expected that only in general hospitals does departmental specialization vary directly with functional specialization, while in psychiatric hospitals this relationship is subject to special conditions. The most important condition of psychiatric hospitals, especially of those under public control, is that they are much larger than general hospitals. Moreover, size is strongly associated with functional specialization, as we have seen in Table 18.

Controlling for the influence of size, then, shows that functional specialization has a positive effect on departmental specialization in all hospital types, although the relationship is not at all uniform (Table 19).

Table 19 shows also that, with functional specialization controlled, departmental specialization tends to be inversely related to organizational size. Only in the voluntary general teaching hospitals representing one of the most complex organizational patterns among all hospital types do we still find a moderately low positive relationship (ry1.2=.23) between size and departmental specialization.

In general, therefore, an increase in size will almost always imply a decrease in departmental specialization. On the other hand, with size controlled, departmental specialization will always tend to be positively related to functional specialization.

This suggests that functional specialization is a *necessary condition* for the development of departmental specialization. But the development of specialized departments is *not a necessary consequence* that results simply from the presence of a high degree of functional specialization. It is therefore possible that organizations may have a relatively high level of functional specialization without necessarily developing the structural differentiation conducive to a high degree of departmental specialization. Such conditions do exist in the large mental hospitals, as we have seen. It can be assumed that in such organizations an increase in size implies largely segmental and parallel specialization rather than departmental specialization.[6] At best, these conditions may entail the development of departmental specialization in a limited form, i.e., only within certain units or subsystems of the larger structure but not in others.

Finally, in regard to the *joint* influence of size and functional specialization on departmental specialization, we observe that the strength of these variables is greater in psychiatric and in the teaching hospitals, as over against the general and the nonteaching hospitals. Thus, if we use the square of the multiple correlation coefficient as an index, size and functional specialization are better predictors of departmental specialization in unifunctional and diversified types, compared to organizations that are multifunctional but not diversified.[7]

Structural coordination derived from departmental specialization

Table 19
Multiple and Partial Correlation Coefficients for Departmental Specialization As Dependent Variable and Size and Functional Specialization As Independent Variables, by Service, Teaching Status, and Control

Partial Correlations Between Departmental Specialization and:	U.S. Hosp.	All 12 Groups	Voluntary				State and Local Governmental				Federal (V.A.)			
			Nonteaching		Teaching		Nonteaching		Teaching		Nonteaching		Teaching	
			Psy	Gen	Psy	Gen	Psy	Gen	Psy	Gen	Psy	Gen	Psy	Gen
(N)	6,825	3,544	30	1,507	13	467	139	956	91	185	23	56	17	60
Size	-.28	-.29	-.20	-.14	-.55	.23	-.57	-.20	-.74	.03	-.49	.02	-.63	-.25
Functional Specialization	.59	.61	.10	.45	.47	.15	.70	.43	.19	.37	.31	.11	.64	.25
Multiple R	.64	.66	.20	.55	.55	.54	.71	.46	.80	.61	.50	.20	.76	.28

is more difficult to obtain in, or less easily "built into," the structure of specialized or diversified organizations. Its presence is therefore tied closely to such structural factors as size and functional specialization. Changes in these aspects of structure will, consequently, tend to have a pervasive effect on the degree of departmental specialization, and on structural coordination. This observation is consistent with the deviant pattern noted in the organizationally specialized voluntary psychiatric hospitals whose smaller size and higher level of functional specialization clearly favors a higher degree of departmental specialization, and thus of structural coordination.

Size and Structure: A Detail

Any discussion of correlations is necessarily abstract since we have to imagine the joint distribution of two or more variables in a pluralistic universe. Let us, therefore, attempt to visualize changes in size by looking at each size category separately so that we can observe changes in structure in slow motion, as it were. I have selected four types of hospitals for this purpose, voluntary general teaching and nonteaching hospitals, and state psychiatric teaching and nonteaching hospitals. As is evident from Table 20, these hospitals are in completely different size ranges.

Among the state hospitals, there are few in the category of under five hundred beds, while all of the voluntary nonteaching general hospitals are in size categories below five hundred beds. Of the voluntary teaching hospitals, forty-three (or about 9 per cent) have more than five hundred beds, and none have fewer than fifty beds.

In examining the effect of size on functional specialization and departmental specialization, let us start with the state psychiatric nonteaching hospitals. Here, functional specialization increases with size in almost linear fashion from .43 to .63 (Table 20). It will be recalled that this does not mean that the larger mental hospitals are more adequately staffed—the personnel/patient ratio does, in fact, *decline* with increasing size in mental hospitals. But the positive relation between size and functional specialization means that a larger proportion of specialized occupational categories are present in larger hospitals, thus contributing to a higher degree of internal functional differentiation and specialization. Obviously, there is a higher level of functional specialization in the teaching hospitals in all size categories.

Table 20
Means of Functional and Departmental Specialization of State Psychiatric and Voluntary General Hospitals, by Size (# of Beds) and Teaching Status

Size (No. of Beds)	Non-Teaching Specialization		(N)	Teaching Specialization		(N)
	Functional	Departmental		Functional	Departmental	
State Psychiatric Hospitals						
Under 500	.43	.48	(11)	.55	.69	(16)
500 - 999	.47	.45	(12)	.57	.56	(3)
1,000 - 1,499	.51	.42	(27)	.67	.49	(9)
1,500 - 1,999	.55	.42	(22)	.63	.48	(6)
2,000 - 2,499	.56	.41	(18)	.67	.45	(7)
2,500 - 2,999	.57	.43	(15)	.72	.49	(45)
3,000 and Over	.63	.46	(23)	.72	.53	(45)
Voluntary General Hospitals						
Under 25	.30	.47	(152)	—	—	—
25 - 49	.39	.50	(435)	—	—	—
50 - 99	.51	.53	(535)	.47	.54	(44)
100 - 199	.63	.55	(333)	.71	.60	(112)
200 - 299	.69	.55	(49)	.78	.63	(142)
300 - 499	.76	.60	(6)	.81	.66	(127)
500 and Over	—	—	—	.84	.69	(43)

In contrast to functional specialization, the degree of departmental specialization, as measured by the Gini index, decreases slightly with increasing size. However, the relationship is somewhat curvilinear, both in teaching and nonteaching psychiatric hospitals. This suggests that the quantitative imbalance among the major departments and personnel categories, i.e., compositional homogeneity, tends to increase with size, generally, but that in exceedingly large organizations (here, over 2,500 beds) a compositional equilibrium is gradually re-established, approaching the initial level of departmental specialization.

The "imbalance" of staff composition with increasing size is due to an increase in subprofessional nursing personnel. Thus, the proportion of aides and attendants tends to increase with increasing size, reaching a high of 57 per cent and 61 per cent, respectively, in the largest size category of the nonteaching and teaching state mental hospitals.

In other words, even though functional specialization increases with size, it is still possible for an organization to become structurally simpler, i.e., if the size increase is accompanied by increasing internal homogeneity, rather than structural differentiation.

The significance of these relationships is underscored when we look at the teaching and nonteaching general hospitals (Table 20). In the general hospitals, similar to the psychiatric ones, functional specialization increases with size. At the same time, however, the degree of departmental specialization also increases with size and functional specialization, indicating that in general hospitals the internal structure becomes more complex as the organization becomes larger.

A generalization which emerges from these findings is that unifunctional, specialized organizations tend to become structurally simpler as they increase in size, since the larger size usually implies a greater degree of internal homogeneity. Under these conditions of increasing size and structural simplification, the dominant mechanisms of control should be bureaucratic with their characteristic emphasis on hierarchical and supervisory forms of coordination.

It is possible that this generalization would also hold under conditions where homogeneity is generated by a size increase in other types of organizational subunits, e.g., in the teaching faculty of a small liberal arts college, or the research staff of a business firm, provided these organizations have a relatively simple task structure. By contrast, in organizations with a multifunctional or diversified task structure, an increase in size is likely to entail not only an increase in functional specialization, but also in structural differentiation conducive to departmental specialization. Such organizations can be expected to have bureaucratized administrative structures only under the condition that departmental specialization is not extensive, and that there is no or only minimal professionalization of the labor force. In other words, one may expect an extensive departmental structure and a professionalized labor force to counteract the process of internal bureaucratization.

We will return to these generalizations and questions as we examine the conditions of bureaucratization in hospitals in greater detail in the following chapters.

Organizational Size: Task vs. Resources

The analysis of the effect of size on the internal division of labor was based, so far, on measures of task size, i.e., number of beds or average daily patient census. Let us now briefly examine the effect of size, in terms of both task and resources, on functional and departmental specialization, and on the number of different medical specialties available in teaching hospitals. It will be remembered that this latter measure comes closest to operationalizing the link between the complexity of the task structure and the internal division of labor, since it can be seen as an aspect of both. For this reason, it has been assumed that the number of medical specialties stands in a relation of mutual dependence with size, rather than being determined unilaterally by size.

In distinguishing between *size of task* and *size of resources* of an organization, we can see now that there is no significant relationship between task size and either the degree of departmental specialization or the number of medical specialties (Table 21).

Only functional specialization is correlated with task size, and only when size is defined on the basis of average daily patient census. But when size is conceptualized in terms of resources and personnel, all relationships tend to be positive.

This finding suggests, first of all, that the number of medical specialties is a determinant of size in the sense that payroll and total expenses increase as a result of the hospital's policy to offer a multiplicity of residency programs, and thus to have the necessary medical specialists available.

Secondly, the degree of functional specialization "interacts" with size in the sense that increasing task size (patient census) increases

Table 21
Correlations Between Organizational Size, Division of Labor, and Number of Medical Specialties, Based on 1,277 Teaching Hospitals (1960)

Size of Task	Internal Division of Labor Specialization Functional	Departmental	No. of Medical Specialties
Number of Beds	.04	-.06	.03
Average Daily Census	.20	-.05	.01
Size of Resources			
Total Payroll, 1960	.26	.20	.45
Total Expenses, 1960	.33	.20	.49
Total Personnel, 1960	.32	.11	.52
Functional Specialization	—	.42	.33
Departmental Specialization	—	—	.35

the differentiation of functions to be performed, as well as the labor force associated with those functions. But as the labor force increases, so do the categories of special technical and professional personnel which, in turn, raises total expenses, especially that part which is allocated for personnel expenditures.

Finally, departmental specialization is moderately sensitive to variations in financial resources as an indicator of size. This would suggest that changes in departmental specialization reflect administrative and policy decisions relatively more than do changes in functional specialization. In other words, while the *amount* of division of labor is tied more closely to the size of the task and the size of the labor force, the *structural patterns* resulting from departmental specialization are more nearly the consequence of the differential allocation of resources and of the underlying policy decisions. It is in this sense that functional specialization is an organizational necessity, while departmental specialization is an administrative device.

Let us now consider the effect of teaching on the internal division of labor in a comparative perspective, i.e., comparing it to the effect of service as well as ownership and control, where relevant, but at the same time controlling for the influence of size.

Division of Labor: A Comparative View

We have already observed the extent to which teaching hospitals have a significantly higher level of functional specialization. Similarly, both teaching and general hospitals are structurally more complex in terms of departmental development. We have also seen that departmental specialization is lowest in the state and local governmental hospitals, but highest in the federal V.A. hospitals.

These relationships are summarized in Table 22, which gives the results of an analysis of variance, with functional and departmental specialization as dependent variables.

With respect to functional specialization, Table 22 shows that the difference between teaching and nonteaching hospitals generates an unusually high F-ratio, while the effect of service is barely significant. For departmental specialization, both teaching and service effects are highly significant. However, since we have already observed the influence of size on both functional and departmental specialization (see Tables 18 and 19), we must take the presence of the significant size differences between psychiatric and general hospitals, as well as between teaching and nonteaching institutions,

Table 22
Effects of Control, Teaching Status, and Service on Functional and Departmental Specialization, Alone and with Size (and Functional Specialization) Controlled

| | Main Effects | | | Interactions | | | Second |
| | | | | First Order | | | |
	Control	Teaching	Service	Control X Teaching	Control X Service	Teaching X Service	Order
			F-Ratios[a]				
Dependent Variables Alone:							
1. Functional Specialization	136.92	1,302.91	10.54	20.96	30.43	27.54	5.25
2. Departmental Specialization	325.02	1,106.31	317.90	12.95	25.16	10.54	.27
With Controls:							
3. Functional specialization with size controlled	281.94	7.71	1,119.49	7.22	58.99	29.94	1.00
4. Departmental specialization with size controlled	261.62	342.70	520.48	7.95	61.54	.23	.58
5. Departmental specialization with size and functional specialization controlled	222.58	371.60	58.71	3.54	34.35	10.59	.13
df₁=	2	1	1	2	2	1	2

[a]The F-Ratios needed for significance at the .01 level: 4.60 (df₁=2), 6.64 (df₁=1); df₂=3,532 (for all effects).

into account. When size is used as a control variable, the results are striking (Table 22, rows 3 and 4). Compared to the situation where functional specialization is analyzed alone, the effects of teaching and service are completely reversed. However, the teaching status of hospitals, i.e., organizational diversification, retains a significant influence, independent of size.

As to the influence of the number of objectives and services (general vs. psychiatric hospitals) on functional specialization, the data lend strong support to the hypothesis that when size is held constant, specialized unifunctional organizations are internally less differentiated than complex multifunctional organizations. The data thus provide empirical confirmation for our initial assumption that the distinction between psychiatric and general hospitals yields a meaningful dimension of task complexity, i.e., that the complexity of the goal and task structure is reflected in the internal differentiation of the organization.[8]

The effects of teaching and service on departmental specialization operate essentially in the same way as those on functional specialization.

When size is controlled (Table 22, row 4), the effect of teaching is reduced, while the effect of service increases. At the same time, we find that the joint teaching/service effect ceases to be significant, indicating independence of these factors relative to each other ($F=.23$).[9]

Finally, when both size and functional specialization are used as control variables, the F-Ratio for the service effect drops, while that of the teaching effect increases slightly. It is of interest that the difference between teaching and nonteaching hospitals should become greater when size and functional specialization are held constant. It suggests that the complexity introduced by diversification is of a different nature from that differentiating unifunctional organizations and multifunctional ones. Put in very simple terms, one could say that a minimum number of jobs, i.e., some minimum of functional specialization, must be present in a given organization before any relationship among the different jobs or, essentially, departmental specialization, can develop. In other words, functional specialization is a necessary condition for departmental specialization.[10]

To shift the perspective to the organizational level, we could say that a number of specialized activities must be present before diversification can develop in an organization.

Ownership and control exercise a significant influence on functional and departmental specialization, which remains when size is

183

controlled. However, controlling for size has a standardizing effect since the F-Ratio increases for functional specialization, but decreases for departmental specialization.

It is interesting to recall in this connection that the V.A. hospitals have a fairly high and constant level of functional specialization, while range and variability is greater among the voluntary hospitals, despite the fact that in this group the size differences are smaller. This suggests that especially voluntary hospitals vary in their staffing policies, while the V.A. hospitals have a more uniform procedure of listing and filling positions. This finding is in line with our earlier suggestion that federal hospitals are more "planned" as organizations than other types.

The smaller differences in functional specialization among the V.A. hospitals, in spite of considerable size differences, suggest also that functional specialization varies directly with size only up to a certain size limit. Once it is reached, the increase in functional specialization levels off.

In general, we can say that although the effect of ownership and control is largely mediated by task complexity (see the significant interaction effects involving "control," Table 22), it nevertheless reaches into the internal structure of hospitals and helps to determine the level of the division of labor.

Summary and Conclusions

In this chapter, I have examined the variations in the division of labor among the twelve hospital types, the effect of size on both functional and departmental specialization, and the joint effect of task complexity and size on these two aspects of the division of labor.

Teaching and general hospitals tend to have a complex internal division of labor, as measured by the degree of functional and departmental specialization. However, since teaching and psychiatric hospitals tend to be larger than their counterparts, the effect of size must be taken into account. Functional specialization varies directly with size, although the strength of this relationship itself varies among the twelve hospital types. Departmental specialization, in turn, varies directly with functional specialization, but is inversely related to size, especially when functional specialization is controlled.

Insofar as departmental specialization provides the basis for structural coordination, we can generalize to the effect that structural coordination decreases as organizational size increases.

The hospital type most characteristic of this condition is the large state mental hospital, which becomes structurally simpler as it becomes larger. However, a detailed examination of the effect of increasing size on structural change reveals that in large mental hospitals the trend toward structural simplification is reversed at a certain size level. Mental hosptials in the size range of between 500 and 2,500 beds tend toward internal homogeneity with increasing size. But when they grow larger than 2,500 beds, there is a tendency for structural balance to be re-established. However, there is no evidence in the present data that the very large mental hospitals again reach the level of internal structural complexity characteristic of the smaller psychiatric hospitals (less than 500 beds).

I have also shown in this chapter that the effect of size depends, in part, on the kind of indicator used to measure size. Thus, a distinction between size of task and size of resources reveals that functional specialization is sensitive to both aspects of size, while departmental specialization varies mainly with size as measured by total payroll and total expenses. Although these findings are based on teaching hospitals only, it appears that functional specialization is an aspect of division of labor which is derived from both the nature and size of the task and, in turn, helps to determine the size of the organizational labor force. Departmental specialization, on the other hand, appears to be more the result of administrative and policy considerations. As an instrument of administrative decision-making, it is therefore a structural device used at the discretion of the administrator. Moreover, decisions which affect the structural arrangements among hospital departments and other subunits necessarily override those which affect specific job titles and individual positions.

In sum, while functional specialization can be seen as a necessary condition for the development of departmental specialization, the latter has priority over the former in terms of administrative decision-making and control. [11] The number of medical specialties present in teaching hospitals represents a conceptual link between task structure and internal division of labor. The number of specialties is also a strong determinant of size when the latter is conceptualized in terms of total expenses and number of personnel.

Finally, the analysis of co-variance of functional and departmental specialization reveals that the difference between psychiatric and general hospitals is accentuated when the effect of size is considered. The variation in departmental specialization, due to the teaching status of the hospital, is increased when the effects of both size and functional specialization are jointly controlled.

In this as well as in the previous two chapters, then, I have examined the broad structural variations among hospitals. We have seen that there are systematic differences between the twelve hospital types in terms of the major analytical dimensions of autonomy and task complexity. The differences between structural patterns have been illuminated by an analysis of the structure and changes in medical technology, and by the analysis of the internal division of labor in hospitals.

On the basis of this analysis of structural variation, I will now, in Part III of this book, examine the modes of coordination in hospitals, especially the interplay between bureaucratic and non-bureaucratic modes. Part II can therefore be seen as an attempt to establish the fact and nature of structural variation among hospitals, as complex organizations, while Part III deals with the consequences of task complexity, autonomy, and internal division of labor for coordination and control.

Notes

1. See Chapter 3 for a detailed description of both functional and departmental specialization.

2. The federal as well as state and local governmental nonteaching psychiatric hospitals have a somewhat higher level of functional specialization than the corresponding general hospitals, a pattern which has already been observed for the differentiation among technical specialties in the previous chapter (Table 15). As before, I assume that the reason is that legal provisions make it mandatory for the less autonomous, public psychiatric nonteaching hospitals to hire personnel for certain technical specialties, regardless of hospital size; such job titles are not necessarily filled in the corresponding general hospitals.

3. This index is useful to the extent that it shows quickly whether the correlations observed in the ungrouped total of 3,544 hospitals tend to be higher, to remain substantially the same, or to be lower when they are computed *within* the twelve "cells" generated by the three-way classification of hospitals.

The overall relationship between any two variables can be assumed to be the result of greater within-group variance if this index approaches zero; or the result of greater between-group variance (or within-group homogeneity) if the index approaches "12", provided that the correlation coefficients do not have values close to the one observed in the ungrouped total. If this latter condition should occur, we would conclude that the dimensions of subclassification do not elaborate, specify, or explain the observed overall relationship. For a description and successful application of this technique, see Leo F. Schnore, "The Statistical Measurement of Urbanization and Economic Development," *Land Economics,* 37 (1961), 239; on the general idea of multivariate analysis involved here, see Paul F. Lazarsfeld, "Interpretation of Statistical Relations as a Research Operation," in Paul F. Lazarsfeld and Morris Rosenberg, eds., *The Language of Social Research* (Glencoe, Ill.: The Free Press, 1955), pp. 115-123.

4. It is conceivable that the absence of any correlation is essentially due to homogeneity. In other words, the high mean level of functional specialization of .74 in this group, the highest among all psychiatric hospitals, suggests that functional specialization is the result of a planned pattern, and that a certain minimum number of job titles are filled regardless of the size of the hospital. See also note 2 above.

5. Since the variables were transformed before the correlation coefficients were calculated, any effect deriving from the curvilinearity of the relationship was probably greatly reduced.

6. On the distinction between segmentation and differentiation, see, for example, Talcott Parsons, *Structure and Process in Modern Societies* (Glencoe, Ill.: The Free Press, 1960), p. 263.

7. The joint effect of size and functional specialization on departmental specialization must be interpreted with caution, since both of these independent variables are highly correlated with one another. It is, consequently, difficult to assign exact weights to the relative contribution each of these variables is making toward the variation in the dependent variable, i.e., departmental specialization. In my judgment, it is nevertheless useful to examine the joint influence of size and functional specialization on other variables, since their association with one another is, in itself, variable, as shown in Table 18. I am grateful to Art Stinchcombe for drawing my attention to the problem in this particular context. For an excellent general discussion of this and related issues, see Robert A. Gordon, "Issues in Multiple Regression," *American Journal of Sociology,* 73 (1968), 592-616; and Hubert M. Blalock, "Correlated Independent Variables: The Problem of Multicollinearity," *Social Forces,* 42 (1963), 233-237.

8. By implication, these findings confirm the validity of the distinction between general and TB hospitals in terms of functional complexity which Anderson and Warkov used as the basis of their study. For Anderson and Warkov it was important to control for size because the V.A. general hospitals are larger, on the average, than the TB hospitals. In the present case, size has to be controlled because the less complex psychiatric hospitals are the larger ones, while the general hospitals are smaller. The only exception occurs among the voluntary teaching hospitals, where the general hospitals are somewhat larger than the psychiatric ones.

9. The same results are obtained when functional specialization instead of size is controlled, confirming not only the close relationship between the two factors, but suggesting also the theoretically important independence of functional and departmental specialization relative to each other.

10. Again, this relationship between the two aspects of the internal division

of labor is all the more important as both are independent measures, the former being based on the proportion of specialized functions, the latter on the relation between categorically defined organizational components.

11. This two-way nexus between the two levels of specialization is similar in conception to Parsons' idea that higher-level action systems exercise cybernetic control over their constituent subsystems, although the former are developmentally (causally) anchored in the latter. It should be obvious, however, that there is no systematic theoretical relationship between the present formulation and the theory of action systems. See Talcott Parsons, "An Outline of the Social System," in Talcott Parsons et al.. eds., *Theories of Society* (New York: The Free Press, 1961), Vol. I, pp. 37-38.

Part III: The Problem of Coordination

8 Professionals in Organizations

Why should the organizational employment of professional workers be problematic? One of the main reasons appears to lie in the widely shared norm that professional work should not, and cannot, be externally regulated. For professionals, at the most, the result of their activities might be externally specified, but not the standards and procedures governing their activities. In business organizations, this is sometimes known as "administration by results"—the unity of operative and regulative rules. This prerogative typically granted to professional practitioners reflects the degree to which they have been successful in turning their "license" into a "mandate."[1] But in the context of an organizational division of labor, and from the point of view of organizational coordination, the license to practice may need to be circumscribed, and the presumed mandate to define "good practice" may become a liability.

These limitations of the prerogatives of the professional work role apply to hospital-based physicians, especially insofar as there has been an increase of specialists as over against general practitioners. But the organizational limitations of the professional role also apply to the many other health professions present in the modern hospital, among them nurses and qualified technical personnel. It is this proliferation of different specialties and the fact of their mutual dependence which is probably the single most important factor in the transformation of occupational roles as each is adapted or forced into the network of the division of labor. It may be useful at this point to restate certain operating definitions used in this study.

Professionalization, first of all, is seen as a continuum ranging from in-service training to apprenticeship to formal training and the development of an occupational subculture. It is not seen as implying a dichotomy of professions (medicine, law) vs. nonprofessions. Professionalization is used here to indicate the degree to which the "production workers" of the organizational labor force have internalized the norms and rules governing their work. It refers to the extent to which operative and regulative rules are integrated with the work process.

As an *organizational* characteristic, professionalization applies therefore not primarily to those who initiate and direct the work process or an aspect of it, e.g., physicians who direct the process of medical care. It applies, in hospitals, mainly to graduate professional nurses who continuously implement the total work process of patient care, including medical care.

Secondly, it should be noted again that from the perspective of organizational objectives and goals, the coordination of specialized activities is not an end in itself. Rather than being a constant factor in human social organization, it must be seen as a set of variables dependent upon the autonomy and task structure of the organization, as well as its internal division of labor and technology. This view implies that certain forms of social organization and task structure may function entirely without external coordination such as supervision and hierarchical authority.[2] Others, such as certain pre-industrial work organizations, may develop hierarchical forms of coordination, depending on the technological complexity of the task.[3] And still others, such as crafts in the building industry or modern "professionalized" armed forces, may employ a labor force whose members can to a large extent make all work-related decisions at the place of work on the basis of specialized knowledge and internalized rules, rather than being dependent on external regulation, supervision, and centralized decision-making.[4]

The hospital is a professional organization to the extent that it employs a labor force with these latter characteristics.[5] The problem of coordination in hospitals is therefore one that is not only determined by variations in autonomy and task structure, technology and division of labor, but also by the additional impact of a professionalized labor force.

That impact is double-edged. On the one hand, generalist professional work, based on the specification of function rather than mere job specialization, tends to be self-coordinating and self-regulating. But once professionals become employees in an organizational context, regulation and coordination, even if only minimal, must of necessity be external. Hence the two most frequent types of conflict involving professionals are: 1) conflict *between* professional and bureaucratic positions and hierarchies (or between bureaucratic and collegial authority structures), and 2) role strain and conflict *within* those status-roles requiring the performance of both professional-technical and administrative-bureaucratic-supervisory work functions, as well as subordination to external authority.

Both types of problems involve relatively specific areas of responsibility and work functions. But in the first case, viz. conflict between generalist-professional and monocratic-bureaucratic authority, both areas remain separate and may become even more polarized. It is a problem that must be dealt with at the level of the organization, not at the level of specific roles and positions. The second type of problem, in contrast, emerges only insofar as administrative-bureaucratic and professional areas of work are fused and integrated in the first place. Consequently, the strain and conflict is to be absorbed by the incumbent of the status-role.

The problem investigated in the present chapter involves both types of conflict due to the dual status of hospital administrators, nurses, and other professionals in the hospital. I will first consider the nature of authority and decision-making in hospitals, particularly in connection with the professionalization of hospital administrators. I will then turn to an analysis of the professional and organizational status of nurses, and explore the nature and consequences of the coordinating functions which graduate professional nurses perform in hospitals.

Authority and Decision-Making in Hospitals

A dominant conception of hospital organization centers about the coexistence of two more or less integrated subsystems, variously referred to as "two lines of authority,"[6] clinical-therapeutic-professional vs. administrative authority systems,[7] and formal vs. informal or "functional" organization.[8] Typically, the focus is on the physician and on the role of the medical-professional practitioner in an organizational or "bureaucratic" setting.[9]

Based on the assumption of an inherent incompatibility between professional and bureaucratic orientations, this role tends to be viewed as problematic and as a source of potential strain and conflict. In organizations where professionals are clearly subordinated to the rank authority of nonprofessional superiors, i.e. where they are required to submit to discipline and supervision, this assumption is probably warranted. However, that condition is not likely to occur in hospitals where physicians carry the formal responsibility for the performance of the actual work functions even though nurses have the de facto responsibility. Nor is it likely to occur in universities as well as certain types of hospitals and medical settings where mixed forms of bureaucratic and professional patterns of authority tend to develop.[10]

A frequent solution, then, is the transference of bureaucratic functions to professionals. Thus, the position of "medical administrator" is often found in teaching hospitals and in psychiatric hospitals. It refers to an M.D. who performs part-time or full-time administrative functions, either in the medical-clinical area or on a hospital-wide basis. The same is true in federal, state, and local governmental hospitals.

It is important to note here that these hospital types also have a higher proportion of salaried physicians than their voluntary nonprofit counterparts. In other words, it could be argued that the higher the proportion of regularly employed medical professionals in a hospital, the more likely will the top administrator also be a medical professional, i.e., a peer rather than a superior. In this way, the friction deriving from the subordination of medical professionals to nonmedical authority would be minimized.

This general hypothesis appears to be borne out by the following comparative figures.

The percentage of hospitals in which the chief administrator is a physician was 79 per cent in all federal hospitals in 1956, 74 per cent in all nonfederal mental hospitals, in contrast to 22 per cent in all nonfederal short-term general hospitals.[11] Similarly, among nonfederal mental hospitals, 88 per cent of the state and local governmental hospitals had an M.D. administrator, in contrast to only 41 per cent of the voluntary nonprofit hospitals. Among the nonfederal, short-term general hospitals, 20 per cent of the state and local governmental hospitals had an M.D. administrator, in contrast to 12 per cent of the voluntary (community) general hospitals.

Among general hospitals, the highest proportion is, of course, found among the proprietary hospitals, with 55 per cent having an M.D. owner-administrator.[12]

The choice of physicians as hospital administrators may reduce conflict between organizational roles and hierarchies, but possibly at the expense of the specificity and clarity of definition of the top executive role itself. In other words, organizational conflict is transformed into role conflict. Its tolerance or resolution is thus shifted to the individual occupying that unenviable position of chief hospital executive. Strain and conflict is absorbed *before* it reaches the level of the organization.

However, both the critical shortage of physicians and the need for trained administrative manpower capable of dealing with the ever-increasing complexity of hospitals seem to indicate that it is basically inefficient to use physicians for administrative functions. Furthermore, the administrator's role in the power structure of the hospital is changing rapidly. The nature of this change lies essentially in a shift of the balance of power from the board and the clinical administrative functions of the medical staff to the non-medical executive role of an administrator.[13]

The role of the hospital administrator, in turn, is becoming not only more salient organizationally, but also more professionalized. Let us briefly look at some of the characteristic aspects of this process of professionalization.

Professionalization of Hospital Administration

Historically, the combination of hospital board power and the prestige of the medical profession have made it difficult for the hospital administrator to come into his own. Yet there can be little doubt that the growing complexity of modern hospitals has led to a de facto expansion of nonmedical administrative authority. To the extent that this trend will continue, it can be expected that professional nonmedical administrators will gradually take the place of the medical administrators even though the social-psychological temptation to have medical professionals supervised only by other medical professionals may remain. On the whole, however, it is clear that structural factors such as autonomy and task complexity of the hospital have an overriding effect on the choice of the top administrator. Let us take a comparative look at the professionalization of nonmedical and nonnursing administrators.

Among the general hospitals in which the chief administrator is neither a physician nor a graduate professional nurse, 30 per cent of the voluntary hospitals and 24 per cent of the state and local governmental hospitals have chief administrative officers who are graduates of a college course in hospital administration.[14] Among mental hospitals, this proportion is 37 per cent for the voluntary and 51 per cent for the state and local governmental hospitals.[15] Among all federal hospitals, 42 per cent of the nonmedical and nonnursing administrators are "professionalized" by this index.[16] It should be noted again that these figures apply for 1956 and are likely to be higher today, especially in the nonfederal general hospitals.

In sum, among state and federal hospitals as well as among mental institutions, the choice of the top executive clearly favors the professionally trained administrator, although he may well be still a "second choice" as over against the M.D. administrator. However, among general hospitals, voluntary nonprofit institutions are the ones which have the largest proportion of professionally trained administrators, and the smallest proportion of M.D. administrators.

Of particular interest in this connection is the question to what extent teaching hospitals, i.e., the elite institutions, set a standard in the choice and characteristics of their top administrators. An analysis of the biographies of teaching hospital administrators suggests that they are, indeed, an elite group in terms of various characteristics of professionalization.[17]

Of the 791 administrators of teaching hospitals listed both in the 1960 Guide Issue of Hospitals and in the Directory of the American College of Hospital Administrators, 16.2 per cent are M.D.'s, 31.0 per cent have some training in hospital administration (19.2 per cent have a master's degree in hospital administration), 16.3 per cent have a diploma or degree in nursing. Since, as we saw, only 12 per cent of all voluntary general hospitals had an M.D. administrator in 1956, we can assume a difference of about 5 or 6 percentage points between teaching and nonteaching hospitals, with teaching hospitals favoring the M.D. administrator.

With respect to the administrator's professional training in hospital administration, the difference is much greater. Taking the 31 per cent who have some training in hospital administration as a proportion of all those who are neither physicians nor nurses (67.5 per cent), we find that 46 per cent of the teaching hospital administrators have some training in hospital administration. Since the average for voluntary general hospitals is 30 per cent, we can assume a difference of about 20 percentage points, with teaching hospitals favoring the pr ssional hospital administrator.

Because of the larger size and the greater prestige of teaching hospitals, this group of administrators is certainly not representative of the universe of administrators of general hospitals. But, in all probability, they do represent a standard of professionalization toward which hospital administration in general is moving. Seen from this perspective, it is significant that of the 791 administrators in 1960, 84 per cent held administrative positions in hospitals before their current positions, 33 per cent having been top administrators in another hospital. The median age of the total group was 49 years in 1960. The typical career pattern of this group is fairly obvious when we see that 73 per cent held administrative positions in their second job before the current one, while almost half (49 per cent) did so in their third most recent previous job. The median number of previous jobs for the whole group is between four and five.

These administrators had been in their present position a median number of 6 years, with 10 per cent having held their present job for more than 15 years. It is noteworthy that the 6-year average length of tenure for this group of hospital administrators is exactly the same as the average for all teaching hospital administrators in 1960.[18]

We have seen that a substantial number of administrators held positions in hospital administration before their current job. Another measure of the career in the field of hospital administration is the extent to which administrators did not come up through the ranks in the same hospital, but held positions in different hospitals.[19] Of the 791 biographies analyzed, 61 per cent show the current hospital administrator to have come from another hospital. The corresponding percentages for the second and third most recent previous jobs are 57 per cent and 43 per cent, respectively.[20] Moreover, 41.6 per cent held *all* of their previous positions in hospitals but only one-tenth of that figure (4.5 per cent) held *all* of their previous jobs in organizations other than hospitals.

In general, these figures indicate that a relatively high proportion of administrators has been professionally mobile in the sense of moving *between* rather than *within* organizations. This mobility can be interpreted in terms of its association with a dominant identification with the field of hospital administration, rather than with a specific hospital.

In other words, rather than being "organization men," this elite group of hospital administrators is composed of persons who are professionals in their own right.

The degree of professional identification, as over against an exclusive orientation toward the employing organization, can also be

197

gauged by looking at the membership in professional associations in contrast to membership in other organizations and associations. Again, the data show a highly professionalized profile for this group. Apart from the fact that all of the 791 administrators are members of *the* professional association, the American College of Hospital Administrators, most are members of two or more *other* professional associations, such as the University Hospital Executive Council or the National Conference of Hospital Administrators. In fact, the median number of such additional professional memberships is three, while the median number of memberships in nonprofessional organizations and associations is only one.

Let us now turn to the analysis of another group of professionals in hospitals, namely nurses, who (not unlike hospital administrators) occupy a dual position in the organization by virtue of being professionals and bureaucrats at the same time.

Professional and Organizational Status of Nursing

In order to discuss the multiple facets of the status and role of nursing, some general remarks about the nurses' work environment are necessary. Probably the most important "significant other" in the nurses' role-set is the physician. Members of the medical staff, such as attending physicians, residents, and interns, and to some extent courtesy and consulting medical staff, have an almost unique position in hospitals compared to the position of professionals in most other organizations. The physician enjoys this special status by virtue of his unrestricted access to the facilities and services as well as power over the personnel of the hospital. Indeed, the hospital is frequently seen as an extension and an instrument of the medical practitioner, particularly since only members of the medical profession may legally "practice medicine."

Yet in the modern hospital, the crucial organizational problem is not so much the integration of professionals into an organizational framework, or the problem of interfering with the professional autonomy and self-regulation of the medical practitioner, but the coordination of a variety of clinical-therapeutic as well as nonmedical organizational concerns. In this perspective, the physician is a specialist among others. He initiates and directs a complex work process but contributes little to its coordination. Moreover, from the point of view of routinization of tasks and procedures, the physician is likely to introduce discontinuities into the work organization and to engage in "episodic interventions" as Habenstein and Christ, following Hughes, have described it.[21]

It is significant that those studies which have concerned themselves with the question of coordination on the operational level of hospital organization have focused not so much on the role of the physician, but rather on the role of the nurse.

There is no question that the administrator plays a vital coordinating role with respect to the medical staff and the board, and with respect to the overall integration of hospital functions on the departmental level. On the level of the patient care unit, however, the administrator, i.e., the administrative function of the hospital as an organization, is represented by the nurse. Here, the "two lines of authority" converge on the position of the head nurse and the staff nurse. Correspondingly, the organizational role of graduate professional nurses in hospitals has at least two distinct facets: the implementation of the therapeutic-clinical aspects of patient care initiated by the physician, and the implementation of the administrative and organizational aspects of patient care deriving from the fact that patients are temporarily "incorporated" into the organizational structure of the hospital.

But these two aspects of the nurse's role at best help to define her organizational status; they do not define her professional status. In order to exercise professional authority independent of the physician and the administrator, the nurse must possess "functionally specific technical competence," [22] universalistic standards of judgment, disinterestedness or affective neutrality, and devotion to "service" or a "collectivity-orientation." [23]

While functional specificity of professional expertise and universalistic judgment based on objective criteria contain elements of what Weber calls "purposive rationality," the devotion to the welfare of the client and to service for the good of the collectivity contains elements of "value rationality," i.e.:

> a rational orientation to an absolute value . . . involving a conscious belief in the absolute value of some ethical form of behavior, entirely for its own sake and independently of any prospects of external success. [24]

An example of such value rationality is the physician's belief in the value of the precepts and standards incorporated in the Hippocratic oath. For nurses it has traditionally been the inspiration to selfless service, in the United States legitimated by the example of Florence Nightingale. This inspiration is an important analytical element of what Habenstein and Christ have called the "traditionalizing" orientation in nursing, in contrast with the more purposive-rational "professionalizing" orientation.[25] Similarly, Reissman and Rohrer call attention to this element in describing their "dedicated" type of nurse for whom the nursing profession and "hospital work had been and continued to be a most important objective."[26] For the "dedicated" nurses, patient care and the "willingness to serve others" were singularly important, all other reasons being inconsequential.[27]

It should be emphasized once again that this value rationality is not in itself a sufficiently defining characteristic of professional status, but it is an important element in the commitment and the sustaining value orientation which is internalized in the process of socialization and formal training and supported by the "community" of colleagues.[28] Closely related to the need for a supportive and protective reference group and to the external and symbolic control it exercises over its members is the legitimation of the professional's formal expertise by the values of the larger society, a legitimation described in terms of the "mandate" of a profession.[29]

Insofar as nursing has developed an independent area of competence supported and protected by a professional membership and reference group and legitimized by the consistency between the value-rational orientation toward serving others and the values of the larger society, it can be said to be a profession.[30]

However, the peculiarity of the nurse's position in the hospital points up the problems inherent in the interpenetration of professional and organizational statuses which accompanies the increasing involvement of professionals in organizational work structures. This problem assumes several forms. In their study of the role definitions of general duty nurses in 51 Missouri general hospitals, Habenstein and Christ found that the professionalizing and traditionalizing orientations are linked to an underlying dimension of professionalism, or a continuum of professional reference-group orientation. This dimension has found expression in the distinction between two career styles, the "homeguard" and the "itinerant." Even among those who qualify as fully professional, some will be swept more completely than others into the mainstream of change and professionalization."[31] While the home-guards form personal attachments and loyalties to the community and the organization, the itinerants, "more fully committed and more alert to the new developments, will move from place to place seeking ever more interesting, prestigeful and perhaps more profitable positions."[32]

In the hospitals studied by Habenstein and Christ, homeguardism is represented by the traditionalizers, although it is basically an aspect of organizational status rather than of professional status.

> Home-guardism includes resistance to formally initiated change, blockage of our short-circuiting chains of formal communication, and the subversion of the formal authority structure to the ends of the home-guard. Generally, much action is rationalized as "for the good of the hospital," or possibly, "for the good of the community."[33]

In reviewing and interpreting various studies of professional reference group orientation, including Gouldner's study of cosmopolitans and locals[34] and Bennis' study of outpatient department nurses,[35] as well as their own work in a welfare agency, Blau and Scott suggest that a crucial factor in professional reference-group behavior is the "opportunity for advancement *within the profession.*"[36]

> Only if it is the *structure of the organization* rather than the *structure of the profession* that restricts opportunities for professional advancement do we expect professional commitment to be accompanied by a cosmopolitan orientation.[37]

Insofar as this general conclusion is derived from the case of nursing, as appears to be true, it provides a plausible interpretation of the negative effect of the nurse's multiple loyalties on her reference-group orientation, and thus on her expected low score on a scale of cosmopolitanism. Bennis and his associates provide the basic empirical model for the restricted opportunity structure of certain professions when they conclude that

> essentially, the group that would gain recognition within the broader professional field must do so through advancing within the administrative or educational areas in the local nursing situation.[38]

The generalizing interpretation advanced by Blau and Scott must be viewed as tentative insofar as their basic strategy is confined to demonstrating an association between contiguous social-psychological attributes, viz. role conceptions and reference group orientations of professionals. By contrast, a crucial characteristic of Hughes' analysis of the home-guard is that its representatives are shown to *act* in certain ways, for example, they do *not* "move from place to place."[39] Moreover,

> those who *stay longer in one place,* whether they have no opportunity

to move, or because they have attachments, *build even more attachments*, becoming less movable and perhaps more resistant to the itinerants and the changes the latter propose and promote. [40]

Consistent with this definition of the home-guard, Habenstein and Christ found that seniority was associated with much less itinerancy. Similarly, these authors found that a majority of the unmarried, older nurses living in the nurses' homes adjacent to the hospitals and holding administrative and supervisory positions in the nursing hierarchy frequently constituted the core of the home-guard.[41]

Bennis and his associates recognized the importance of this variable of itinerancy, but they conceptualized and operationalized it in terms of mobility rather than seniority in the present job or what could be called a nurse's "institutional age" or working years. Although having moved once, a given nurse might still have a high number of working years in her present job, and thus may have become a "local." Failure to control for the outpatient nurses' seniority may well be one reason for the negative findings of Bennis et al., namely that cosmopolitans turn out to have certain local characteristics. [42]

Equally consequential in the case of nurses may be the failure to control for marital status. Married working nurses, regardless of their professional orientation, may experience inter-hospital mobility which is related to their husbands' rather than their own careers. Unmarried nurses, on the other hand, are more likely to be *both* more professionally oriented and more attached to a specific work group or hospital.

Finally, the slight relation between education and reference group orientation reported by Bennis et al. might have been stronger if *joint* controls for marital status and age had been applied. [43]

The concern with reference-group orientation alone may therefore lead to erroneous conclusions, since the structural and career determinants of both cosmopolitanism and professionalism may affect these orientations differentially. Already Merton, in his description of local and cosmopolitan influentials, states that most of the differences between these two types "seem to stem from their difference in basic orientation." Significantly, Merton adds in a footnote that

> nothing is said here of the objective *determinants* of these differences in orientations. To ascertain these determinants is an additional and distinctly important task, not essayed in the present study.[44]

Thus Gouldner's typology of cosmopolitans and locals is developed from interviews based on a sample of college faculty members but without controlling for seniority. In fact, Gouldner states that the sample "was supplemented by a list of new faculty members who had joined the staff that year."[45] Since Gouldner's "principal objective was that of concept construction," he proceeded to develop his typology on the basis of the interrelations of his three key independent social-psychological variables: commitment to skill, organizational loyalty, and inner-outer reference-group orientation.[46] Again, as in the case of Bennis et al., failure to control for seniority renders the interpretation of the empirical data problematic. It should be clear that these criticisms are not primarily concerned with the validity and usefulness of the typological distinction between cosmopolitans and locals, but rather with the problematic question of what constitutes a professional reference group, especially in the case of nurses.

It is important to note that compared to the relatively adequate fit between Gouldner's data and theory, Bennis and his associates are confronted with a more complex situation in that certain nurses have *both* professional and organizational orientations. In other words, we are dealing here with two different dimensions rather than with the opposite poles of one continuum.

Thus, Bennis' conclusions transcend the unidimensionality of the local-cosmopolitan scale. Without clearly specifying the new dimensions, Bennis et al. suggest four types: 1) work-group and skill-oriented nurses (the original cosmopolitans); 2) administratively oriented nurses (the original locals); 3) the "interested" (personal and professional); and 4) the "uninterested."

In view of the distinction between professional and organizational orientation as two separate dimensions rather than types, Bennis' data and conclusions exhibit a strikingly close affinity to the multidimensional conceptual framework proposed by Goldberg, Baker, and Rubenstein.[47]

In sum, Bennis' cosmopolitans rank high on *both* personal-professional and organizational dimensions suggested by Goldberg et al., while the opposite is true of Bennis' fourth type, the "uninterested," which is clearly a residual category. Types two and three represent the "pure" types of administrative (local) and personal-professional orientations, respectively.

What conclusions can be drawn from these studies? The main elements of the hospital nurse's professional identity are not predominantly the traditional nursing expertise and the consensus on role definitions within the community of nursing professionals.

Membership in professional nursing associations is low, and is moreover influenced by a host of extra-professional factors, including type of control and ownership of the hospital in which the nurse is employed, and the absence or low visibility of rewards and benefits. [48] Formal training and specialization are undergoing continuous change and redefinition and thus contribute indirectly to the differentiation of the nurse's role structure, as well as to the increasing scope and complexity of her role-set in the hospital. The transformation of the nurse's role is the dominant theme of research and writing in this area.

The two main elements of the nurse's role which appear to legitimate her claim to professional status are a pervasive service orientation and the specification of functions which are partly taken over from the physician and the administrator, partly constituted by an independent area of competence, and partly assumed by virtue of a central position in the organization of work. At the risk of subverting the analytical separation of professional, historical, organizational, informal, formal, and functional elements in the nurse's role, one could say that the graduate nurse derives professional authority from a combination of professional and nonprofessional functions. The crucial feature of this combination is that nurses perform both functional-coordinating and administrative-coordinating tasks, and that the line of demarcation between these two areas cannot be clearly drawn.

To the extent that the administrative functions are part of a formal hierarchy, the nurse's role exemplifies in an unexpected way Weber's concept of legal-bureaucratic authority which is based on both rank and expertise. But since the specification of functions, rather than of procedures, presupposes independent judgment and the application of internalized technical norms and standards, the nurse's role involves, in addition, a measure of discretion and responsibility characteristic of professional service. I will describe this latter facet of nursing in the following section.

Coordinating Functions of Professional Nurses

Professional nurses exercise coordinating functions on the level of work organizations in two ways: as administrators, supervisors, and lower level representatives of the nonmedical administrator of the hospital and as "line" workers who are responsible for the implementation of medical directives and the provision of "independent" nursing care of the patient. In an apt summary of the nurse's functions, Habenstein and Christ state: The nurse's " . . . vertical functional reach extends far above and below the formal nominal definition of what her work consists [of]." Furthermore,

> the horizontal reach of her functions is more likely than not to extend across services than remain within any one of them . . . her relative scarcity in a disadvantaged ratio to auxiliary assistance *increases* the range of her duties, *increases* her chances for error, *increases* the number and kind of interpersonal on-the-job contacts. [49]

The formal job description of the general staff nurse does not include a specification of the "horizontal" and "vertical reach of her functions," except for an indication that she "may supervise non-professional personnel of the unit" and that "some aspects of [her] job are similar" to those of the head nurse.[50] The emphasis is slightly shifted in the job description of the general head nurse who

> supervises and administers nursing service of a single patient-care unit . . . and among many other functions . . . provides for nursing care of patients in the unit and cooperates with other members of the medical care team and personnel of other departments in providing for patients' total needs. [51]

The explicit recognition of cooperation with other personnel groups turns into a broad mandate to coordinate the multiplicity of services converging on the patient care unit if we consider the sociological consequences of the nurse's responsibility for the continuity of space, time, and function.[52]

In his analysis of the formal and informal exigencies of the nurse's role, Mauksch shows that the continuity of the nurse's presence on the patient care unit has important consequences for her pivotal role in the coordination of patient care. By distinguishing between the formal organizational "care structure" of the hospital and the medical-clinical "cure-structure," as well as the territorial and functional characteristics of the administratively defined patient care units, Mauksch points out that the head nurse (and, also to some extent, the staff nurse) coordinates not only between care and cure structure, but also between specialized functions and demands within each of these two subsystems.[53] Thus the nurse is

> first, by virtue of her nursing function the person who performs those bedside tasks which are nursing care rather than medical therapy, and which therefore are part of the hospital's direct responsibility and her profession's prerogative. Secondly, by virtue of the absence of an administrative hierarchy, the nurse has become the administrator of

the territorial unit, the partient care area . . . Thirdly, by virtue of the growing specialization and diversification of the tasks that are volved in patient care, and by virtue of the continuity of time, she has become the mediator and coordinator of the various functionaries who, with but episodal responsibility for their specialties, come and go on the nursing care unit, without assuming any responsibility for overall coordination and continuity.[54]

These conclusions are supported by an abundance of evidence based on the observation and analysis of nursing work functions.[55]

Assuming, then, that job titles correspond roughly to functions performed, and that the proportion of graduate professional nurses is an indicator of the degree of professionalization of the nonmanagerial labor force, it is relevant to compare that proportion for different types of hospital autonomy and task complexity. By the same token, it is useful to compare simultaneously the proportion of subprofessional nursing personnel for different hospital types, since both professional and subprofessional groups are in many ways complementary and interdependent. This interdependence is, in part, expressed in the variation of the size of these groups relative to each other.

Professionalization: A Structural Variable in Hospitals

It is not difficult to understand the key role of nursing services in hospitals when we see that, on the average, over half of the total hospital labor force is concentrated in that category (Table 23, row 1). These mean percentages, based on the total number of personnel, include of course both professional and subprofessional nursing personnel. There is a considerable degree of variation among the different hospital types, ranging from a mean of almost 60 per cent in state and local governmental nonteaching general hospitals to almost 30 per cent in the V.A. teaching general hospitals. The significance of this variation emerges clearly when we differentiate between professional and subprofessional nursing personnel and compare the relevant proportions *between* and *within* the 12 hospital types (Table 23, rows 2 and 3).

First of all, the proportion of graduate professional nurses varies significantly *between* hospital types (Table 23, row 2). The lowest average is 5 per cent in state nonteaching psychiatric hospitals, while the highest is 27 per cent in voluntary nonteaching general hospitals. The most obvious difference exists between the psychiatric and the

Table 23
Mean Per Cent (Relative Size) of Various Categories of Nursing Staff and Degree of Differentiation Among Subprofessional Personnel

	U.S. Hosp.	All 12 Groups	Voluntary				State and Local Governmental				Federal (V.A.)			
			Nonteaching		Teaching		Nonteaching		Teaching		Nonteaching		Teaching	
			Psy	Gen	Psy	Gen	Psy	Gen	Psy	Gen	Psy	Gen	Psy	Gen
(N)	6,825	3,544	30	1,507	13	467	139	956	91	185	23	56	17	60
1. Total Nursing Staff (of Total Personnel) (sum of rows 2 and 3)	54	55	51	58	40	47	57	59	54	46	43	33	42	32
2. Professional (of Total Personnel)	22	23	13	27	12	23	5	22	8	18	8	15	8	14
3. Subprofessional (of Total Personnel)	32	32	38	31	28	24	52	37	46	28	35	18	34	18
4. Nonadministrative Professional (of Total Nursing Staff, row 1)	28	31	14	34	18	43	5	25	11	33	16	39	17	41
5. Differentiation of Subprofessional Nursing Personnel (Gini index, based on 4 categories)	.42	.43	.40	.43	.32	.55	.28	.42	.27	.52	.26	.27	.27	.28

207

general hospitals, i.e., the latter have a much higher level of professionalization. The differences vary further among different types of control. Voluntary hospitals have the highest proportion of nurses in all four types, while among the general hospitals the lowest proportion is found in the V.A. institutions.

Finally, teaching hospitals have a somewhat lower proportion of professional nurses in all categories, compared to their nonteaching counterparts, except for the state psychiatric teaching hospitals.

However, *within* hospital types, the difference between the size of the professional relative to the subprofessional components is itself variable. In addition, the proportion of professional nurses in administrative and supervisory positions is also variable; or to put it another way, the hierarchical structure of the nursing department is not constant.

One may take all these variable factors into account by calculating the percentage of professional nurses in nonadministrative positions as a proportion of the total nursing staff (Table 23, row 4). The results reveal not only the even more salient extent of professionalization of general hospitals as over against psychiatric hospitals, but they also bring into clear focus the advantage which teaching hospitals have in this respect as compared to nonteaching hospitals. Moreover, we can see now that *both* voluntary nonprofit (i.e., "autonomous") hospitals and the externally "controlled" V.A. hospitals have equally high levels of professionalization, as compared to the state and local governmental hospitals.

In general, then, our understanding of the functions of professional nursing is enhanced if we know what role subprofessional nursing personnel play in a given type of hospital. This category includes licensed practical nurses, aides, attendants, orderlies, and other subprofessional nursing personnel.

In Table 23, row 3, we can see how the relative size of the subprofessional nursing component varies among the different hospital types. Similar to professional nursing, the strongest effects are due to service and control. Psychiatric hospitals, of course, have a particularly large component of aides and attendants, with the nonteaching state mental hospitals ranking highest (52 per cent). This proportion decreases in the V.A. and the voluntary psychiatric hospitals, although the subprofessional nursing component remains the largest relative to the others. In addition, teaching constitutes a sizeable influence, with the exception of the V.A. hospitals.

In considering the joint distribution of the professional and subprofessional nursing components in different types of hospitals, we can assume that the number of professional nurses available determines the need for, or the limitations on, the number of subprofessional nursing personnel, especially since professional nurses can be considered a "scarce resource."

In other words, it may be argued that the proportion of aides and attendants would rise if psychiatric and general hospitals would recruit still fewer professional nurses. A structural consequence of this would be an increase in the *compositional homogeneity* and a corresponding decrease in the internal differentiation of the hospital.

As expected, the correlations between professional and subprofessional components are negative ($r = -.56$ for the 3,544 hospitals in all 12 groups). This inverse relationship is strongest among the voluntary and local governmental nonteaching hospitals ($r = -.65$), and weakest among the corresponding V.A. hospitals ($r = -.05$), suggesting crudely the relative extent of substitution of subprofessional for professional nursing personnel in these types of hospitals.

Substitution is, of course, only one of several ways of looking at the critical supply-demand situation with respect to professional nurses. The need for flexibility in the face of scarcity may also lead to a positive process of delegation of nursing functions to subprofessional nursing personnel and to the consequent differentiation of this group into levels and subspecialties. Alternatively, it is possible to have a large, relatively undifferentiated group of aides and attendants supervised by a few professional nurses.

Let us briefly look at the degree of differentiation of the subprofessional nursing group. Calculating the distribution of subprofessional nursing personnel among four categories [56] by means of the Gini coefficient of concentration [57] yields a measure of differentiation among nursing levels *below* that of staff nurse (Table 23, row 5). The closer the coefficient approximates 1.0, the more even is the distribution among the four categories and the greater therefore the degree of delegation; the smaller the coefficient, the greater the extent of supervision of many aides and attendants by a few nurses.

The evidence indicates that there is, in fact, a higher degree of differentiation among subprofessional categories of nursing personnel in general hospitals as compared to psychiatric ones. This tendency is even stronger among nonfederal general teaching hospitals. The data lend support to the interpretation that the extent of "downward" multilevel delegation of nursing functions is higher in general hospitals. By contrast, in psychiatric hospitals as well as in the V.A. system, professional nurses perform essentially supervisory functions with respect to a relatively large contingent of more or less undifferentiated subprofessional nursing personnel, such as aides and attendants.

In general, we can probably assume that both substitution and differential delegation are used in hospitals to alleviate the shortage of professional nurses.

Finally, the general negative effect of hospital size on professionalization ($r = -.43$ for all 12 groups) accentuates the differences between psychiatric and general hospitals and between teaching and nonteaching institutions in the expected direction. This simply means that it is relatively more difficult for larger hospitals to recruit and maintain an adequate professional nursing staff, particularly for large mental hospitals. But teaching hospitals, too, suffer from this trend, although the negative effect of size is partially offset by the fact that teaching hospitals offer a professionally more attractive environment to nurses in other respects. In other words, in addition to size, there are a host of more or less "hidden" (i.e., structurally less visible) factors such as quality, working conditions, work load, general atmosphere, etc. which determine the relative attractiveness to professional nurses of teaching general hospitals as well as small psychiatric hospitals.[58]

In sum, hospitals are strictly speaking not "professional" organizations, but rather "professionalized" to a certain degree. Insofar as graduate professional nurses coordinate the work processes of the hospital on the operational level, they do so not only as team-leaders and informal supervisors of practical nurses and aides, but most of all as professionally trained workers with an extraordinary degree of discretion and independent judgment.

Professionalization and Coordination

On the basis of the preceding analysis, it is argued that staff and head nurses engage in what March and Simon have called "coordination by feedback," i.e., communications aiming towards adaptation in contingency situations, in contrast to "coordination by plan," achieved through the scheduling of process-specialization and other forms of standardization.[59]

Given the pre-coordination of activities and the relative stability and predictability of the situation, March and Simon do "not expect any particularly close relation between the coordinative mechanisms and the formal organizational hierarchy."[60] While supervisory and administrative nurses can rely on a measure of formal authority in nonroutinized situations, the lower level professional nurse initiates and legitimates as well as processes information without the use of formal sanctions.[61] Thus, she provides coordination by feedback mainly on the basis of her professional status, i.e., on the basis of a considerable amount of discretion. It is significant that March and Simon note in the context of their discussion of the division of labor and coordination that "specialization and the structure of sub-programs is as much sociological as it is technological. The organization depends to a great extent upon the *training* that employees bring to it." [62] Furthermore, the professional nurse's crucial position in the network of communication and coordination increases her opportunity and capacity for the "absorption of un-certainty" which in turn has consequences for organizational decentralization of authority and the "influence structure of the organization." [63]

The important point here is that the staff nurse makes decisions on the basis of professional expertise which contribute to organizational coordination. On the level of the patient care unit, then, coordination by feedback is directly related to the availability of graduate professional nurses. [64]

Conclusions

In this chapter, I have analyzed the professionalization of hospitals in terms of two key groups: hospital administration and nursing service. The professionalization of hospital administrators indicates the degree to which those responsible for hospital-wide coordination of activities have a certain "generalist" expertise and orientation, independent of their functional specialties such as medical or nursing practice, or even business administration, for that matter. Professional hospital administrators are thus specialized "generalists." The importance of their overall coordinating function increases to the extent that hospitals change from doctor-centered institutions to multifunctional, diagnostic, and therapeutic service centers. While "medical administrators" still satisfy the principle of collegial authority and facilitate the absorption of organizational conflict on the level of roles and their individual incumbents, the professionalization of hospital administration indicates a movement toward greater rationalization of the control structure and of the processes of coordination in hospitals. This trend is particularly visible in teaching hospitals. But it stands to reason that teaching hospitals, in this as well as other respects, are pace-setters for the large spectrum of nonteaching hospitals of all types.

The professionalization of hospitals was further analyzed in terms of the key role of nursing services. Professional nursing practice is undergoing a remarkable process of differentiation, both horizontally and vertically. As a result, nurses do not only perform the traditional functions of giving bedside care and implementing medical decisions within various medical-nursing specialties. Nurses also assume the de facto responsibility for coordinating medical and para-medical activities on the operating level of the hospital, i.e., in the patient care unit. It is this aspect of the nurse's role which is characterized by a high level of discretion. Professional nurses thus contribute significantly to the process of coordination at the work level of the hospital.

I will now turn to an analysis of the relative complementarity between professional and bureaucratic modes of coordination. This will be done by considering two classical elements of bureaucracy as they appear in hospitals: nursing administration as the major bureaucratic-hierarchical structure in hospitals and the administrative-clerical staff at the disposal of the hospital administrator.

Notes

1. Everett C. Hughes, *Men and their Work*, (Glencoe, Ill.: The Free Press, 1958), pp. 78-87.
2. For an excellent analysis of the absence of authority and external coordination among the Fox Indians, see Walter B. Miller, "Two Concepts of Authority," in James D. Thompson et al., eds., *Comparative Studies in Administration* (Pittsburgh, Pa.: University of Pittsburgh Press, 1959), pp. 109-110. But we need not go to pre-industrial work activities to get an appropriate example. Modern work organizations, too, may involve built-in coordination of activities in situations of complex interaction, such as the one described by Temple Burling in *Essays on Human Aspects of Administration*, New York State School of Industrial and Labor Relations (Cornell University, Bulletin 25, August 1953), pp. 10-11, as quoted by Erving Goffman, *Behavior in Public Places* (New York: Free Press Paperback, 1963), pp. 90-91:

What is actually happening is that the changing needs of the patient, as they develop in the course of the operation, determine what everybody does. When a surgical team has worked long enough together to have developed true teamwork, each member has such a grasp of the total situation and of his role in it that the needs of the patient give unequivocal orders. A small artery is cut and begins to spurt. In a chain-of-command organization the surgeon would note this and say to the assistant, "Stop that bleeder." The assistant, in turn, would say to the surgical nurse, "Give me a hemostat," and thus, coordinated effort would be achieved. What actually happens is that the bleeder gives a simultaneous command to all three members of the team, all of whom have been watching the progress of the operation with equal attention. It says to the surgeon, "Get your hand out of the way until this is controlled." It says to the instrument nurse, "Get a hemostat ready," and it says to the assistant, "Clamp that off." This is the highest and most efficient type of cooperation known. It is so efficient that it looks simple and even primitive. It is possible only where every member of the team knows not only his own job thoroughly, but enough about the total job and that of each of the other members to see the relationship of what he does to everything else that goes on.

This illustration of internalized coordination is, of course, reminiscent of George Herbert Mead's famous description of social behavior as a game, based on each player's ability to take the roles of the other players and to organize them into a "generalized other." George H. Mead, *Mind, Self, and Society* (Chicago: University of Chicago Press, 1934), pp. 152-164.
3. See, e.g., Stanley H. Udy, Jr., *Organization of Work* (New Haven, Conn.: Human Relations Area File Press, 1959), pp. 36-41.
4. Arthur L. Stinchcombe, "Bureaucratic and Craft Administration of Production," *Administrative Science Quarterly,* 4 (1959), 168-187; Morris Janowitz, *The Professional Soldier* (Glencoe, Ill.: The Free Press, 1960), pp. 21-75.
5. See also Amitai Etzioni, *Modern Organizations* (Englewood Cliffs, N.J.: Prentice Hall, 1964), pp. 81-82.
6. Harvey L. Smith, "Two Lines of Authority: The Hospital's Dilemma," in E. Gartley Jaco, *Patients, Physicians, and Illness* (Glencoe, Ill.: The Free Press, 1958), pp. 468-477.
7. Alfred H. Stanton and Morris F. Schwartz, *The Mental Hospital* (New York: Basic Books, 1954); William Caudill, *The Psychiatric Hospital as a Small Society* (Cambridge, Mass.: Harvard University Press, 1958).
8. Jules Henry, "The Formal Structure of a Psychiatric Hospital," *Psychiatry,* 17 (1954), 139-151; Richard T. Viguers, "Who's on Top? Who Knows?" *The Modern Hospital,* 86 (1956), 51-54.
9. Joseph Ben-David, "The Professional Role of the Physician in Bureaucratized Medicine: A Study in Role Conflict," *Human Relations,* II (1958), 255-274; George Bugbee, "The Physician in the Hospital Organization," *New England Journal of Medicine,* CCLXI (1959), 896-901; see also his "Administration and the Professional in the Hospital," *Hospital Administration,* VI (1961), 26-33; Robert N. Wilson, "The Physician's Changing Hospital Role," *Human Organization,* XVIII (1959), 177-183;

Mary E. W. Goss, "Patterns of Bureaucracy Among Hospital Staff Physicians," in Freidson, pp. 170-194; Robert K. Merton, et al., eds., *The Student-Physician* (Cambridge, Mass.: Harvard University Press, 1957), pp. 71-79; Howard S. Becker et al., *Boys in White* (Chicago: University of Chicago Press, 1961), pp. 341-363; Amitai Etzioni, "Interpersonal and Structural Factors in the Study of Mental Hospitals," *Psychiatry*, XXIII (1960), 13-22; George Reader and Mary E. W. Goss, "Medical Sociology with Particular Reference to the Study of Hospitals," *Transactions of the IVth World Congress of Sociology* (London: International Sociological Association, 1959), II, 139-152; Rose L. Coser, "Authority and Decision-Making in a Hospital," *American Sociological Review*, XXIII (1958), 56-63; Eliot Freidson, "Client Control and Medical Practice," *American Journal of Sociology*, LXV (1960), 374-382; Mark Lefton et al., "Decision-Making in a Mental Hospital: Real, Perceived, and Ideal," *American Sociological Review*, XXIV (1959), 822-829; Amitai Etzioni, "Authority Structure and Organizational Effectiveness," *Administrative Science Quarterly*, IV (1959), 43-67.

10. Goss, "Patterns." Goss's concept of "advisory bureaucracy" or "semi-bureaucracy" contains elements of Gulick's "coordination by ideas" and Weber's "collegial authority" and "democratic administration"; see also Demerath's idea of a mixed collegial-bureaucratic administration or "collegialized management," in Nicholas J. Demerath et al., *Power, Presidents, and Professors* (New York: Basic Books, 1967), pp. 16-40, 215-238.

11. Louis Block, *Hospital Trends,* a publication of Hospital Topics (n. d.), pp. 178, 150, 120.

12. Ibid., p. 121.

13. See, e.g., Robert C. Hanson, "The Systemic Linkage Hypothesis and Role Consensus Patterns," *American Sociological Review*, XXVII (1962), 304-313; Robert W. Hawkes, "The Role of the Psychiatric Administrator," *Administrative Science Quarterly*, VI (1961), 89-107; Paul J. Gordon, "The Top Management Triangle in Voluntary Hospitals," *Journal of the Academy of Management*, IV (1961), 205-214; Charles Perrow, "The Analysis of Goals on Complex Organizations," *American Sociological Review*, XXVI (1961), 854-866; Harold L. Wilensky, "The Dynamics of Professionalism," *Hospital Administration*, VII (1962), 6-24; Edith M. Lentz, "Hospital Administration—One of a Species," *Administrative Science Quarterly*, I (1957), 444-463; Frederick L. Bates and Rodney F. White, "Differential Perceptions of Authority in Hospitals," *Journal of Health and Human Behavior*, II (1961), 262-267; Laura G. Jackson, *Hospital and Community* (New York: Macmillan, 1964).

14. Block, op. cit., p. 121.

15. Ibid., p. 150.

16. Ibid., p. 178.

17. The assistance of Carolyn Block in coding the biographical data is gratefully acknowledged.

18. See Ch. 5, note 30.

19. Everett C. Hughes, op. cit., p. 136, has contrasted this itinerant career pattern of professionals with that of the home-guard. A. W. Gouldner ascribes a cosmopolitan orientation to the itinerants, a local orientation to the home-guard, in his "Cosmopolitans and Locals," *Administrative Science Quarterly*, II (1957-58), 281-306, 444-480.

20. It should be noted here that 42 per cent of the administrators did not have more than three previous jobs, and 94 per cent did not have more than seven previous jobs.

21. Robert W. Habenstein and Edwin A. Christ, *Professionalizer, Traditionalizer, and Utilizer* (2nd ed.; Columbia: University of Missouri, 1963), p. 48; Everett C. Hughes, op. cit., p. 74; Hans O. Mauksch, "The Nurse: A Study in Role Perception" (unpublished Ph.D. dissertation, Department of Sociology, University of Chicago, 1960). On nursing as a profession, see Fred Davis, ed., *The Nursing Profession* (New York: Wiley, 1966).

22. Talcott Parsons, "The Professions and Social Structure," *Essays in Sociological Theory* (rev. ed.; New York: The Free Press of Glencoe, 1964), p. 38.

23. Ibid., pp. 41-44.

24. Max Weber, *The Theory of Social and Economic Organization*, Talcott Parsons, ed., (New York: Oxford University Press, 1947).

25. Habenstein and Christ, op. cit., pp. 45-47.

26. Leonard Reissman and John H. Rohrer, *Change and Dilemma in the Nursing Profession* (New York: Putnam, 1957), p. 170.

27. Ibid., p. 171.

28. William J. Goode, "Community Within a Community: The Professions," *American Sociological Review*, XXII (1957), 194-200.

29. Hughes, op. cit., pp. 78-87; see also his "Professions," Daedalus, XCII (1963), 655-668.

30. See also Esther L. Brown, *Nursing for the Future* (New York: Russell Sage, 1948), chs. 4 and 6; also her *Newer Demensions of Patient Care* (New York: Russell Sage, 1962), Part II, pp. 105-108.

31. Hughes, *Men*, p. 136.

32. Ibid.

33. Habenstein and Christ, op. cit., p. 48.

34. A. W. Gouldner, loc. cit.

35. Warren G. Bennis et al., "Reference Groups and Loyalties in the Out-Patient Department," *Administrative Science Quarterly*, II (1958), 481-500.

36. Peter H. Blau and W. Richard Scott, *Formal Organizations* (San Francisco: Chandler, 1962), p. 70.

37. Ibid., p. 71 (italics mine).

38. Bennis et al., op. cit., p. 497.

39. Hughes, *Men*, p. 136.

40. Ibid. (italics mine).

41. Habenstein and Christ, op. cit., pp. 49-52, 56-58.

42. Bennis, et al., op. cit., pp. 495-496.

43. On the importance of type of nursing education for professional,

bureaucratic, and service orientation among nurses, see Ronald G. Corwin, "The Professional Employee: A Study of Conflict in Nursing Roles," *American Journal of Sociology*, LXVI (1961), 604-615.

44. Robert K. Merton, *Social Theory and Social Structure* (rev. ed.; Glencoe, Ill.: The Free Press, 1957), p. 394.

45. Gouldner, op. cit., p. 293.

46. Ibid., pp. 292-294.

47. Louis C. Goldberg et al., "Local-Cosmopolitan: Unidimensional or Multidimensional?" *American Journal of Sociology*, 70 (1965), 704-710.

48. Habenstein and Christ, op. cit., pp. 111-114.

49. Ibid., p. 155.

50. U.S. Employment Service, *Job Descriptions and Organizational Analysis for Hospitals and Related Health Services* (Washington, D.C.: U.S. Government Printing Office, 1952), pp. 312-313.

51. Ibid., p. 326.

52. Hans O. Mauksch, "Nursing Dilemmas in the Organization of Patient Care," *Nursing Outlook*, V (1957), 31-33.

53. Mauksch, "The Nurse: A Study," pp. 130-150.

54. Ibid., p. 141.

55. See, e.g., Everett C. Hughes et al., *Twenty Thousand Nurses Tell Their Story* (Philadelphia: Lippincott, 1958). In addition to the works already cited, see particularly National League of Nursing Education, *A Study of the Nursing Service in Fifty Selected Hospitals* (New York: United Hospital Fund, 1937); Faye G. Abdellah and Eugene Levine, "Effect of Nurse Staffing on Satisfactions with Nursing Care," Hospital Monograph Series, No. 4 (Chicago: American Hospital Association, 1958). My own participant observation and analysis of certain aspects of nursing education and service in a large metropolitan voluntary general teaching hospital strongly support the conclusions arrived at in other similar studies; see, e.g., Wolf V. Heydebrand and Mary E. Keeney. "Institutional Factors in the Clinical Evaluation of Student Nurses," paper presented at the 38th Annual Institute of the Society for Social Research, University of Chicago, 1961; Wolf V. Heydebrand, "Some Observations Regarding the Problems of Teaching in Clinical Nursing," unpublished manuscript, 1961; and his "Criteria and Determinants in the Evaluation of Clinical Performance in Nursing: A Research Report" (Presbyterian St. Luke's Hospital School of Nursing, Chicago, 1961). (Mimeographed.)

56. Licensed practical nurses, aides and attendants, orderlies, and other sub-professional nursing personnel. Note, in this connection, also the fact that the differentiation of nursing functions has occurred, in part, as a result of the delegation of medical functions "downward" to professional nurses (see especially Chapter 6, Table 12), even though the proportion of professional nurses in the hospital labor force has been declining since 1935.

57. For the calculation of the Gini coeffecient of concentration, see the general description presented in Chapter 3 under the heading "Departmental Specialization."

58. See also George W. Albee, *Mental Health Manpower Trends* (New

York: Basic Books, 1959), pp. 160-180; Harry W. Martin and Ida H. Simpson, *Patterns of Psychiatric Nursing* (New York: American Nurses' Foundation, 1956); Richard L. Simpson, *Attendants in American Mental Hospitals* (Chapel Hill: Institute for Research in Social Science, University of North Carolina, 1961). National Commission on Community Health Services, *Health Manpower* (Washington, D. C.: Public Affairs Press, 1967), pp. 110-118. On measures of "negative effectiveness" such as job satisfaction and the related problem of turnover rates, see also Chris Argyris, *Diagnosing Human Relations in Organizations: A Case Study of a Hospital* (New Haven, Conn.: Yale University Press, 1956); and Everett C. Hughes et al., op. cit.

59. James G. March and Herbert A. Simon, *Organizations* (New York: Wiley, 1958), pp. 160-161.

60. Ibid.

61. Mauksch, "The Nurse: A Study", p. 142.

62. March and Simon, op. cit., p. 161.

63. Ibid., pp. 164-165.

64. Basil S. Georgopoulos and Floyd C. Mann, *The Community General Hospital* (New York: MacMillan, 1962), pp. 277, 282. Coordination by feedback includes an important subtype which Georgopoulos and Mann have called "corrective coordination." "Corrective coordination always takes place with reference to specific problems and after the problem has occurred." In view of the fact that their study of ten general nonteaching hospitals is organized around the concept of organizational coordination, it is unfortunate that Georgopoulos and Mann have not included this important type of coordination in their study. Following March and Simon in their distinction between the two major types of coordination, the authors assume that overall coordination is not likely to be effective unless it is rational and planned. Thus they state that the

> assumption that the system is well coordinated, until specific problems concerning the articulation of activities arise . . . easily leads to a patch-work kind of coordination rather than to more rational, more positive and more thorough and encompassing coordination plans.

Because of its character as corrective coordination and "because of its relatively high prevalence . . . this type of coordination is easier to grasp but more difficult to operationalize." Given the framework within which this particular study was conducted, this statement is probably correct. But it is not surprising that Georgopoulos and Mann found a relatively low correlation between their measures of coordination and the proportion of nursing staff members who are registered nurses. In particular, the rank order correlation between the proportion of registered nurses and the general, patient care centered type of coordination was lowest among the four measures of coordination used, while it was somewhat higher for the "programmed," "regulatory" (administrative) type of coordination.

Similarly, the rank order correlations between the proportion of nursing staff members who are registered nurses and an administrative-communicative type of coordination within the nursing department ("lack of difficulty in finding out what happened on the job since last at work") was moderately high, while it was not significant for the other types of coordination used. It should be noted also that hospital size was inversely related to the measures of coordination, although not on a significant level.

9   Bureaucratic and Professional Coordination

In this chapter, I shall show that bureaucratic and professional modes of coordination may coexist in the same organization rather than being alternative or mutually exclusive modes of administration and control. Being characteristic features of modern organizations, they interpenetrate in various ways.

One of the most obvious forms of interpenetration between bureaucratic and professional coordination is what I would like to call the "bureaucratization of professionals." Certain professional nurses, for example, become part of the bureaucratic-administrative hierarchy to the extent that they are formally vested with the authority delegated by the hospital administrator. The extent of delegation can be gauged by analyzing the bureaucratic-hierarchical structure of nursing administration in hospitals.

Insofar as nurses perform both professional-technical and bureaucratic-hierarchical functions, it is of considerable theoretical and practical interest to understand the extent of interrelation between these two structural elements.

The second type of relationship between professional and bureaucratic modes of coordination to be investigated here concerns their potential conflict on the organizational level, in contrast to the potential conflict between the bureaucratic and professional facets of a given role. In other words, I will be concerned here with the question as to what extent professionalization counteracts bureaucratic-hierarchical modes of coordination. Thus, I will show, first, that the coexistence of both modes is possible at certain levels, specifiable for each mode. Secondly, I will show that, independent of the fact of coexistence, both may be dynamically interrelated. For example, an increase of professionalization may lead to conflict with bureaucratic-hierarchical coordination, especially where the latter is elaborate and highly developed. Conversely, the negative relationship between both may be minimal if they coexist on a relatively low level, as measured by the relevant proportions for each hospital, or the mean proportions for each of the twelve hospital types.

Of course, bureaucratization does not exhaust itself in the building of chains of command and in the process of hierarchical delegation. Thus, a further aspect of internal bureaucratization to be investigated here concerns the relative size of the administrative-clerical staff in hospitals. Here, I intend to determine, first, the extent to which the relative size of the administrative-clerical staff has increased between 1935 and 1959. But in addition to this historical comparison, I shall demonstrate the relative stability of the effect which structural factors such as autonomy, task structure, and size have on internal bureaucratization. Finally, I intend to show that the relationship between the administrative-clerical staff and professionalization parallels that between hierarchy and professionals, but that it varies with the underlying structural conditions defined by task complexity and division of labor.

Bureaucratization of Professionals

In contrast to the "informal" assumption of administrative and coordinating functions on the part of graduate professional nurses, in general, nursing is also formally recognized as the executive arm of hospital administration.[1] The formal job description of the general nurse supervisor, for example, specifies that

> she directs and supervises nursing service of a group of patient care units . . . and coordinates services rendered by nursing personnel with those rendered by personnel of other departments. . . . In addition, she supervises . . . professional nursing and non-professional personnel of the unit. . . . The nursing supervisor is responsible for the *administrative* and *technical* supervision over the nursing program of the group. [2]

Similarly, the assistant director and director of nursing service "coordinates activities of various hospital departments, promoting and maintaining harmonious relationships among personnel supervised, medical staff [sic], patients, and others."[3]

These broad administrative responsibilities and the combination of administrative and technical functions in upper echelon nursing positions imply the kind of mixture of administrative and technical authority which Weber described as typical for legal-bureaucratic administration. Whereas staff and even head nurses lack the formal authority to coordinate the diverse services converging on the patient care unit, nurses in supervisory and administrative positions perform distinctly hierarchical coordinating functions, while remaining members of a "functional" department. However, the stress and strain frequently depicted as inherent to the role of the nurse as a consequence of "multiple subordination," lack of clear role definition, and conflict between professional and bureaucratic demands is not characteristic of formal administrative and supervisory nursing positions as much as it is of the positions of head and staff nurse. It is on these lower levels that coordination of the work process is required but not formally authorized, and therefore potentially stressful.

We have seen that, formally, professional nurses in administrative and supervisory positions have as subordinates both subprofessional nursing personnel as well as staff and head nurses. The total hierarchy may have as many as nine or ten levels, if we count assistant directors of nursing or assistant supervisors, etc. as separate levels. However, let us for the moment disregard the question of the number of hierarchical levels and assume that there is a distinct line of demarcation separating the levels of the head nurse and below from those of the supervisor and above. Combining all nursing positions of supervisory rank and above, regardless of level, and calculating this number as a proportion of the total nursing staff yields an administrative-supervisory ratio. This ratio or proportion is a rough measure of the average span of control insofar as the hierarchy in question is telescoped into two levels: subordinates and their superiors.

A comparison of the different hospital types shows that the administrative-supervisory ratio varies according to definite patterns: it tends to be somewhat higher in general hospitals as compared to psychiatric ones, and lower in teaching than in nonteaching ones. (Table 24, row 1).

Table 24
Mean Administrative-Supervisory Ratio Within Total Nursing Personnel and Within Professional Nursing Staff, and Correlation Between Hospital Size and Administrative-Supervisory Ratio (Professional)

	U.S. Hosp.	All 12 Groups	Voluntary				State and Local Governmental				Federal (V.A.)			
			Nonteaching		Teaching		Nonteaching		Teaching		Nonteaching		Teaching	
			Psy	Gen	Psy	Gen	Psy	Gen	Psy	Gen	Psy	Gen	Psy	Gen
(N)	6,825	3,544	30	1,507	13	467	139	956	91	185	23	56	17	60
1. Administrative-Supervisory Ratio (Total Nursing Staff)	.13	.11	.12	.12	.13	.06	.04	.12	.04	.07	.02	.06	.02	.03
2. Administrative-Supervisory Ratio (Professional Nursing)	.30	.27	.45	.27	.45	.13	.44	.33	.27	.18	.15	.13	.12	.10
3. Correlation Between Size and Administrative-Supervisory Ratio (Row 2)	-.34	-.29	-.12	-.39	.12	-.44	-.16	-.28	-.05	-.56	-.17	-.38	-.48	-.23

Voluntary hospitals are an exception to both patterns in addition to having the highest ratios as compared to state and local governmental and V.A. hospitals.

In interpreting these patterns, we can assume that the amount of external supervision and control increases with the number of supervisors per subordinates. However, before drawing any definite conclusions, it is necessary to consider two other factors which influence the administrative-supervisory ratio: the size of the hospital, and the number and width of hierarchical levels. The number of levels, moreover, tends to increase with size since a larger staff invites, if not requires, a greater degree of delegation of control to intermediate levels in the hierarchy of authority.

To take these factors into account, let us first examine the administrative-supervisory ratio *within* the professional nursing staff. Since the ratio of professional to subprofessional nursing personnel is highly variable, the question arises as to what extent administrative-supervisory positions are concentrated at the *upper levels* of the total nursing hierarchy, i.e., to what extent professional nursing is bureaucratized.

This refined administrative-supervisory ratio yields a somewhat different picture of the bureaucratic structure of nursing (Table 24, row 2). Since psychiatric hospitals have a comparatively small proportion of professional nurses, the extent to which nurses assume formally administrative-supervisory functions becomes doubly salient. In other words, the degree of bureaucratization of professionals is comparatively much higher in psychiatric than in general hospitals and tends to be higher in nonteaching as over against teaching hospitals. The degree of complexity of the hospital task structure can thus be shown to militate against the bureaucratization of nursing as the key department in hospitals, a department which typically provides the administrative line structure extending from the hospital administrator to the operating level, viz. the patient care unit.

Furthermore, the degree of external control does *not* foster the bureaucratization of professionals, contrary to what one might expect on the basis of stereotypes about governmental bureaucracies. The more "autonomous" voluntary hospitals tend to have the highest levels of bureaucratization, while the "externally controlled" V.A. hospitals have the lowest levels.[4]

The effect of size differences between hospital types underlines these patterns and tends to accentuate their importance. Increasing size tends to reduce the administrative-supervisory ratio within professional nursing, in general (Table 24, row 3). This negative effect of size on the bureaucratization of professionals is especially pronounced in general hospitals. In other words, increasing size facilitates delegation of authority to lower levels, especially where the complexity of the task structure is defined by multiple services.

As noted above, the use of the administrative-supervisory ratio as a measure of bureaucratization imposes a two-level hierarchical conception on a potentially multilevelled authority structure. Let us therefore look at a structural measure of delegation which takes into account the relative span of control at each of the levels of the hierarchy. In this way it becomes possible to look at the shape of the organizational pyramid as a whole.

Structural Aspects of Delegation of Authority

A discussion of delegation of bureaucratic authority in hospitals requires a brief consideration of two aspects of the notion of authority structure: decision-making and supervision.

When we are speaking of the authority structure of an organization, we may refer to a simple, two-level arrangement of super- and subordination, on the one hand, or to a multilevel structure involving as many as ten or twenty levels extending between the operational or work level and the top executive or the governing board. For either of these two extremes, i.e., two vs. twenty levels, it is assumed that the "lower" level or levels carry out the actual work functions, operations, and "production" activities, while the upper level or levels perform the functions of regulation, coordination, direction, and innovation. If the total spectrum of activities of an organization could be specified in terms of rules (i.e., in terms of specific means in relation to specific ends), one could say that lower-level activities are concerned with the application of *operative rules*, while each higher level *relative to a lower one* is concerned with the application of *regulative rules*. Moreover, a highly skilled or professional worker's activities are "self-regulated" in that he has internalized both operative and regulative rules while for an unskilled worker both types of rules must be externally specified and their application supervised. The single professional worker is what is known in social work and certain other work settings as a "director-worker" or a "self-supervising workman."[5]

A two-level hierarchy implies that regulative functions are being performed which are external to the work process. But we cannot yet easily separate supervision from goal-setting since both aspects tend to be involved at the "superordinate" level more or less

224

simultaneously. The supervisor-director has to supply operational goals to the worker, and at the same time control, supervise, facilitate, audit, or review their implementation, depending on the worker's degree of discretion. Besides, the work group may be heterogeneous in occupational composition and thus operate more like a team than a chain gang.

It is only when there are three or more levels in a hierarchy that different types of *regulative rules* become visible and "operational," and that the separation of supervision and goal-setting becomes pragmatically feasible and analytically meaningful. While supervision can, of course, be defined as a form of routine decision-making, it is the well-known distinction· between "critical" and "routine" decision-making, or between policy and administrative decisions, which becomes relevant here.

If an administrative-supervisory ratio is used to measure the degree of bureaucratization, it is difficult to interpret its meaning unless there is a clear indication whether span of control, and thus supervisory authority, is involved (or rather, centralization or decentralization of decision-making authority).[6]

If the two-level structure implied by a ratio involves a supervisory relationship, a small ratio may indicate a wide "average" span of control, i.e., many supervisors per workers, and thus "close supervision."

If, on the other hand, we conceptualize the two levels in terms of decision-making, a small ratio becomes an indicator of "concentration of power" while a large ratio implies decentralization and dispersion of authority. The result is frequently a confusion of meanings and a simplification and reduction of the notion of authority *structure* to "average span of control" or "decentralization."[7]

The concepts of delegation and decentralization of authority are often referred to by invoking the image of a flat organizational pyramid, while a centralized hierarchy is described in terms of a steep pyramid.[8]

This stereotypical image requires considerable empirical correction. In an attempt to transcend the conceptual limitations of the administrative-supervisory ratio as a measure of bureaucratization, I have developed a structural measure of hierarchical differentiation. This measure provides a single index of hierarchical structure, taking into account the number of levels and the relative size of each level. If the number of levels is fixed, it is still possible to describe the distribution of personnel among the levels so as to obtain an index of the degree of steepness and flatness of the organizational or departmental pyramid.

Let us assume that a given organizational pyramid has four levels. For example, in the professional nursing hierarchy in hospitals, the first of the four levels would be the top administrative and supervisory nursing personnel, i.e. 1) director of the nursing and assistant directors, if any. The second level would be 2) nursing supervisors. The third level would be represented by 3) head nurses, and lowest "operating" level by 4) staff nurses on the patient care units.[9]

The distribution of professional nurses among these four levels can be described much like the left and right halves of a population pyramid. But we can also transform this pyramid into a cumulative distribution or a J-curve by combining the two halves of the pyramid. This amounts to turning a positively skewed distribution with four class intervals from a horizontal to a vertical position, so that it would be skewed "downward". Such a downward skew would reflect the degree to which the lowest level is occupied by the largest number of personnel, while relatively fewer personnel would be located at the higher levels.

Let us assume, for example, that a given hospital has 1) two top echelon nursing administrators (the director of nursing and an assistant director), 2) three nursing supervisors, 3) three head-nurses, and 4) twenty-two staff nurses on patient-care units. Such a distribution would be heavily skewed to the right or downward, with a weighted mean of 3.5 (see Figure 2, position A).

By contrast, a pyramid with 1) one top administrator, 2) four supervisors, 3) twelve headnurses and 4) thirteen staff nurses would have a quite different shape. As a distribution, it would be less skewed, with a weighted mean of 3.2 (see figure 2, position B).

The assumptions underlying this reasoning are that the organizational hierarchies to be compared have a pyramidal shape, that the hierarchical levels are equidistant, that the degree of variation occurs within a certain limited range (i.e. that the skew is greater than zero and positive)[10], and that the number of hierarchical levels is constant.

Such a distributional measure can, of course, be applied to organizational hierarchies with a much larger number of levels, and there is no reason why it could not be adapted so as to take variable numbers of levels into account.

The indicator adopted for the purpose of measuring the hierarchical distribution of personnel among four organizational

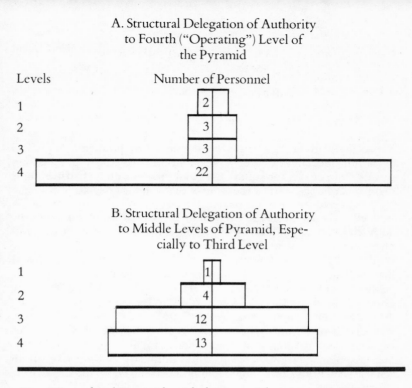

A. Structural Delegation of Authority to Fourth ("Operating") Level of the Pyramid

Levels   Number of Personnel

1   2
2   3
3   3
4   22

B. Structural Delegation of Authority to Middle Levels of Pyramid, Especially to Third Level

1   1
2   4
3   12
4   13

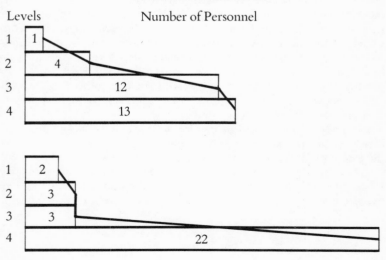

Two Hierarchical Pyramids with the Same Administrative-Supervisory Ratio (.20) but with Different Distributions of Personnel Among Four Hierarchical Levels

Levels   Number of Personnel

1   1
2   4
3   12
4   13

1   2
2   3
3   3
4   22

227

levels in hospitals is the measure of *relative skewness*

$$\text{Beta} \quad 1 = \frac{m_3^2}{m_2^3}$$

where m_2 and m_3 are the second and third moments (standard deviation and skewness) of a distribution involving four class intervals.[11] In effect, the squared skew of this four-class distribution is divided (standardized) by the cube of the standard deviation.

As expected, there is a considerable degree of variation among the twelve hospital types as to the extent of delegation of bureaucratic authority from the administrator downward to the level of the staff nurses on the patient care units.

While none of the hospital types have an inverted pyramidal structure, or even a perfectly diamond-shaped form, the shape of the pyramid varies from a "flat" extreme among the V.A. teaching general hospitals (B = + 3.99) to a relatively "steep" form among the state psychiatric teaching hospitals (B = + .91). In general, if the elaboration of formal positions and levels indicates anything about organizational arrangements for the exercise of delegated authority, then psychiatric hospitals delegate less authority to lower levels than general hospitals, and nonteaching hospitals less than teaching hospitals.

In other words, in the less complex hospital types the supervisory levels become larger relative to their subordinate levels, indicating not only a higher degree of bureaucratization of nurses, but also the fact that there is more delegation to the intermediate levels rather than to the operational (staff) level of the nursing hierarchy. Conversely, in the more complex general teaching hospitals, there tends to be maximum delegation to the operational level of the nursing hierarchy, with relatively fewer nursing supervisors and administrators staffing the upper levels of the hierarchy. Finally, it is again noteworthy that the federal V.A. hospitals rank highest on this structural measure of delegation.

In sum, the patterns of delegation follow closely those suggested above, where the administrative-supervisory ratio was used.[12] But the extent of delegation now becomes much more visible. In part this is so because the measure of relative skewness is much more sensitive to the variability of hierarchical structure than a ratio involving two hypothetical levels.

Table 25
Extent of Delegation of Bureaucratic Authority Among Four Levels of the Professional Nursing Hierarchy, As Measured by the Degree of Relative Skewness

		Voluntary				State and Local Governmental				Federal (V.A.)			
U.S. Hosp.	All 12 Groups	Nonteaching		Teaching		Nonteaching		Teaching		Nonteaching		Teaching	
		Psy	Gen	Psy	Gen	Psy	Gen	Psy	Gen	Psy	Gen	Psy	Gen
(N) 6,825	3,544	30	1,507	13	467	139	956	91	185	23	56	17	60
+2.02	+2.27	+1.12	+2.19	+1.56	+3.30	+1.64	+1.91	+.91	+2.56	+2.83	+3.00	+3.10	+3.99

More importantly, the measure can be seen as an empirical validation of the assumption that a low level of bureaucratization of professionals (a small administrative-supervisory ratio) implies the delegation of bureaucratic-administrative authority, i.e., the dispersion of hierarchical authority toward the operating level. Although the present data do not permit the distinction between supervisory and executive decision-making authority, the preceding analysis suggests that bureaucratic authority structures with several hierarchical levels facilitate downward delegation of authority, depending on the size of the hierarchical levels relative to each other. Thus, a "flat" multilevel hierarchy may, in fact, not only permit but require a high degree of discretion at the operating level. A highly bureaucratized professional staff, on the other hand, with relatively wide top hierarchical levels, suggests a high degree of hierarchical coordination. It can therefore be assumed that decentralization of decision-making tends to be closely related to a high degree of delegation of authority in a multilevel structure and conversely, that centralization associated with top-level bureaucratization manifests itself in a large administrative-supervisory ratio.

While the use of relative skewness of the distribution of personnel among hierarchical levels provides a *structural* measure of delegation of authority, to be validated by more refined measures on actual decision-making as it applies to hierarchical structures as a whole, there are still other problems of conceptualization and measurement which require our attention. One of them has to do with the fact that *activities* rather than whole hierarchies may be centralized or decentralized, as Leibenstein has suggested.[13] This idea implies that within the same hierarchy, some activities or work groups may be described as hierarchically undifferentiated, while others may have several levels among which authority is distributed. Furthermore, both may be more or less autonomous within the larger hierarchy.

The second problem concerns the possibility of multiple hierarchies, as distinguished from a single multidivisional or multidepartmental hierarchy. The present use of relative skewness as a measure of delegation generalizes from one functional unit, viz. nursing, to the organization as a whole. While nursing can, in fact, be treated as the administrative line structure of the hospital, it would be still more desirable methodologically to take into account *both* functional and hierarchical differentiation in organizations. Thus, a composite index made up of the centralization or delegation scores of all functional subunits, activities, or clusters of activities would constitute a more nearly adequate measure of organizational delegation, which could then be related to actual decision-making patterns.

After having demonstrated that both professional and bureaucratic modes of coordination do, in fact, *coexist* in the same organization, I will now turn to an analysis of their *interrelation*, and to the question of their potential conflict on the organizational level.

Hierarchical Coordination

Given the tendency for the more complex general and teaching hospitals to be more professionalized *and* to facilitate the downward delegation of bureaucratic-administrative authority, the question arises as to what extent these patterns support and condition each other. The nature of hospital work processes and the importance of nursing within them suggests that the greater the degree of professionalization, the greater the extent of delegation of authority so as to maximize the amount of discretion at the operating level. This expectation is, in fact, borne out by our data (Table 26). Regardless of whether we use, as a measure of bureaucratization, the administrative-supervisory ratio (row 1), or its conceptual opposite, viz. the extent of downward delegation across four levels in the nursing hierarchy (row 2), professionalization does in fact reduce the degree of bureaucratic-hierarchical coordination. This relationship, which is moderate to weak in some of the hospital types, becomes stronger and more uniformly negative when hospital size (average daily patient census) is controlled.[14] However, there are two types of exceptional patterns which require comment: the voluntary psychiatric hospitals and the four federal V.A. hospital types. Why does professionalization *not* constitute a strong antidote to bureaucratization in these hospital types? Conversely, why is the extent of delegation of bureaucratic authority only weakly or even negatively related to professionalization?

The answer lies not so much in the complexity of the task structure of these hospital types, but in the relative complexity of their internal division of labor, especially the differentiation of subunits. It will be remembered from the analysis in Chapter 7, Table 17, that both voluntary and V.A. psychiatric hospitals have comparatively high levels of departmental specialization. While I will demonstrate the actual effect of this internal structural complexity on the relation between professionalization and bureaucratization in the next chapter, we can here anticipate the argument by considering the implications of the "deviant" relationships in Table 26.

Table 26

Correlation Between Professionalization and Two Measures of Bureaucratization:
1) Bureaucratization of Professionals, and
2) Extent of Delegation of Bureaucratic Authority Among Four Levels

	U.S. Hosp.	All 12 Groups	Voluntary				State and Local Governmental				Federal (V.A.)			
			Nonteaching		Teaching		Nonteaching		Teaching		Nonteaching		Teaching	
			Psy	Gen	Psy	Gen	Psy	Gen	Psy	Gen	Psy	Gen	Psy	Gen
(N)	6,825	3,544	30	1,507	13	467	139	956	91	185	23	56	17	60
1. Bureaucratization of Professionals (Ratio)	-.32	-.30	-.03	-.38	-.45	-.24	-.40	-.36	-.35	-.23	-.01	-.03	-.17	-.21
2. Extent of Delegation of Authority (Relative Skewness)	.23	.22	.13	.26	-.34	.23	.23	.25	.32	.22	-.00	.04	-.04	.06

Administration and supervision within the professional nursing hierarchy is, as a rule, directed toward both professional *and* subprofessional personnel. But the smaller the proportion of sub-professional personnel and the greater the degree of functional specialization and differentiation of the total labor force, the more will nursing become a self-contained specialty among others. One consequence of this development is the fact that the administrative-supervisory ratio in nursing becomes smaller, and that supervision is not primarily directed toward the subprofessional nursing per-sonnel, but tends to be limited to professional nursing functions. At the same time, nonadministrative and nonsupervisory professional nurses assume the more informal responsibilities of team-leadership among an increasingly differentiated subprofessional nursing group. Supervision thus becomes "professional supervision." As a result, the conflict between professional and bureaucratic modes of coordination is reduced.

An increase in professionalization may actually be unrelated to the question of bureaucratization or delegation, as seems to be the case among the V.A. hospitals and the voluntary psychiatric non-teaching hospitals. Indeed, professionalization in the case of the small but internally very complex voluntary psychiatric teaching hospitals may lead to the simultaneous development of a professional hierarchy such that there is a large supervisory nursing staff but very little delegation as a result of professionalization. Here, professionalization appears to foster the concentration of professional nurses at the supervisory level. Furthermore, growth as indicated by a size increase also tends to lead to the bureaucratization of professionals in these relatively small hospitals, as Table 24, row 3, shows. This relationship appears to reflect the *increase in the number of separate administrative patient care units* for which additional supervisory nursing personnel must be hired.

There will be occasion to return to an analysis of the voluntary psychiatric teaching hospitals which, as a group, provide a methodologically important "negative case" for my general argument.

Let us now turn to an analysis of the other aspect of internal bureaucratization, namely the development and relative size of the administrative-clerical staff in hospitals.

Autonomy, Task Complexity, and Administration

According to the earlier theoretical discussion of the determinants of internal bureaucratization presented in Chapters 2 and 4, the administrative-clerical staff can be seen as an instrument of organization-wide communication and coordination at the disposal of the administrator-executive. The extent to which hospitals and other organizations make use of a specialized administrative staff raises two related questions: what are the historical and developmental factors which give rise to an administrative-clerical staff, and to what extent do both managerial considerations as well as the complexity of the task structure and the internal division of labor determine the relative size of this administrative apparatus. To study the developmental question properly, it would be necessary to investigate the emergence of administrative functions over time, i.e., from the point at which the organization is established. Some of the guiding assumptions for such an investigation would be that there are certain stages in organizational development which require different kinds and amounts of coordination, that increasing task complexity requires increasing bureaucratic-administrative control, and that an increase in size as such may contribute to economies of scale, thus reducing the relative magnitude of "administrative overhead."[15]

While the present data do not permit a diachronic analysis, it is possible to study the differences between two points in time for which comparable data exist, i.e., 1935 and 1959. It will also be possible to draw certain inferences as to the effect of structural factors on the relative size of the administrative-clerical staff in hospitals. Among these factors, I will give special consideration to ownership and control, certain aspects of the task structure such as the number and diversity of organizational objectives, and such factors as size, age, and internal division of labor.

Let us first turn to the historical comparison of the effect of certain structural factors on the administrative-clerical staff.

A Historical Comparison: 1935 and 1959

The 25 years of hospital growth and development after 1935 are generally characterized by an increase in numbers and in the average size of hospitals, a significant increase in the number of personnel per 100 beds, far-reaching advances in medical technology, and a decline in the relative proportion of medical and nursing personnel.[16] These changes reflect, on the whole, the growing internal complexity of hospitals, especially of general hospitals.[17]

The decline of the proportion of medical and nursing personnel parallels the growing diversity of occupational specialties which has come to dominate the hospital scene. While the relative weight and salience of medical and nursing personnel in the total spectrum of hospital occupations has decreased, these two groups gained in functional importance by virtue of a gradual shift from generalist to specialist definitions of the scope of their work role.

The growth of internal structural and technical complexity between 1935 and 1959 has led to a corresponding increase in specialized administrative functions, as measured by the proportion of business and clerical personnel. Let me single out three factors which have influenced the level and growth of this type of internal bureaucratization in hospitals: ownership and control, the complexity of the task structure, and organizational size.

External Control and Internal Bureaucratization. The administrative "response" to structural complexity is by no means automatic, as we can see from the fact that within all three service categories of general/special, TB, and psychiatric hospitals, there are systematic differences between the four types of hospital ownership and control (Table 27). Thus, while there has been a moderate increase between 1935 and 1959 in the relative size of the administrative-clerical staff in all three service categories, it is uniformly largest among the federal V.A. hospitals. Indeed, these hospitals are now far more bureaucratized than others. But this is as far as the familiar stereotype about public and governmental bureaucracies will go. In point of fact, the state and local governmental hospitals do not exhibit the same growth patterns as the federal governmental hospitals, nor do they reach a particularly high level of administrative specialization in 1959. The proprietary hospitals, on the other hand, have a comparatively large administrative-clerical staff, but have shown almost no increase in bureaucratization between 1935 and 1959.

The data presented in Table 27 reveal two remarkable tendencies in the bureaucratization of hospitals: first, a historical trend of slightly increasing bureaucratization, with ownership and control exercising a differential influence; second, a certain degree of structural stability in the effects of type of service, i.e., of the relative complexity of the task structure. Let us look at these structural effects in more detail.

Complexity of Task Structure and Bureaucratization. If we consider the data shown in Table 27 as representing different populations of hospitals, we may look at the various possible

Table 27

Change in Relative Size of Administrative-Clerical Staff: A Comparison of 1935 and 1959, by Type of Service and Ownership and Control

	Number of Hospitals		Average Size		Personnel/100 beds		% Personnel in Business and Clerical Positions	
	1935	1959	1935	1959	1935	1959	1935	1959
All Hospitals	5,836	6,490	177	241	45	120	6.8	8.2
General and Special	4,733	5,777	91	147	77	127	7.2	8.4
Federal (V.A. & P.H.S.)[a]	153	180	220	372	57	121	7.7	13.7
State and Local Govt'l.	569	1,234	181	170	64	125	6.4	7.5
Voluntary Nonprofit	2,469	3,428	101	153	89	135	7.0	8.1
Proprietary	1,542	935	30	49	59	100	9.4	9.6
Tuberculosis	506	272	140	235	45	76	6.0	6.3
Federal (V.A. & P.H.S.)	19	12	218	340	55	103	6.7	12.0
State and Local Govt'l.	299	222	173	247	46	75	5.5	5.8
Voluntary Nonprofit	119	32	95	135	43	79	7.2	7.3
Proprietary	69	6	51	108	37	52	9.2	9.1
Psychiatric	597	441	892	1,484	18	68	5.6	6.9
Federal (V.A. & P.H.S.)	27	43	979	1,538	35	68	7.4	11.6
State and Local Govt'l.	324	240	1,502	2,382	16	46	5.3	5.7
Voluntary Nonprofit	48	66	210	145	42	111	6.4	8.0
Proprietary	198	92	47	78	65	92	5.9	7.1

[a]Includes only Veterans' Administration and Public Health Service Hospitals, i.e., excludes military hospitals.

Source for 1935: Adapted from E. H. Pennel et al., "Business Census of Hospitals, 1935," *Public Health Reports* (Washington, D.C.: U. S. Government Printing Office, 1939), Supplement No. 154, p. 32, Table 26.

Source for 1959: Data from the present study, specially adapted for purposes of comparison, based on the 1959 Annual Survey of Hospitals by the American Hospital Association.

comparisons in terms of multiple replication. For example, the differences in the relative size of the administrative-clerical staff tend to be of the same order, whether we compare types of ownership within service categories, or the latter within the former, or both as between 1935 and 1959. Thus, general and special hospitals, i.e., those offering more than one major type of medical service, have a larger administrative-clerical staff than TB or psychiatric hospitals within each of the four types of ownership and control, both in 1935 and in 1959.[18]

The differences between TB and psychiatric hospitals are less clear-cut, but we may note that the increase in bureaucratization between 1935 and 1959 has been relatively larger among psychiatric hospitals than TB hospitals, a shift reflected also in the more than 300 per cent increase of the personnel/bed ratio.

If the multiplicity of services has a positive effect on the relative size of the administrative-clerical staff, this must be true also of other aspects of the task structure; for example, the *diversity* of objectives as measured by the distinction between teaching and nonteaching hospitals, medical education vs. nursing education, education vs. research, and various combinations of all of these. To illustrate the effect of these different types and degrees of task complexity on bureaucratization, let us look at a specific group of hospitals, namely state and local governmental hospitals in 1959.

The scale of increasing complexity—from the "unifunctional" psychiatric hospitals to variously diversified teaching general hospitals affiliated with medical and/or nursing schools—can have no more than face validity at this point. But even if we grant the unsystematic and highly selective character of this scale of complexity of the task structure, it is not difficult to see that the *greater the number of different structural elements* contained in a given organization, *the larger is the relative size of its administrative-clerical staff.* Clearly, structural diversity within the same organization generates administrative specialization.

Let us now turn to a consideration of organizational size as a factor in bureaucratization.

Effect of Size on Bureaucratization. In the comparisons considered up to this point, there is an unknown amount of influence of hospital size on the relative size of the administrative-clerical staff. Let us therefore look at the effect of task structure over time when size is controlled (Table 29).

The result of the historical and structural comparison within fixed size categories reveals, again, two opposite tendencies. First, Table

Table 28

Relative Size of Administrative-Clerical Staff by Degree of Complexity of Task Structure Among State and Local Governmental Hospitals (1959)

Degree of Complexity of Task Structure	Hospital Type	(N)	% Personnel in Business and Clerical Positions
Low One or Few Major Objectives	Psychiatric Tuberculosis	(240) (222)	5.7 5.8
Medium Many Major Objectives	General and Special	(1,234)	7.5
	General Only	(956)	7.6
Many and Diversified Objectives	General Teaching	(185)	7.9
High	[State General Teaching Only]		
Multiple Diversification (Affiliations)	With Nursing School	(8)	7.6
		(2)	8.3
	With Nursing and Medical School	(25)	9.6

29 shows that in each of the three service categories, the largest hospitals have experienced the greatest increase in bureaucratization, while there is a decline among the small hospitals. In other words, the larger the hospital, the greater the proportional increase in administrative-clerical functions between 1935 and 1959. This observation indicates that the largest hospitals have become disproportionately more complicated from the point of view of internal structure and administration, even though the advancement of medical technology during the same period has favored the smaller hospitals.[19] This suggests that one may interpret

Table 29

Change in Relative Size of Administrative-Clerical Staff, 1935 and 1959, by Type of Service and Size (# of Beds)

	# of Hospitals		% Personnel in Business and Clerical Positions	
	1935	1959	1935	1959
General and Special	4,733	5,777	7.2 [a]	8.4
Under 25 beds	1,282	423	9.6	9.4
25 to 49 beds	1,150	1,391	9.2	8.5
50 to 149 beds	1,540	2,246	7.2	8.0
150 and over	761	1,717	6.9	8.5
Tuberculosis	506	272	6.0	6.3
Under 50 beds	135	24	9.4	8.1
50 to 149 beds	231	117	6.5	5.9
150 and over	140	131	5.7	6.4
Psychiatric	597	441	5.6	6.9
Under 50 beds	144	48	8.4	7.4
50 to 499 beds	189	144	7.4	7.8
500 and over	284	249	5.3	6.3

Source for 1935: Adapted from Pennel et al., op. cit. (Table 27).

Source for 1959: Adapted from data for the present study.

[a] The percentage of the total payroll for administrative-clerical personnel in 1935 (i.e., the "administrative overhead") tends to follow a similar pattern in relation to type of service and size as the percentage of personnel (Pennel et al., op. cit., p. 34, Table 30).

the growing bureaucratization in terms of increasing departmentalization and, generally, increasing complexity of the division of labor, rather than just an increase in technological complexity.

The second conclusion to be derived from Table 29 concerns the changes in the effect of size on the *level* of bureaucratization. Within each service type, the level of bureaucratization is highest in the smaller hospitals. Moreover, bureaucratization tends to decrease with increasing size. However, this is true only for 1935. In 1959, the largest size categories show a slightly higher level of bureaucratization. The 1959 psychiatric hospitals deviate from this pattern in that the curvilinear relationship between administrative-clerical staff and size is inverted: bureaucratization increases with size, but only up to a point (about 500 beds). When mental hospitals become larger than that, there is a definite decline in the relative size of the administrative-clerical staff.

Of course, one must not overlook here the fact that ownership and control play an important role, both historically and structurally. This means, first, that the inverse relationship between administrative component and size applies mainly to the state mental hospitals rather than to the much smaller private psychiatric hospitals. Among all psychiatric hospitals, only the latter have become smaller on the average, while at the same time becoming more numerous, as Table 27 shows.

Secondly, the smaller, private psychiatric hospitals have become internally much more complex, compared to the large state institutions, as I have shown in Chapter 7. Therefore, we can see again that the administrative-clerical staff has grown as a result of *structural changes*, i.e., changes in the level of internal complexity which, in voluntary psychiatric hospitals, approximates that of nonteaching general hospitals. Internal complexity thus may help to articulate the complexity of the task structure, and both task structure and internal division of labor must be seen as powerful determinants of bureaucratization.

There is, however, a residual question as to the general tendency of bureaucratization to decline with size in middle-sized organizations, but to increase again slightly in very large organizations. Since the 1935 data do not permit a comparison beyond certain size categories, let us briefly look at the effect of size in four specific hospital types in 1959, with size categories broken down in greater detail. (Table 30).

The comparison between the state mental teaching and non-teaching hospitals shows the same tendency of declining bureaucratization with increasing size which we observed before. But now we can see that even in the state mental hospitals there is a slight upswing in the largest size category of 3,000 beds and over. Furthermore, while the difference between teaching and non-

Table 30
Mean Per Cent of Personnel in Business and Clerical Positions in State Psychiatric and Voluntary General Hospitals, by Teaching Status and Size

Size Number of beds	Nonteaching		Teaching	
		State Psychiatric Hospitals		
		(N)		(N)
Under 500	7.4	(11)	10.4	(16)
500 - 999	6.9	(12)	7.1	(3)
1,000 - 1,499	6.2	(27)	5.3	(9)
1,500 - 1,999	4.7	(22)	5.9	(6)
2,000 - 2,499	5.2	(18)	4.3	(7)
2,500 - 2,999	4.5	(15)	4.0	(11)
3,000 and over	4.7	(23)	4.9	(45)
		Voluntary General Hospitals		
Under 25	7.7	(152)	—	—
25 - 49	8.0	(435)	—	—
50 - 99	8.2	(535)	9.9	(44)
100 - 199	8.2	(333)	8.6	(112)
200 - 299	7.8	(49)	8.8	(142)
300 - 499	5.9	(6)	8.6	(127)
500 and over	—	—	8.6	(43)

teaching hospitals is pronounced in the smaller size categories, the level of bureaucratization tends to become similar in the very large institutions, regardless of teaching status.

The voluntary general hospitals, on the other hand, show an altogether different pattern for nonteaching as compared to teaching hospitals. While in the latter the level of bureaucratization declines slightly with increasing size but eventually levels off, the former exhibit a pattern similar to that observed for the small psychiatric hospitals (see Table 29); the relative size of the administrative-clerical staff increases with size, but then drops below the initial level with further size increases.

Given this pattern of variation in the level of bureaucratization among different size categories, I will now turn to an analysis of the overall relationship between bureaucratization and task complexity on the basis of the 1959 data, controlling for size and treating size as a continuous variable rather than in terms of discrete categories.

First of all, while the mean proportion of personnel in business and clerical positions is about 8 percent for all hospitals, as I have noted above, it varies from a low average of 5.6 percent in nonteaching state mental hospitals to a high of 17.6 percent in the V.A. nonteaching general hospitals (Table 31, row 1).

Taking into account this time the teaching-nonteaching distinction, these data show once again that there is a significant difference between the three types of ownership and control, with the federal V.A. hospitals contributing the largest share. Similarly, there is a significant difference in the expected direction between psychiatric and general hospitals. As shown above, the negative effect of size on bureaucratization is most pronounced among the psychiatric hospitals (Table 31, row 2). Finally, the difference between teaching and nonteaching hospitals is not significant unless size is controlled (Table 32, rows 1 and 2).

These findings strongly confirm those by Anderson and Warkov, whose study was based on 49 V.A. general and TB hospitals.

In fact, the present data provide a framework for multiple replication by virtue of the inclusion not only of two other types of ownership and control, but also of an additional type of "functional complexity" implied by the teaching/nonteaching comparisons, in addition to the ones between psychiatric and general hospitals.

The results of controlling for size in the analysis of covariance presented above imply (but do not demonstrate) the negative relationship between size and the relative size of the administrative-clerical staff.[20]

A closer examination of this relationship within each of our 12 hospital types reveals that the negative effect of size on bureaucratization is most pronounced among psychiatric hospitals.

Since we have seen already that the degree of departmentalization significantly decreases with size in psychiatric but not in general hospitals,[21] we can conclude that the level of internal structural complexity has an important intervening effect on the level of bureaucratization in hospitals.[22]

In sum, the following preliminary conclusions can be stated with respect to the variation in the relative size of the administrative-clerical staff in hospitals. First, the level of bureaucratization varies directly with the degree of complexity of the task structure such that general hospitals are more bureaucratized than psychiatric ones, and teaching hospitals more than nonteaching hospitals when size is controlled. The degree of bureaucratization tends to decrease with growing size, particularly in the "unifunctional" psychiatric hospitals. But even though such organizations tend to become structurally somewhat simpler as they grow larger, we can observe a slight upswing in the level of bureaucratization in the very large size categories. This indicates that the direct effect of size is most pronounced in very large as well as very small organizations, but mediated by a number of factors and thus more indirect in middle-sized organizations.

The effect of ownership and control on internal bureaucratization is exceedingly strong, particularly where type of control can be conceptualized in terms of "external bureaucratization," as in the V.A. hospitals. Since these hospitals are linked to a larger federal agency, the Veterans' Administration, by hierarchical as well as administrative-coordinative channels, one may well interpret their higher level of bureaucratization in terms of external control. For example, we know that the manager of a V.A. hospital is responsible to the chief medical director of the Veterans' Administration; that he is appointed by the administrator of the Veterans' Administration; and that personnel are appointed to their positions under the rules and regulations of the U.S. Civil Service Commission. It is likely that detailed annual reports have to be submitted; perhaps intermittent reports have to be written. The question remains whether these activities do, in fact, require a larger administrative staff, and whether quite similar activities are not also performed by other public and even by voluntary hospitals in relation to their governing boards.

Another consideration in explaining the large administrative component of V.A. hospitals is the fact that they have a special patient population which, though more homogeneous than that of other hospitals, requires nevertheless a more comprehensive, "total

Table 31

Relative Size of Administrative-Clerical Staff (Mean Per Cent of Personnel in Business and Clerical Positions) and Its Correlation with Size, by Service, Teaching Status, and Control

	U.S. Hosp.	All 12 Groups	Voluntary				State and Local Governmental				Federal (V.A.)			
			Nonteaching		Teaching		Nonteaching		Teaching		Nonteaching		Teaching	
			Psy	Gen	Psy	Gen	Psy	Gen	Psy	Gen	Psy	Gen	Psy	Gen
(N)	6,825	3,544	30	1,507	13	467	139	956	91	185	23	56	17	60
1. Relative Size of Administrative-Clerical Staff	8.3	8.2	8.4	8.1	7.6	8.8	5.6	7.6	5.6	7.9	12.3	17.6	11.2	16.8
2. Correlation Between Size and Administrative Staff	-.13	-.01	.05	.01	-.63	-.10	-.33	.00	-.66	-.24	-.27	-.14	-.18	-.08

Table 32
Effects of Control, Teaching Status, and Service on Relative Size of Administrative-Clerical
Staff: Alone, and with Size Controlled

| | Main Effects | | | Interactions | | | Second |
| | | | | First Order | | | |
	Control	Teaching	Service	Control X Teaching	Control X Service	Teaching X Service	Order
			F-Ratios[a]				
Dependent Variable:							
Relative Size of Administrative-Clerical Staff							
Alone:	469.19	3.48	167.22	4.64	15.69	2.61	.87
With Size Controlled:	464.24	19.78	59.28	5.38	12.62	6.61	.61
$df_1=$	2	1	1	2	2	1	2

[a] F-Ratios needed for significance at the .01 level:
4.60 ($df_1=2$), 6.64 ($df_1=1$); $df_2=3,532$ (for all effects).

245

institutional" form of care. Thus, during their already longer average stay, servicemen and veterans receive many legal, occupational, and welfare services which, in turn, require the maintenance of files and frequent communication with outside agencies.

Finally, one must not overlook the fact that even though V.A. hospitals are probably more uniform and standardized than local governmental or voluntary hospitals, they are therefore not necessarily less complex, or overbureaucratized. In other words, planning and centralized administration need not find expression only in a larger administrative component. On the contrary, pre-coordinated activities may require less administrative and clerical personnel. At the same time, planning and pre-coordination may imply a higher degree of division of labor and functional specialization such that functions are more rationally subdivided and personnel more efficiently allocated. We will explore this question more fully later on, but we may note here that the V.A. hospitals are not only more "bureaucratized" than the other types, but they are also among the most complex technologically and organizationally, as well as comparable in quality to the best nongovernmental hospitals.

Let us now turn to a brief consideration of the effect of professionalization on the relative size of the administrative-clerical staff, parallel to the earlier discussion of the effect of professionalization on the hierarchical authority structure and on the extent of delegation of authority.

Professionalization and the Administrative-Clerical Staff

According to the hypothesis that professionalization of the labor force constitutes an alternative to bureaucratic modes of coordination and administration, one should find the relative size of the administrative-clerical staff to be inversely related to professionalization. This relationship should parallel the inverse correlation between professionalization and the administrative-supervisory ratio in nursing discussed earlier in this chapter. Moreover, the two measures of internal bureaucratization, i.e., the administrative-supervisory ratio and the relative size of the administrative-clerical staff, should be positively related.

Generally, the simple correlation data do not indicate a particularly strong or consistent relationship between professionalization and the relative size of the administrative-clerical staff, nor between the latter and the administrative-supervisory ratio (Table 33).

We may note a moderate positive relationship between professionalization and the relative size of the administrative-clerical staff in the state and local governmental as well as the voluntary psychiatric teaching hospitals, and in the V.A. psychiatric nonteaching hospitals. There is, furthermore, a moderate inverse relationship between the relative size of the administrative-clerical staff and the administrative-supervisory ratio in the voluntary psychiatric teaching hospitals. On the whole, however, the zero-order correlations do not and perhaps cannot be expected to tell us very much, for the following reasons.

From our previous analysis of professionalization, we know that an increase in professional nurses has the effect of reducing both the subprofessional nursing component as well as the administrative-supervisory ratio. Therefore, the effect of these two variables must be taken into account if we want to gauge the relative contribution of professionalization to administrative-clerical functions in hospitals. Similarly, size needs to be controlled since we know of its overall negative effect on the relative size of the administrative-clerical staff. [23]

The analysis of the effect of professionalization on the relative size of the administrative-clerical staff, controlling for these other variables, shows that effect to be generally negative, and much stronger than that observed in the simple correlations (Table 34).

We can conclude from this analysis that an increase in the proportion of professional nurses contributes to a decrease in the administrative-clerical component, holding constant not only size but also the subprofessional nursing component and the administrative-supervisory ratio. Thus, moderate support can be claimed for the hypothesis that a professionalized labor force provides an alternative to bureaucratic modes of administration. In the case of the administrative-clerical staff in hospitals, we can probably assume a certain extent of mutual causation. In other words, professional nurses will take over administrative-clerical functions and thus reduce the need to hire additional clerical personnel in situations where task complexity and internal differentiation would require it. Conversely, policies of employing an adequate administrative-clerical staff may forestall the use of valuable nursing manpower for the performance of administrative and clerical tasks. There is much evidence from this and other

Table 33
Correlations Between Relative Size of Administrative-Clerical Staff and 1) Professionalization (% Graduate Professional Nurses) and 2) Administrative-Supervisory Ratio in Nursing, by Service, Teaching Status, and Control

	U.S. Hosp.	All 12 Groups	Voluntary				State and Local Governmental				Federal (V.A.)			
			Nonteaching		Teaching		Nonteaching		Teaching		Nonteaching		Teaching	
			Psy	Gen	Psy	Gen	Psy	Gen	Psy	Gen	Psy	Gen	Psy	Gen
(N)	6,825	3,544	30	1,507	13	467	139	956	91	185	23	56	17	60
1. Administrative Staff and Professionalization	.06	.03	.02	-.09	.37	-.01	.01	.01	.38	.07	.50	-.13	-.14	-.03
2. Administrative Staff and Administrative-Supervisory Ratio	-.32	-.30	-.03	-.38	-.45	-.24	-.40	-.36	-.35	-.23	-.01	-.03	-.17	-.21

248

hospital studies that the diffuse, generalist employment of nurses tends to prevail in community general hospitals and in the large state mental hospitals. In V.A. hospitals, on the other hand, the proportion of professional nurses is generally much smaller than in the other types, but, due to a large administrative-clerical staff, it is conceivable that professional nurses may devote more time to nursing-specific functions.[24]

An interesting additional finding emerges from the generally negative effect of the sub-professional component on the relative size of the administrative-clerical staff (Table 34, row 3). Thus, one may interpret the subprofessional nursing component in terms opposite those of functional and departmental specialization, i.e., in terms of the relative absence of internal differentiation and complexity. If this is valid, then an increase in subprofessional nursing personnel indicates growing *compositional homogeneity* of the hospital labor force. Such an increase should, therefore, entail a decline in the relative size of the administrative-clerical staff.

It will be noted that this interpretation of the subprofessional nursing component as a measure of compositional homogeneity provides a test of one part of the Anderson-Warkov hypothesis that "the relative size of the administrative component decreases as the number of *persons performing identical tasks* in the same place increases."[25] I have already shown that the administrative component increases with the degree of complexity of the task structure which is, of course, Anderson and Warkov's complementary hypothesis. [26] The phrase "persons performing identical tasks" refers originally to low task complexity (viz. TB hospitals). Assuming that aides and attendants, etc., perform "identical tasks," one may use their proportion here as a direct measure of compositional homogeneity, or "low internal complexity" although the Gini coefficient of concentration or the proportion of specialized functions are more adequate measures of internal complexity.

But a focus on homogeneity would also, in part, explain the inverse variation between size and the administrative component (Table 34, row 4). This inverse relationship implies that the administrative component decreases as the compositional homogeneity of the organization increases. If the homogeneity is produced by increasing organizational size, or by structural and compositional changes in the labor force, the result will tend to be similar: to simplify the internal structure and to facilitate coordination and relieve the hospital of certain administrative-clerical tasks. Fur-

Table 34

Influence of Professionalization on Administrative-Clerical Staff: Partial Regression Coefficients (b*), Regression Errors, and Squared Multiple Correlation Coefficients (R^2), for Relative Size of Administrative-Clerical Staff (Dependent Variable) and Professionalization, Administrative-Supervisory Ratio, Sub-Professional Component, and Size (Independent Variables), by Service, Teaching Status, and Control

	U.S. Hosp.	All 12 Groups	Voluntary				State and Local Governmental				Federal (V.A.)			
			Nonteaching		Teaching		Nonteaching		Teaching		Nonteaching		Teaching	
			Psy	Gen	Psy	Gen	Psy	Gen	Psy	Gen	Psy	Gen	Psy	Gen
(N)	6,825	3,544	30	1,507	13	467	139	956	91	185	23	56	17	60
1. Professionalization	-.17ª (.02)	-.36ª (.02)	-.14 (.20)	-.32ª (.03)	.15 (.32)	-.14ª (.05)	-.22ª (.09)	-.12ª (.04)	-.16 (.11)	-.11 (.09)	.26 (.22)	-.12 (.13)	-.38 (.35)	.10 (.15)
2. Administrative-Supervisory Ratio	-.04 (.01)	-.07 (.02)	.08 (.18)	-.06 (.03)	-.29 (.27)	-.03 (.05)	-.12 (.09)	.04 (.04)	.00 (.00)	-.08 (.10)	-.14 (.19)	.09 (.14)	-.47 (.32)	.28 (.14)
3. Subprofessional component	-.31ª (.01)	-.50ª (.02)	-.39 (.20)	-.34ª (.03)	.31 (.27)	-.24ª (.05)	-.35ª (.08)	-.23ª (.04)	-.38ª (.13)	-.17ª (.08)	-.48ª (.24)	-.51ª (.15)	.34 (.29)	-.36ª (.16)
4. Size	-.21 (.01)	-.21 (.02)	.00 (.00)	-.07 (.03)	-.57 (.26)	-.22 (.06)	-.36 (.08)	-.02 (.03)	-.47 (.12)	-.33 (.10)	.05 (.22)	.13 (.15)	-.71 (.36)	.22 (.18)
Multiple R^2	.09	.16	.13	.07	.55	.05	.25	.03	.49	.08	.41	.27	.31	.12

[a] A regression coefficient, in order to be considered statistically significant, should be at least twice its error. The regression error is given in parentheses underneath each coefficient.

250

thermore, such tasks are probably also performed by sub-professional nursing personnel, especially in the large mental hospitals.

Summary and Conclusions

In this chapter I have described hospitals in terms of various measures of internal bureaucratization, and I have shown that professionalization serves to counteract, though not to displace, bureaucratic modes of coordination.

Bureaucratization exists in hospitals in at least two forms: as a combination of goal-setting and supervisory authority as well as downward delegation of that authority through the levels of a hierarchical structure, and as a specialized administrative-clerical staff geared toward organization-wide coordination. To the extent that the administrative-supervisory ratio in nursing serves as an indicator of the external enforcement of operative rules, it competes with the internalized application of operative rules, i.e., with the self-regulation and discretion of a professionalized labor force. The complexity of the task structure facilitates downward delegation of authority and maximizes professional discretion at the operating level. Therefore we may conclude that bureaucratic and professional modes of coordination coexist in hospitals, each mode at a particular level within a particular type of task structure. But in their dynamic interrelation within a given hospital type, certain elements of competition or structural conflict may be observed. Professionalization tends to reduce the administrative-supervisory ratio, and to facilitate the downward delegation of bureaucratic authority, as measured by the relative skewness of the distribution of professional nurses among four hierarchical levels.

The historical comparison of hospital structure shows a slight increase in the relative size of the administrative-clerical staff between 1935 and 1959. Yet there is a remarkable structural stability insofar as external control, task structure and size generally retain the strength and nature of their influence on administrative specialization. V.A. hospitals, in particular, have developed a relatively large administrative apparatus due to external bureaucratization and control, internal complexity, and the special requirements of their patient population. But in addition to external control, the complexity of the task structure is one of the most powerful determinants of the relative size of the administrative-clerical staff. Thus, general teaching hospitals with multiple diversification such as nursing school affiliation and medical research (university and medical school affiliation) rank highest in administrative specialization because they have the largest number of different structural elements which need to be coordinated. State psychiatric nonteaching hospitals, on the other hand, are "unifunctional" organizations, at least from this comparative perspective. Even though they may be large and have many subunits, such subunits tend to be structurally similar so that growth in size leads to an increase in structural and compositional homogeneity. In these hospital types, therefore, the relative size of the administrative-clerical staff remains small and tends to decrease with growing size, with the exception of the very large size categories, where a slight increase in administrative specialization can be observed.

The voluntary psychiatric hospitals, finally, illustrate that "low task complexity" may be accompanied by a relatively high degree of internal structural complexity. It is here that the level of bureaucratization is not only comparatively high but tends to increase with professionalization and the subprofessional component, although these relationships are below the level of statistical significance.

In general, both professionalization and the sub-professional nursing component tend to have the effect of reducing the relative size of the administrative-clerical staff, but for opposite reasons. Professionalization contributes to organizational coordination at the operational level, and thus removes or bypasses some of the complexities of work organization emerging from an increasing internal division of labor. As a result, it is possible to keep the administrative overhead relatively lower than would otherwise be possible. The subprofessional component, on the other hand, has a negative effect on administrative specialization because it serves to increase the compositional homogeneity of the organizational labor force, and thus causes hospitals to become structurally simpler. Although structural and compositional homogeneity do not represent the conceptual opposite of departmental and functional specialization, an increase in homogeneity nevertheless has the effect of requiring less administrative-clerical coordination.

It cannot be decisively argued here to what extent this reduction in bureaucratization is due to managerial choice based on economic or "internal" political considerations. However, in addition to the obvious influence of ownership and control, task complexity and internal structure do exercise a considerable influence on administrative specialization which cannot be easily explained by managerial discretion alone.

The influence of internal structural complexity, especially of departmental specialization, has up to this point been largely inferred from the previous analysis of division of labor rather than analyzed directly. I shall therefore, in the following chapter, continue the analysis of bureaucratic modes of coordination by simultaneously taking into account the two major intervening factors: professionalization and departmental specialization. In the context of that analysis, both of these variables will be interpreted as nonbureaucratic modes of coordination, in contrast to the bureaucratic ones of the administrative-supervisory ratio and the relative size of the administrative-clerical staff.

Notes

1. See, e.g., Virginia H. Walker, *Nursing and Ritualistic Practice* (New York: Macmillan, 1967), pp. 101-168; Herman Finer, *Administration and the Nursing Services* (New York: Macmillan, 1952), pp. 3-24; Malcolm McEachern, *Hospital Organization and Management* (Chicago: Physicians' Record Co., 1957), Ch. 9.
2. U.S. Employment Service, *Job Descriptions and Organizational Analysis for Hospitals and Related Health Services* (Washington, D. C.).
3. Ibid., pp. 304, 308.
4. All these differences are statistically significant in an analysis of variance. The F-Ratio for the administrative-supervisory ratio in professional nursing is $F = 236.04$ for the difference between teaching and non-teaching hospitals, $F = 86.62$ for the differences among types of ownership and control, and $F = 62.60$ for the difference between psychiatric and general hospitals.
5. For an excellent description of the "composite work role" and other aspects of an incipient socio-technical system, see Eric L. Trist et al., *Organizational Choice* (London: Tavistock, 1963), pp. 32-33; for an implicit distinction between operative and regulative rules see A. W. Gouldner, *Patterns of Industrial Bureaucracy* (Glencoe, Ill.: Free Press, 1954), p. 163.
6. Ratios or proportions of personnel in administrative, managerial, supervisory, or clerical positions, or the A/P ratio involving administrative and other salaried employees vs. production workers, have been used as direct measures of centralization. See Reinhard Bendix, *Work and Authority in Industry* (New York: Harper Torchbooks, 1963), p. 216; see also the discussion of the "MPO ratio" (managers, professionals, and officials) in Amos Hawley's "Community Power and Urban Renewal Success," *American Journal of Sociology*, 68 (1963), 424; also Arthur Stinchcombe, "Bureaucratic and Craft Administration of Production," *Administrative Science Quarterly*, 4 (1959), 184. Stinchcombe, however, distinguishes between goal-setting and supervision. In general, one can probably state that bureaucratization need not imply centralization. If an

organization is bureaucratized in that it has many hierarchical levels, it may, in fact, be decentralized in that decision-making authority tends to be delegated to lower levels.

7. Political scientists and political sociologists who think about organizations and societies in terms of such concepts as "elites and masses," elites vs. nonelites or "lower participants," ruling class, or power structure, often find themselves in the dilemma of imposing a simplistic, two-level conception of power on a more or less complex structure. The problem is aggravated if an organization or society has, in fact, twofold or multiple hierarchies rather than just one, i.e., if it is both horizontally and vertically differentiated into more than two levels and two semi-autonomous subunits. See, for example, Harold Lasswell, *Politics* (New York: Meridian Books, 1958), p. 13; C. Wright Mills, *The Power Elite* (New York: Oxford University Press, 1956); William Kornhauser, *The Politics of Mass Society* (New York: The Free Press, 1959); Amitai Etzioni, *A Comparative Analysis of Complex Organizations* (New York: The Free Press, 1961), pp. 3-22; Amos Hawley, loc. cit.; Dorwin Cartwright, "Influence, Leadership, Control," in James G. March, ed., *Handbook of Organizations* (Chicago: Rand McNally, 1965), pp. 1-47. A significant correction of this "ratio" concept of power structure is its definition as a system of delegated (legitimate) powers, or the definition of power in terms of "chains of contingent activities"; see Arthur L. Stinchcombe, *Constructing Social Theories* (New York: Harcourt, Brace, and World, 1968), pp. 151-155; see also William H. Starbuck, "Mathematics and Organization Theory," in March, op. cit., pp. 373-382; and James S. Coleman, *Introduction to Mathematical Sociology* (New York: The Free Press, 1964), pp. 430-468. For hospitals, the complicated nature of their authority structure has long been recognized; see, e.g., Harvey L. Smith, "Two Lines of Authority," in E. Gartley Jaco, ed. *Patients, Physicians, and Illness* (Glencoe, Ill.: The Free Press, 1958), pp. 468-478; Hans O. Mauksch, "The Organizational Context of Nursing Practice," in Fred Davis, ed., *The Nursing Profession* (New York: Wiley, 1965), pp. 109-137; Walker, op. cit., pp. 154-160; and Gerald D. Bell, "Determinants of Span of Control," *American Journal of Sociology*, 73 (1967), 100-109.

8. Peter Blau and W. Richard Scott, *Formal Organizations* (San Francisco: Chandler, 1962), pp. 168-169.

9. I am following here the work classification of professional nurses suggested by Habenstein and Christ's study; see Robert W. Habenstein and Edwin A. Christ, *Professionalizer, Traditionalizer, Utilizer* 2nd. ed. (Columbia: University of Missouri, 1963), pp. 115-120.—A similar measure was constructed for the medical-nursing hierarchy (the "clinical" hierarchy) in teaching hospitals, with the upper two levels represented by medical residents and interns, rather than nursing administrators. I have not discussed this measure further in the present context since it is applicable in its current form only to teaching hospitals. But it should be noted that Patricia Kendall devised a corresponding index to measure the structural-hierarchical characteristics of residency programs in teaching hospitals,

identifying three types of hierarchical "shapes": pyramid, semi-pyramid, and parallelogram. The pyramidal shape represents the centralized end of the continuum, engendering competitiveness among residents, whereas the parallelogram implies decentralization and leads to cooperativeness; cf. Patricia Kendall, "The Learning Environments of Hospitals", in Eliot Freidson, ed. *The Hospital in Modern Society* (New York: Free Press, 1963), pp. 213-215.

10. A symmetric distributic would have a skewness of zero and would correspond to a diamond-shaped organizational hierarchy, indicating a relatively wide expansion of the middle levels of the organization. A negative skewness would indicate the case where there is more personnel at the upper than at the lower levels, a situation sometimes observable in academic departments and, generally, in professional organizations.

11. The computation follows the procedures given in Frederick E. Croxton and Dudley J. Cowden, *Applied General Statistics*, 2nd ed. (Englewood Cliffs: Prentice Hall, 1955), pp. 229-232.—A more direct measure of the hierarchical pyramid in terms of the properties of the normal curve would be one involving the fourth moment, as Paul Lazarsfeld has suggested to me in personal communication. The fourth moment measures the degree of kurtosis of a distribution, e.g. whether it is leptokurtic (steep) or platikurtic (flat) and could therefore be directly adapted to measure the shape of the organizational pyramid.

12. Although the language of centralization and decentralization tends to oversimplify hierarchical phenomena, it suggests it self especially where managerial ratios or data on actual decision-making are used. Thus, the above generalization that delegation of authority is associated with decentralization of decision-making was applied in a study of 150 public personnel agencies (civil service commissions), where a small managerial ratio was interpreted as implying centralization of decision-making, a large ratio decentralization. Peter M. Blau, et. al., "The Structure of Small Bureaucracies," *American Sociological Review*, 31 (1966), 182-185. One of the projects of the Comparative Organization Research Program, a study of some 250 state and local finance departments, made it possible to show that decentralization of decision-making is moderately associated with an increase in the number of hierarchical levels, although the findings still apply only to selected levels (e.g., first line supervisor, middle managers, division head) rather than to the whole hierarchical structure. For detailed reports on this project, see Peter M. Blau, "The Hierarchy of Authority in Organizations," *American Journal of Sociology*, 73 (1968), 457-465, and Marshall W. Meyer, "Two Authority Structures of Bureaucratic Organization," *Administrative Science Quarterly*, 13 (1968), 211-228; see also Wolf V. Heydebrand, "The Study of Organizations," *Social Science Information*, 6 (1967), 72-74.

13. Harvey Leibenstein, *Economic Theory and Organizational Analysis* (New York: Harper, 1960), pp. 256-262.

14. The correlations in row 2 of Table 26 are generally positive since relative skewness measures delegation.

15. Ernest Dale, *Planning and Developing the Company Organization Structure* (New York: American Management Association, 1952), pp. 21-119; Mason Haire, "Biological Models and Empirical Histories of the Growth of Organizations," in Mason Haire, ed., *Modern Organization Theory* (New York: Wiley, 1959), pp. 272-306; William H. Starbuck, "Organizational Growth and Development," in March, op. cit., pp. 451-533; Theodore Anderson and Seymour Warkov, "Organizational Size and Functional Complexity," *American Sociological Review*, 26 (1961), 23-28; Louis R. Pondy, "A Discretionary Model of Administrative Intensity," *Administrative Science Quarterly*, March, 1969. Pondy provides a strong argument for an interpretation of "administrative intensity" in terms of the marginal costs and benefits which derive from regulation and coordination. This interpretation is tied to a broader theoretical framework which tends to favor the element of discretion and managerial choice in regulation and coordination, in contrast to a focus on the technological and task determinants of coordination. In my own analysis, the variation of the relative size of the administrative-clerical staff by ownership and control indicates that managerial policies constitute, indeed, a significant influence, a conclusion which halfway meets Pondy's argument for a greater share of managerial determinism on political-administrative, if not on economic, grounds. However, the complexity of the task structure does have a strong influence on internal structure and coordination, as I have shown, and must therefore be given considerable weight in an explanation of administrative specialization and other forms of bureaucratization. Furthermore, there is some evidence from the data on teaching hospitals that hospital age has a slight negative effect on the relative size of the administrative-clerical staff (r = -.15), suggesting the influence of extra-managerial, structural factors on the growth pattern of the administrative staff.

16. See Chapter 6, Table 12 and Chapter 8, note 56.

17. Note that among TB and mental hospitals, the increase in size has occurred at the expense of a decrease in numbers, i.e., of growing concentration; see Table 27.

18. The one exception here, voluntary TB hospitals in 1935, does not, in my judgment, constitute a significant enough deviation from the general pattern so as to require special explanation.

19. See Chapter 6, Table 13.

20. It will be noted that in our data it was not necessary to control for size in order to support the Anderson-Warkov hypothesis, since the less complex psychiatric hospitals are, as a rule, larger than the more complex general hospitals. When size is controlled, the difference between psychiatric and general hospitals (service effect) remains highly significant (Table 32, row 2). But now the control of size has the effect on the teaching/nonteaching difference which Anderson and Warkov found in relation to the difference between TB and general hospitals. With size controlled, the teaching hospitals have a larger administrative component than the nonteaching hospitals. The influence of type of control is not significantly affected by holding size constant, i.e., the differences between voluntary, state and local

governmental, and V.A. hospitals remain significant.

21. See Chapter 7, Table 18, row 2.

22. Solely for reasons of simplifying the presentation and discussion of the results as much as is possible under the circumstances, I want to deal with the effect of departmentalization on bureaucratization in the next chapter.

23. It should be noted here that any curvilinear effect of size is significantly reduced by the fact that size is used here in its transformation to a logarithmic scale (see Appendix F: Transformation of Scales).

24. This does not necessarily mean they devote more time to patient care as such; see, e.g., Faye G. Abdellah and Eugene Levine, *Effect of Nurse Staffing on Satisfaction with Nursing Care*, Hospital Monograph Series, No. 4 (Chicago: American Hospital Association, 1958); Walker, op. cit., pp. 169-187; see also the pattern of variation in Table 34, row 1 and Table 23, rows 2 and 4.

25. Anderson and Warkov, *American Sociological Review*, 26 (1961), 27 (italics mine).

26. Ibid.

10 Complexity and Nonbureaucratic Coordination

Coordination in modern organizations is made problematic by three types of complexity: that of the organizational environment, the organizational task structure, and internal division of labor. In this chapter, I will suggest a way of relating these three aspects of complexity. I will also show that on all three counts, increasing complexity generates not hierarchical but lateral modes of coordination through "horizontal" communication and interaction between subunits. In short, the more complex organizations become, and the more complex their interrelations insofar as they become environments for each other, the more likely will nonhierarchical modes of coordination predominate, the less likely will bureaucratic-hierarchical modes of coordination and control be adequate.

There are many nonhierarchical forms of coordination which are relevant here and need to be investigated. Examples are the various mechanisms of participation, representation, negotiation, and decision-making embodied in such roles as that of ombudsman and other linker roles, in joint committees and conferences, and in different mediation and arbitration structures. However, I will focus here only on some aspects of nonbureaucratic coordination, notably those deriving from the functional interdependence of subunits within organizations, the role of professionalization in providing coordination by feedback, and the extent of external relations between organizations and their environment. Specifically, I will argue that the functional interdependence of specialized departments and subunits can be interpreted as giving rise to lateral modes of coordination, and that the internal structural complexity of organizations is itself a factor that both generates problems of coordination and contributes to their resolution.

Accordingly, I will first examine the joint effect of departmental specialization and professionalization on bureaucratization in its two major manifestations: administrative specialization (the relative size of the administrative-clerical staff) and hierarchical coordination (the administrative-supervisory ratio). In doing so, I will deal with some of the implications for organizational theory of the work of Anderson and Warkov and of Stinchcombe, as well as with Weber's concept of bureaucracy.

In this connection I also want to note again two conditions which are of particular importance for this analysis: first, the *level* of internal structural complexity of an organization at a given point in time, in contrast to the pattern of structural relationships; and second, the nature of professionalization, i.e., whether professional work takes the form of "general practice" or approaches the expertise of the "specialist".

Following the analysis of the joint effect of departmental specialization and professionalization on bureaucratization, I will propose a distinction between types of hospitals in terms of dominant or prevalent modes of coordination. This way of looking at hospital types leads to an "empirical classification" of hospitals, i.e., to a "theoretically grounded" typology of hospital organization.

Finally, I will examine one prototypical pair of hospitals: the "closed" institution and its more important countertype, the "open" organization. As the language suggests, these prototypes are viewed as implying certain criteria of evaluation, a question which I will touch on briefly later in this and the final chapter.

Departmental Specialization, Interdependence, and Lateral Coordination

In my analysis of structural variation among hospitals, departmental specialization as measured by the Gini coefficient of concentration has emerged as the theoretically and empirically most powerful indicator of internal division of labor, i.e., of internal structural complexity.[1] Departmental specialization was shown to reach its highest level in those hospitals which have the most complex task structure, viz. general teaching hospitals. Since these hospitals are among the most professionalized, as well as among those with the relatively largest administrative-clerical staff and the smallest administrative-supervisory ratio, the question arises as to the intervening effect of departmental specialization and professionalization on both of these aspects of bureaucratization. Presumably, departmental specialization should serve to increase both bureaucratization and professionalization, but professionalization has, as I have shown, a negative effect on bureaucratization. Let us look at the data in question.

The simple (zero-order) correlations between departmental specialization and professionalization as well as bureaucratization give a foretaste of the nature of this fairly complex set of relationships (table 35).

First of all, we see that professionalization is not directly related to departmental specialization if we look at all U.S. hospitals or the combined 12 groups (Table 35, row 1, columns 1 and 2). But among the twelve groups, there are certain significant variations in this relationship.[2] Thus in psychiatric hospitals, professionalization tends to be positively related to departmental specialization, but the correlation tends to be lower or even negative in general hospitals.

Similarly, the relative size of the administrative-clerical staff tends to be positively related to departmental specialization in the psychiatric hospitals, but the relationship becomes negative in the more complex teaching hospitals and in most of the V.A. hospitals (Table 35, row 2).

Clearly, the relationship between professionalization and bureaucratization on the one hand and internal structural complexity on the other appears to depend on the *level* of internal complexity at which this relationship is being considered. Thus, whether we use as indicators of the complexity level the degree of complexity of the task structure, or the degree of complexity of the internal division of labor, both professionalization and the relative size of the administrative-clerical staff tend to be negatively related to departmental specialization in those hospitals where the level of complexity is relatively high.[3]

The relationship between hierarchical coordination (the administrative-supervisory ratio) and departmental specialization presents a somewhat different picture (Table 35, row 3). First of all, the relationship in the hospital universe and the combined 12 groups is moderately negative. Secondly, most of the correlations within the groups, while also negative, are lower.

The generally negative character of the relationship between the administrative-supervisory ratio and departmental specialization suggests that hierarchical coordination decreases as a result of departmental specialization. The greater the internal structural complexity of hospitals, the smaller the administrative-supervisory ratio, and the greater the extent of delegation of bureaucratic authority.[4]

Let us now turn to a multivariate analysis of this relationship, using the relative size of the administrative-clerical staff and the administrative-supervisory ratio as dependent variables, respectively, with departmental specialization, professionalization, and size as the independent variables (Table 36).

The results of this analysis generally clarify and strengthen the findings based on the simple correlations, as shown above in Table 35, as well as those discussed earlier in Chapter 9, especially Tables 26, 33, and 34.

The upper panel of Table 36 (Panel A) shows the joint effect of departmental specialization, professionalization, and size on the relative size of the administrative-clerical staff.

First, we note the fact that the relationship between departmental specialization and the administrative staff changes from moderately positive to zero and moderately negative as the internal complexity of the organizational types increases. The state mental hospitals are among the least complex, but it is here where an increasing degree of departmental specialization contributes to an increase in the relative size of a specialized administrative staff. Again, it is among voluntary psychiatric teaching and the V.A. hospitals where the inverse relationship between departmental specialization and bureaucratization is most pronounced.

Corresponding to this change from a positive to a negative relationship is an almost perfectly "parallel" (but opposite) change in the relation between professionalization and bureaucratization as we move from the less to the more internally differentiated organizational structures. Thus it is also in regard to the voluntary psychiatric teaching and the V.A. psychiatric hospitals that the previously observed positive relationship between professionalization and bureaucratization reappears.

As to the lower half of Table 36 (Panel B), the moderate negative relationship between the administrative-supervisory ratio and departmental specialization, especially in the more complex

Table 35

Correlations Between Departmental Specialization (Gini Coefficient of Concentration) and 1) Professionalization; 2) Relative Size of Administrative-Clerical Staff; and 3) Administrative-Supervisory Ratio, by Service, Teaching Status, and Control

	U.S. Hosp.	All 12 Groups	Voluntary				State and Local Governmental				Federal (V.A.)				Within Group Homogeneity
			Nonteaching		Teaching		Nonteaching		Teaching		Nonteaching		Teaching		
			Psy	Gen	Psy	Gen	Psy	Gen	Psy	Gen	Psy	Gen	Psy	Gen	
(N)	6,825	3,544	30	1,507	13	467	139	956	91	185	23	56	17	60	
1. Professionalization	.01	.03	.26	.15	-.04	-.17	.24	.16	.63	-.20	.58	-.35	.36	.18	0
2. Administrative-Clerical Staff	.09	.21	.11	.06	.04	-.10	.23	.06	.55	-.20	.24	-.13	-.60	-.16	8
3. Administrative-Supervisory Ratio	-.37	-.37	-.07	-.25	-.31	-.27	-.28	-.22	-.21	-.44	.14	-.18	.04	-.16	11

[a]Number of groups with a correlation coefficient lower (in absolute numbers) than that of the combined 12 groups (Col. 2); see Ch. 7, Note 3.

Table 36

Joint Effect of Departmental Specialization, Professionalization, and Size on Two Measures of Bureaucratization: Regression Coefficients (b*) and Multiple R^2's for the Relative Size of Administrative-Clerical Staff (Upper Panel) and Administrative-Supervisory Ratio (Lower Panel) As Dependent Variables, Respectively, and Departmental Specialization, Professionalization, and Size As Independent Variables, by Service, Teaching Status, and Control

	U.S. Hosp.	All 12 Groups	Voluntary				State and Local Governmental				Federal (V.A.)			
			Nonteaching		Teaching		Nonteaching		Teaching		Nonteaching		Teaching	
			Psy	Gen	Psy	Gen	Psy	Gen	Psy	Gen	Psy	Gen	Psy	Gen
(N)	6,825	3,544	30	1,507	13	467	139	956	91	185	23	56	17	60
A. Relative Size of Administrative-Clerical Staff As Dependent Variable														
1. Departmental Specialization	.14	.23	.12	.06	-.09	-.08	.31	.06	.22	-.09	-.25	-.16	-.86	-.17
2. Professionalization	-.01	-.03	.00	-.09	.12	-.04	-.27	-.01	-.14	.00	.63	-.22	.14	-.03
3. Size	-.16	-.09	.07	.00	-.60	-.07	-.37	-.01	-.58	-.19	-.12	-.20	-.46	-.11
4. Multiple R^2	.03	.05	.02	.01	.42	.02	.19	.00	.45	.06	.29	.08	.58	.04
B. Administrative-Supervisory Ratio As Dependent Variable														
5. Departmental Specialization	-.19	-.18	-.09	-.08	-.36	-.14	-.11	-.09	-.11	-.21	.27	-.15	-.03	-.12
6. Professionalization	-.46	-.47	-.10	-.34	-.55	-.33	-.47	-.36	-.47	-.44	-.23	-.20	-.52	-.30
7. Size	-.42	-.42	-.18	-.34	-.20	-.42	-.32	-.28	-.33	-.58	-.15	-.41	-.74	-.34
8. Multiple R^2	.36	.32	.03	.28	.33	.30	.26	.22	.17	.51	.08	.18	.44	.16

teaching hospitals, lends support to the hypothesis that hierarchical coordination is not a result of increasing internal structural complexity, but rather of the homogeneity and routinization of work processes. These findings suggest a specification of Weber's assumption of hierarchical, monocratic authority as essential for the effective discharge of complex administrative tasks. Where complex problem-solving is capable of routinization, standardization, and "seriability," hierarchical administrative patterns may, indeed, be more effective and therefore more prevalent, as for example, in large mental hospitals. However, where the task complexity is generated by multiple and diverse objectives and services, as is the case in general teaching hospitals or, for example, in pre-industrial work organizations with diffuse, multiple objectives,[5] non-bureaucratic, "associational" forms of administration involving lateral coordination will predominate. I have already indicated that Weber has dealt with these alternative forms of administration in terms of his concept of "democratic administration" and the "principle of collegiality." This principle limits or modifies monocratic authority insofar as it involves the separation of powers, consultation and cooperation among a plurality of individuals or advisory collegial bodies, mutual veto powers, and voting.

In general, the empirical findings derived from the analysis of hospital structure force us to reconsider the implications of a complex division of labor for specific modes of coordination as well as for overall organizational coordination. We can assume that in the organization of patient care in modern hospitals the specialization of functions and especially of departments implies a high degree of interdependence.

Interdependence provides a basis for coordination insofar as work functions represent phases or elements of an interdependent work flow. Interdependence among people, among specific activities, and among specialized departments raises countless problems of coordination and mutual adjustment. Structuring the resolution of these problems on the interpersonal and subunit level implies coordination on the organizational level insofar as the organization is a "going concern".[6]

Let us briefly look once again at the Gini coefficient of concentration in order to relate the logic of this measure of departmental specialization to the empirical findings.

Logical Implications of the Gini Index

It will be remembered from the discussion in Chapter 3 that the Gini coefficient measures the evenness of distribution of the organizational labor force among a number of departments or personnel categories. Specifically, it measures the deviation from a theoretical distribution in which all categories are of equal size. In other words, it is an idicator of the quantitative weight of a number of groups relative to each other, independent of a mean or an arbitrary origin. In the present case, the total hospital labor force was divided into seven departments or categorical components. These seven components were selected on the basis of a kind of "natural logic" inherent to hospital organization. They include 1) salaried physicians and medical house staff, 2) graduate professional nurses, 3) practical nurses, aides, and attendants, 4) technical personnel, 5) maintenance personnel, 6) business and clerical personnel, and 7) "other," personnel (mainly new technical specialists).

Expressing these components as percentages of the total hospital labor force and arranging them according to size rank yields a profile of the occupational composition of the hospital. Let us assume the hypothetical case where all 7 categories are of equal size, i.e., each being one-seventh or a little over 14 per cent of the total labor force. If p_i is any one of the $n = 7$ percentages, then the total hospital labor force is $p = n \, p_i$, or the sum Σp_i over all seven categories (see Figure 2a).

The completely even distribution in Figures 2a, when plotted in terms of a Lorenz curve, corresponds to the triangle $nP/2$, i.e., the area under the diagonal which divides the total area nP into halves[7] (Figure 2B). The Gini coefficient for the distributions in Figures 2a and b has the value of 1.0, calculated by the formula

$$\frac{2\Sigma c_i - 1}{n}$$

where c_i is the cumulated percentage in a given category and Σc the sum of the cumulated percentages, summed over all $n = 7$ categories.

To illustrate the possible variation of the Gini coefficient, let us now look at two extreme empirical examples of hospital structure, chosen from among the 12 hospital groups: the state and local governmental nonteaching psychiatric hospitals, and the V.A. general teaching hospitals. The psychiatric nonteaching hospitals have a mean Gini index value of .43 which summarizes the following "structural profile" (Figure 3a):

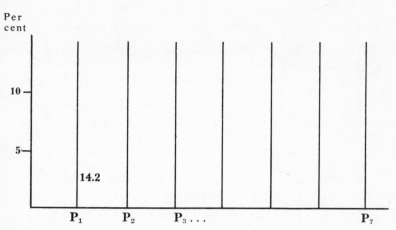

Figure 2*a*
Theoretical Distribution: All Seven Categories Are of Equal Size

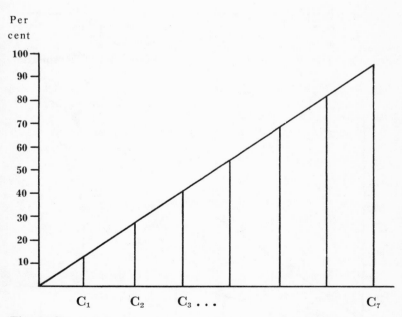

Figure 2*b*
The Lorenz Curve for a Completely Even Distribution
(Gini Coefficient G=1.0)

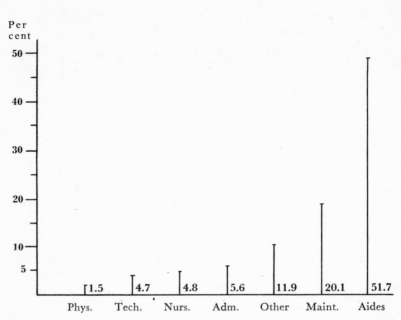

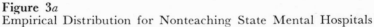

Figure 3a
Empirical Distribution for Nonteaching State Mental Hospitals

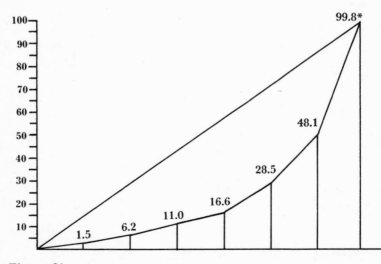

Figure 3b
Lorenz Curve for a Very Uneven Distribution (G=.43)

Graphically, the profile of this "simple" hospital type appears as a considerable deviation from the diagonal, as Figure 3b shows.

In contrast, the structural profile of the V.A. general teaching hospitals, with a mean Gini value of .72, looks as follows (see Figure 4a).

Clearly, the structural difference between these two hospital types is illustrated by the graphic representations, if not by the values of the Gini coefficient.

I shall now investigate in what sense the degree of departmental specialization can be interpreted in terms of "structural coordination." What is the logical implication of measuring the structural balance or imbalance of an organization in terms of its component parts?[8]

If a given population is distributed among categories or classes, then the percentage of the total population in a given category equals the probability of a unit to be in that category. The probability of the joint occurrence of two units from the same category equals the product of their relative frequency, i.e., p^2, where p is the proportion in a given category. If in a given population homogeneity of units exists by virtue of the fact that a large number of units are in one category, then their "joint occurrence" is the probability that they belong to the same category. Interpreted sociologically, joint occurrence is the interaction or interrelation between two units drawn randomly. Thus, the sum of the squared probabilities, $\Sigma\ p^2$, will yield a measure of compositional homogeneity, or the likelihood that members of a given category will *not* interact with those of another category. The term $1 - \Sigma\ p^2$ would therefore indicate the degree of heterogeneity in population, together with the likelihood of interaction among the members of different categories.

It must be noted, of course, that interaction thus interpreted holds only for a randomly selected pair of units. One could argue that in organizations just the opposite is the case, i.e., that interaction is highly structured and the relationship between actors is formally defined. Furthermore, "joint occurrence" (interpreted as interaction or interdependence) assumes the existence of an aggregate population, with no spatial, temporal, ecological and social restrictions imposed on it. This assumption, again, is not necessarily warranted since people work in specific areas defined in terms of space (offices, wards, wings, floors, buildings, etc.), time (e.g., shifts), and other categories of work organization (communication, authority, etc.).

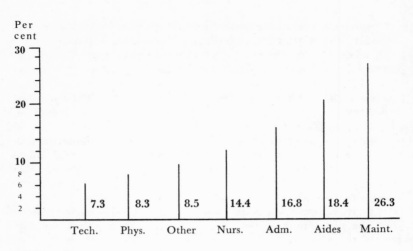

Figure 4*a*
Empirical Distribution for V.A. General Teaching Hospitals

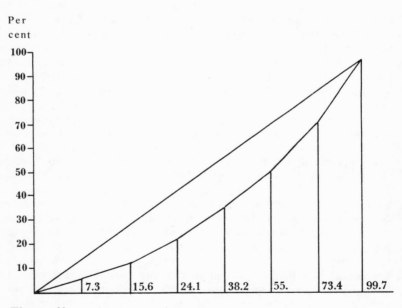

Figure 4*b*
Lorenz Curve for a Slightly Uneven Distribution (G=.72)

However, one can adduce at least two sets of factors which support the original assumption. One factor refers to the realities of informal organization, the other to the work flow which is formally organized in terms of functional interdependence.

The first factor is the tendency of workers in the same category to interact more frequently with each other than with those from other categories. In the relevant literature, this fact is usually observed in relation to social class and status groups, peer group formation, and the emergence of subcultures, i.e., in relation to the importance of the "informal organization." A classical example specific to hospitals is a study of the patterns of interaction and communication among various personnel categories in a hospital.[9] Wessen found that members of personnel categories, such as doctors, nurses, and attendants, tended to interact more frequently with each other than with members of other categories. In hospitals and other work organizations this tendency is, of course, reinforced by uniforms and other symbols characteristic of the various categories.

The second factor which supports the notion that "joint occurrence" can be interpreted in terms of a social relationship has to do with the structural-ecological relationship between what Hawley has called "categoric units." In the tradition of the ecological interpretation of the division of labor, Hawley states that the symbiotic relationships among categoric units are "due directly to the specialization of functions in the community."[10] While the *internal* relations of the categoric group tend to be commensalistic (and thus potentially competitive), symbiotic patterns, including cooperative and exchange relationship, tend to characterize the more autonomous corporate units. In contrast, the relationship *between* categoric units or associations of "functionally homogeneous individuals" is determined in part by their *size relative to each other.* If one categoric unit dominates, in terms of size, the total division of labor in a system, we could say that the level of functional specialization as well as the degree of interdependence are relatively low, since functional homogeneity, including the relationships between like-structured subunits or individuals, would predominate.

To the extent, then, that the probability of joint occurrence of, or interrelation between, individuals of the *same unit* decreases, or is replaced by relationships among individuals of *different units*, the heterogeneity and differentiation of the whole "community" or organization increases together with the interdependence of specialized functions.[11]

In sum, the interpretation of departmental specialization in terms of interdependence and the emergence of lateral coordination assumes that in hospitals we are dealing with functionally dissimilar groups of personnel whose work is interdependent. The larger one or two of the groups, the smaller the others and the lower the absolute level of interaction and interdependence between groups. Thus, if over 50 per cent of the hospital personnel are aides and attendants, as is true in the state mental hospitals, the likelihood of interaction among members of different groups is drastically reduced, even though the interaction is formally structured and not random. An increase both in the number of groups and in the size of groups relative to each other will increase their relative autonomy and interdependence. Substantively, this idea is similar to Coleman's conflict prevention model in communities. Here, too, the assumption is that of an "ongoing process' as evidence for the successful solution of problems of coordination on the subsystem levels of social structure, i.e., the absorption of stress and conflict at a given level, thus reducing the probability that conflict is shifted to the next higher level. An example I have discussed earlier is the putative preference among organizations of role conflict over group or departmental conflict and, in general, over conflict at the level of the whole organization.

Given the positive effect of the level of internal structural complexity for the lateral coordination among more or less autonomous units, how does this process affect professionalization, and how do both of these nonbureaucratic modes of coordination relate to the bureaucratic ones? The answer, as I shall argue in the next section, depends in large part on the transformation of the character of professionalization from general practice to a more task-specific, specialist form.

From "Generalist" to "Specialist": The Changing Functions of Professionals

We have seen that professionalization tends to increase with departmental specialization in the psychiatric hospitals, but that in general hospitals this relationship is either zero or negative (Table 35). Interpreted in terms of *levels*, this means that both departmental specialization and professionalization are dependent on each other as long as they appear on a comparatively low level, as is true in psychiatric hospitals. As the internal division of labor becomes more complex, professionalization also reaches a higher level, but at the same time it becomes more independent of (or even counteracts) the division of labor. One could say that job specialization and person specialization are more likely in conflict with each other at higher levels of specialization, but not when both are in a rudimentary form or at an incipient stage of development.[12]

The interaction between departmental specialization and professionalization is particularly salient with respect to the administrative-clerical staff, as I have shown in Table 36, Panel A. Both variables affect this aspect of bureaucratization in opposite directions, depending on the *level* of departmental specialization, i.e., on the degree of internal structural complexity. This finding is of particular importance for the conclusions of both the Anderson-Warkov and Stinchcombe studies.

The Anderson-Warkov hypothesis, it will be remembered, suggests that the crucial intervening variable between size and bureaucratization is "functional complexity" or the degree of role specialization, i.e., a combination of task complexity and division of labor (Figure 5).

The Stinchcombe hypothesis, on the other hand, focuses on the effect of professionalization on bureaucratization by considering two different production settings: mass production (high job specialization and routinization) and the building industry involving craft-type subcontractors (high worker specialization and nonroutinization, including seasonal variation) (Figure 6).

By considering the *joint effect* of departmental specialization and professionalization under conditions of high and low structural complexity (departmental specialization), it is possible to evaluate the Stinchcombe and Anderson-Warkov models simultaneously (Figure 7).

By way of summarizing these complex relationships, let me suggest a theoretical interpretation based on variations in the *level* of internal structural complexity (departmental specialization) as well as on the distinction between generalist and specialist variants of professionalization.[13]

As I have noted in Chapter 4, the specification of professional work goals involves a combination of different, technically heterogeneous functions carried out by the same worker. This archetype of crafts and professional roles is characteristic of much hospital work, particularly of the nurse's role. Professionalization thus understood has generally been found to be closely associated with complex task performance and self-regulation.

Professional nurses in nonadministrative positions perform professional functions to the extent that they have internalized the norms governing their work, assume responsibility for the continuity

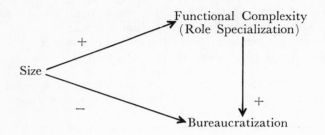

Figure 5
The Anderson-Warkov Hypothesis

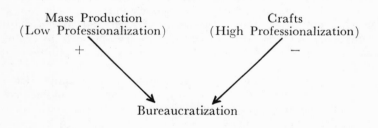

Figure 6
The Stinchcombe Hypothesis

of total patient care, and exercise discretion independently of either the functional authority of physicians or the rank authority of nursing supervisors and administrators. We have also seen that this kind of role specification is contingent on the balance between the professional and the subprofessional components. The larger the subprofessional component, the less prevalent is professional coordination and the more prevalent is hierarchical coordination (in the present case, mainly the bureaucratization of professionals).

Let us now look once again at this generalized pattern from the perspective of the two special conditions: a low level of departmental specialization, implying low internal structural complexity, and a high level of departmental specialization, indicating high structural complexity (see Figure 8).

If a given hospital has a high level of compositional homogeneity and task routinization, and generally, a low level of internal structural complexity, this pattern is characterized by inverse relationships between professionalization and hierarchical coordination on the one hand and the relative size of the administrative-clerical staff on the other. For this "simple" structural pattern, then, one may accept Stinchcombe's hypothesis that a (generalist) professionalized labor force constitutes an alternative to bureaucratic administration.[14]

The "simple" structural pattern (Figure 8A) also shows the positive effect of departmental specialization on the relative size of the administrative-clerical staff, suggesting a further confirmation of the Anderson-Warkov hypothesis. Thus, with respect to the administrative-clerical staff, the Anderson-Warkov and the Stinchcombe hypotheses are compatible and hold jointly under conditions of low internal structural complexity.[15]

By contrast, in hospital types with a more complex internal structure, the opposite of the Stinchcombe and Anderson-Warkov hypotheses holds. The administrative-clerical staff tends to be inversely related to departmental specialization, but positively to professionalization (Figure 8B).

We can interpret this reversal as the result of the interaction between division of labor and professionalization. As the internal division of labor becomes more complex, the nature of professional work is transformed by becoming more task-specific, differentiated, and specialized. Professional work becomes an integral part of the division of labor and thus contributes to the very complexity which it helps to integrate and coordinate under conditions of lower structural complexity.[16]

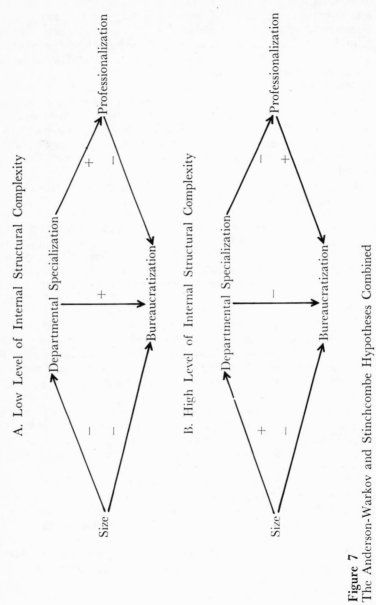

Figure 7
The Anderson-Warkov and Stinchcombe Hypotheses Combined

276

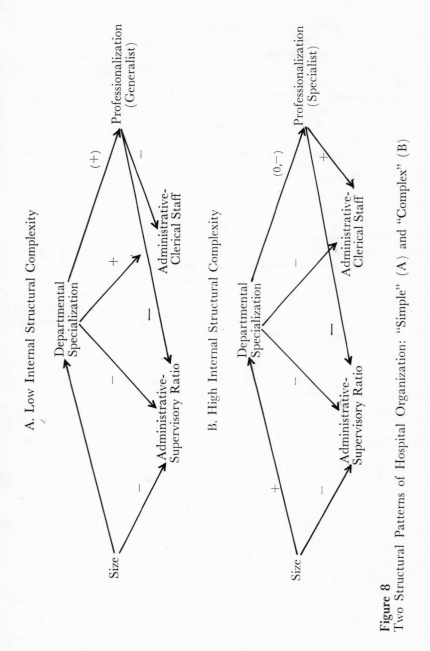

Figure 8
Two Structural Patterns of Hospital Organization: "Simple" (A) and "Complex" (B)

Since professional work itself becomes functionally more specific, it contributes relatively less to organizational coordination. This two-fold loss of coordination, therefore, increases the need for the regulation of specialists, i.e., for a larger administrative-clerical staff. Once this process has advanced to the point where professionals are highly specialized, departmental development based on the new professional specialities may, once again, be expected to reduce the need for bureaucratic-administrative forms of coordination.[17]

In short, the interpretation advanced here suggests a differentiation of the concept of professionalization in at least two directions. First, specialist professional work is more narrowly task-specific than its generalist ancestor. While the latter involves the notion of a total work process in which the product is completed by, and visible to, the worker, specialist work is much more fragmented, if not truncated. It approximates job specialization rather than person specialization, although the latter is at a relatively high level.

Second, general practice, apart from its independent economic base and the elements of entrepreneurship, is "free" in the sense that it provides its own communication system and hierarchy of work rules rather than requiring external rules and controls. Of course, every skilled task-performance involves a measure of autonomy and discretion. But the scope of specialist practice—unless it is conducted as a "private practice"—is considerably more narrow, its decision-making more routinized, and its definition of the product more dependent on the definition and participation of others in the work process. Professional specialists are therefore also more dependent on administrative services which provide communication, coordination, and regulation, not to mention protection from the potential encroachment of others on their power and status privileges.

The necessity to coordinate specialists gives rise to administrative-clerical services more likely than to a bureaucratic hierarchy. Conversely, the bureaucratization of professionals (where it occurs to any degree) does not by definition, nor in all organizational contexts, imply hierarchical coordination; it also contains elements of administrative-clerical specialization.[18]

From this perspective, the increasing bureaucratization of professionals implies closer ties between their administrative tasks and their specialized work functions. This process parallels the transformation of professional work from the specification of goals to the specification of procedures, i.e. to a form of technical specialization. This means that the frame of reference of professional work ceases to be the occupational structure or the larger social system and becomes, instead, an organization or a class of organizations.[19] Such a transformation implies further that professional behavior, in the sense of self-regulation through reference group membership, is shifting toward a type of collectivity orientation in which organizational and personal-professional loyalties tend to coincide.[20] This does not mean that cosmopolitans would become locals, but that the distinction is superseded by new forms and combinations, especially in those highly complex organizations which are able to combine professionally specialized and organizational-administrative concerns. Such a development would restrict the usefulness and quality-control function of professional reference and peer groups, reducing them to mere interest groups. In modern professional organizations, this would imply a new post-Weberian form of integration of professional-technical expertise and organizational position, if not rank.[21]

In spite of the similarity, there are certain differences between this modern form of bureaucratic professionalism and Weber's concept of legal-bureaucratic administration. First, one may expect a greater degree of role specialization among such modern professionals, a difference which is comparable to that between professional specialists and technicians. Secondly, one would expect the elaboration of a stratification system among professionals, as well as the formation of professional elites, operating within, and on the basis of, correspondingly stratified organizational systems. Third, while the scope of any given organizational system may be smaller than the large, monolithic, public bureaucracy envisaged by Weber, it is now possible to discern a wide variety of organizations and occupational groups which constitute an organizational market structure as well as a system of stratification within certain classes and types of organizations.[22]

These considerations certainly apply to the most advanced and complex types of hospitals where hierarchical and "purely" professional types of coordination are giving way to structural and administrative-regulative modes, i.e., where professional specialization becomes part of the overall specialization of functions and of the generally more differentiated and diversified organization of work. The development suggested here for hospitals and other professional organizations has certain implications for a new conception of organizations, which I will explore especially in the last chapter.

I will now return to a systematic comparison of the twelve empirical hospital types in terms of the *levels* of each of the modes of coordination, bureaucratic and nonbureaucratic. The purpose is to define and distinguish the patterns of coordination characteristic of different hospital types, and to develop an empirical classification of types of hospital organization.

The "Withering Away of Bureaucracy"?: A Typology of Hospital Organization

In the previous chapters, I have sought to analyze the separate effects of autonomy, task structure, and size on the internal division of labor and professionalization and of these latter two variables on the two bureaucratic modes of coordination: the administrative-supervisory ratio, and the relative size of the administrative-clerical staff. This analysis has, in effect, treated departmental specialization and professionalization as intervening variables with respect to the bureaucratic modes of coordination. But insofar as departmental specialization and professionalization can be seen as contributing to overall organizational coordination, they can be reconceptualized as modes of coordination, albeit nonbureaucratic ones. I have also shown that the nonbureaucratic modes of coordination interact in their influence on bureaucratization, i.e., they influence each other while influencing the bureaucratic modes of coordination.

Let us, for the moment, disregard this complex pattern of structural relationships and consider only the *level* at which the two bureaucratic and the two nonbureaucratic modes of coordination occur in the twelve hospital types. For purposes of presentation, I will call the administrative-clerical staff "administrative" coordination, departmental specialization "structural" coordination, professionalization "professional" coordination, and the administrative-supervisory ratio "hierarchical" coordination.

The *level* of each of the four modes of coordination is defined in terms of the means of the respective variables (Table 37). Dividing each of the four sets of twelve means into "high" (+) and "low" (—) categories yields the following classification[23] (Table 38).

Table 38 represents an "empirical classification" of organizations in the sense that the different hospital groups are classified simultaneously along several dimensions or variables.[24]

The result is a multivariate description of formal organizations which is limited only by the specific range of values assumed by the variables, given the valid and thus comparable measurement of the organizational dimensions and concepts. Since the present data are standardized for the universe of hospitals, comparative concepts such as "high" and "low," and "more" or "less" can be expressed numerically on a true scale. This would not necessarily be true for all variables if, for example, hospitals, universities, business firms, and governmental agencies were to be classified in a multivariate space.

The six types of hospital organization shown in Table 38 represent an empirical classification in terms of the four modes of coordination only. But since the complexity of the task structure and the size of the hospital groups are known, and since the internal structural complexity is given by the level of departmental specialization (structural coordination), the new empirical types have a considerable degree of consistency and plausibility. I shall briefly describe each one in turn.

Type I

This type is organizationally specialized (unifunctional), has a comparatively low level of internal structural complexity and a high degree of compositional homogeneity and is very large. Its main coordinating mechanism consists of a bureaucratized professional nursing staff. If hospitals are seen as professional organizations, this type represents a very low level of professionalization. The type subsumes both nonteaching and teaching psychiatric hospitals, most of them operated by the health departments of state governments. It fits the well-known descriptions of "state mental hospitals" as well as Goffman's "asylums" or "total institutions." One may call this type a "large specialized custodial" organization.

Type II

This type has a low-to-intermediate level of internal structural complexity. In terms of task structure, it is a functionally diffuse but nondiversified organization. Its main coordinating mechanisms are a high degree of professionalization and, at the same time, a high degree of bureaucratization of professionals. This type includes mainly the state and local governmental as well as the voluntary nonteaching general hospitals, i.e., the small community general hospital. Numerically, it represents the modal type of hospital organization with almost 2,500 cases, i.e., over one-third of all U.S. hospitals. I will refer to this type as a small "multifunctional service" organization.

Type III

This type is organizationally specialized and has a comparatively high level of professionalization and bureaucratization of professionals. There are two subtypes distinguishable in terms of complexity of task structure and internal structure.

Table 37
Mean Levels of Four Modes of Coordination: Means of Administrative-Supervisory Ratio (Hierarchical), % Graduate Professional Nurses (Professional), Degree of Departmental Specialization (Structural), and Relative Size of Administrative-Clerical Staff (Administrative), by Service, Teaching Status, and Control

Mode of Coordination	U.S. Hosp.	All 12 Groups	Voluntary				State and Local Governmental				Federal (V.A.)			
			Nonteaching		Teaching		Nonteaching		Teaching		Nonteaching		Teaching	
			Psy	Gen	Psy	Gen	Psy	Gen	Psy	Gen	Psy	Gen	Psy	Gen
(N)	6,825	3,544	30	1,507	13	467	139	956	91	185	23	56	17	60
Hospital Number:			1	2	3	4	5	6	7	8	9	10	11	12
Hierarchical	.30	.27	.45	.27	.45	.13	.44	.33	.27	.18	.15	.13	.12	.10
Professional	.22	.23	.13	.27	.12	.23	.05	.22	.08	.18	.08	.15	.08	.14
Structural	.53	.54	.52	.52	.61	.63	.43	.50	.51	.63	.56	.65	.58	.72
Administrative	.08	.08	.08	.08	.08	.09	.06	.08	.06	.08	.12	.18	.11	.17

Table 38
Relative Prevalence of Modes of Coordination for Organizational Type

| Hospital Number | Modes of Coordination | | | | Organizational Type |
	Adminis-trative	Struc-tural	Profes-sional	Hier-archical	
5, 7	−	−	−	+	I. Large Specialized Custodial
2, 6	−	−	+	+	II. Small Multifunctional Service
3, (1)	−	+	+	+	III. Small Specialized Thereapeutic
4, 8	−	+	+	−	IV. Large Diversified Service
10, 12	+	+	+	−	V. Large Complex Service
9, 11	+	+	−	−	VI. Large Specialized Service

The diversified subtype has a relatively high level of internal complexity, including medical-technological complexity. It consists of the voluntary teaching psychiatric hospitals as Stanton and Schwartz, Caudill, and Strauss et al. have described them.

The nondiversified subtype has a low-to-intermediate level of internal complexity. But it has a relatively high level of professionalization and bureaucratization of professionals, both constituting its major modes of coordination. In this respect, it is similar to Type II. However, this subtype consists of the voluntary nonteaching psychiatric hospitals.

Generically, one may refer to Type III as a "small specified therapeutic" organization.

Type IV

This type has a high level of internal structural complexity. Its main coordinating mechanisms are a high degree of professionalization and a high level of "structural coordination." While bureaucratic forms of coordination are present in this structural type, they are not highly developed.

This type includes both state and local governmental as well as voluntary teaching general hospitals. They are among the most complex, technically best equipped hospitals. I will refer to this type as a "large diversified service" organization.

Type V

While structurally very similar to Type IV, Type V is distinguished by its large, specialized administrative-clerical staff. The level of internal structural complexity is relatively very high. The prevalent modes of coordination, in addition to the administrative-clerical staff, are professionalization and structural coordination. This type includes the teaching and nonteaching V.A. general hospitals. One may call it a "large planned service" organization.

Type VI

Type VI comprises specialized service organizations having a comparatively high level of internal structural complexity. The main modes of coordination are structural and administrative, in contrast to the prevalence of professional and hierarchical modes of Type III. This type includes the teaching and nonteaching V.A. psychiatric hospitals. I call this type a "large specialized service" organization.

If one apples Sumner's distinction between crescive and enacted institutions to these organizational types, Types V and VI would more nearly approximate the planned "enacted" organization, while Type II has more "crescive" characteristics. It should be clear that in terms of a formal definition, all formal organizations are "enacted" institutions. Yet if taken in analytical terms, Sumner's distinction implies that enacted institutions are rational, planned social structures, while crescive institutions are organismic, adaptive, "naturally" evolved social structures.[25]

The above typology constitutes a confirmation of two basic hypotheses of this study concerning the relation between task complexity and the modes of coordination.

The typology shows, first, that the greater the degree of complexity of the task structure, the greater the number of different mechanisms of coordination. Technically, this hypothesis receives support only if we accept the equivalence of "presence" and "prevalence." The four modes of coordination we have identified are present in all hospitals regardless of degree of complexity. However, only one mode predominates in Type I, while two modes predominate in Types II, IV, and VI, and three modes predominate in Types III and V.

We can generalize by saying that specialized (unifunctional) organizations tend to have one or two dominant modes of organization, while nonspecialized or multipurpose organizations tend to have two or more modes of coordination. It should be noted that Types I to III have a relatively simple task structure and a low level of internal complexity compared to IV, V, and VI. Furthermore, Types I, II, and III all have a high level of hierarchical coordination, while none of the other types do (Table 38).

The second hypothesis for which there is support in this typology is that specific types of task structure and internal complexity tend to give rise to specific modes of coordination. Eight of the twelve hospital types investigated here have a relatively high level of professionalization. In one sense, this simply means that one characteristic that distinguishes most hospitals from other types of organizations is that they are "professional" organizations. This ratio of two-thirds is, of course, quite arbitrary since it depends entirely on the number of specific hospitals types and the number of dimensions used for their classification. But although it is probably not unrepresentative of the hospital universe to have a high level of professionalization, there are without question a considerable number of hospitals which cannot be classified as "professional" organizations or which have very low levels of professionalization.

More specifically, we can say that multifunctional organizations, i.e., general hospitals, tend to have a high level of professionalization which operates as a coordinating mechanism complementary to hierarchical and administrative coordination. Similarly, among specialized organizations, whether diversified or not, the bureaucratization of professionals is a dominant mode of coordination, while this is not true for the internally complex diversified organizations.

It is interesting to note that the two forms of bureaucratization, i.e., the bureaucratization of professionals and the administrative-clerical staff, do not co-exist on equally high levels. Where one predominates, the other is less developed, and vice versa. This does not mean, however, that their relationship is always and necessarily inverse.

Finally, departmental specialization is somewhat more likely to operate as a coordinating mechanism in diversified than in nondiversified organizations. This observation, of course, raises the difficult question to what extent diversification can only develop (or be developed) because there is a sufficient degree of interdependence of functions in the first place. I will not be able to give a satisfactory answer to this question within the framework of this study. But the problem can be investigated through an elaboration and refinement of the dimension of task diversification as well as on the basis of various measures of interdependence and of lateral modes of interaction and communication, measures which differ from the ones employed here by being more direct and specific.

I shall now consider the third type of complexity which affects the modes of coordination in hospitals, namely the complexity of the organizational environment.

The "Open Organization": Internal Structure and External Environment

In the preceding sections of this chapter I have sought to demonstrate, within certain limits, the *systemic* nature of the relationships between internal structural patterns and the modes of coordination. For example, a major portion of the variation in the relative size of the administrative-clerical staff can be accounted for by variations in hospital ownership and control, complexity of task structure, size, departmental specialization, and professionalization (see Table 36, Panel A). Similarly, departmental specialization and professionalization interact in their effect on administrative coordination.

Let me shift the focus of attention, for the moment, from the separate independent variables to their joint effect, i.e., to the variation in the size of the squared multiple correlation coefficient

(R^2), which can be taken as a measure of the proportion of variance in the dependent variable (here the administrative-clerical staff), "explained" or "accounted for" by the variation in the independent variables.

The differences in the size of the R^2 in the upper half of Table 36 are clearly related to autonomy and task structure, in addition to size and departmental specialization. First of all, it is obvious that the R^2 is largest in the psychiatric hospitals. But among the six psychiatric types, the explanatory value of the internal structural variables as signified by the R^2 is greatest for the federal V.A. hospitals (.58 and .29), somewhat lower for the state and local governmental psychiatric hospitals (.45 and .19), and lowest for the voluntary psychiatric hospitals (.42 and .02). If we interpret the size of R^2 as a measure of the extent to which a hospital possesses "system" characteristics, i.e., where internal factors can be explained by other factors of internal structure, then it is plausible to conclude that the "planning" and standardization of the Veterans' Administration is a determinant of the "systemic" characteristics of its hospitals. Conversely, the more "autonomous" voluntary hospitals seem, in this perspective, more "open" toward the environment.

However, here one must again be aware of the two aspects of the concept of autonomy, namely resources and the power to make decisions for the organization. In this study, most of the findings relating to autonomy have revealed a strong difference between the federal V.A. hospitals, on the one hand, and the voluntary and state and local governmental hospitals, on the other. Upon closer examination one finds that most of the differences tend to occur between the V.A. and the voluntary hospitals, with the public state and local governmental hospitals sometimes falling in the middle, sometimes ranking with the voluntary hospitals (sometimes even lower). This variability in the characteristics of hospitals with "medium dependency" suggests that the two dimensions of organizational autonomy, economic and political autonomy, should be measured independently. Federal V.A. hospitals rank low in de jure legal-political autonomy, but high in de facto economic autonomy, since budgets are prepared on the basis of relatively high standards of patient care. Conversely, voluntary hospitals rank relatively high on both dimensions, assuming that community chest and other financial support is as much "guaranteed' as is the budget submitted by the V.A. hospital administrator.

By contrast, the public state and local governmental hospitals have relatively low de jure as well as relatively low de facto operating autonomy, i.e., they tend to rank low in terms of both resources and decision-making autonomy.[26]

In sum, while it is plausible to interpret the gradual increase in the magnitude of R^2 from voluntary to public to federal psychiatric hospitals in terms of a scale of increasing "systemness" of hospital structure, corresponding to an underlying scale of decreasing autonomy, we must refrain from drawing definite conclusions for conceptual and empirical reasons.

The conceptual reason is that federal hospitals are less autonomous than others only in a formal, legal sense. Being regulated on a higher administrative level assures them both a certain measure of economic-financial viability and independence, as well as freedom to maintain high standards of quality and performance. To do so in the face of budgetary constraints is probably one of the most difficult problems of state and local governmental hospitals, a situation which is significantly similar to that of proprietary hospitals, a type with a theoretically high degree of autonomy.

The empirical reason against a unidimensional interpretation of "openness" in terms of autonomy is given by the fact that only psychiatric hospitals exhibit this responsiveness to "external control," and only with respect to the relative size of the administrative-clerical staff (Table 36, Panel A). Among general hospitals, the R^2 tends to approach zero, regardless of ownership and control. We may conclude therefore that "external control" has a consistent effect at best in those types of organizations which are predisposed by their task structure to assume the characteristics of a "closed" system.

Let me take this argument one step further and, from an "external" perspective, examine the fact that internal structural factors are relatively potent predictors of the administrative apparatus in psychiatric hospitals, but not in general hospitals.

The systematic differences in the size of the R^2's suggest that the psychiatric hospitals, as specialized organizations, are more isolated from, and less interdependent with, their environment. This isoloation could easily be explained by the special requirements of the clientele, i.e., the psychiatric patient population. By contrast, the multifunctional general hospitals seem to be more dependent on the external environment, if only in terms of exchange of services, patient turnover, and greater involvement in the "health metabolism" of the community. One of the clearly "external" factors in our data is size of community, or the degree of urbanization and complexity of the organizational environment.

Complexity of the Organizational Environment

In order to test the idea that general hospitals, particularly teaching hospitals, are more extensively "associated" with the external environment than psychiatric hospitals, let us examine the simple correlations between size of community and six "internal" organizational variables, i.e., size of organization, functional specialization, departmental specialization, professionalization, the administrative-supervisory ratio, and the relative size of the administrative-clerical staff (the latter four, redefined as modes of coordination, are presented in Table 39).

The results support the hypothesis that the "external" factor of community size is more important in the case of general hospitals and teaching hospitals than for psychiatric hospitals. In twenty-one out of thirty-six comparisons between general and psychiatric hospitals, the correlations for general hospitals are higher. In twenty-two out of thirty-six comparisons between teaching and nonteaching hospitals, the correlations are higher in the teaching hospitals.

Clearly, this procedure does not constitute a statistical test; nor does a correlation necessarily indicate a greater degree of interdependence between the organization and its environment. However, in the absence of other truly "external" variables, community size may be understood as representing a variety of factors, such as availability of services, complexity of the labor market, and presence and "density" of other organizations.

It is interesting to note in this connection that for the 1,200 teaching hospitals in 1960 the complexity of the environment as measured by size of community has a positive effect on the number of internships offered ($r = .11$), the number of residencies offered ($r = .15$), the number of different types of residencies, i.e., the degree of medical complexity ($r = .18$), and the likelihood of a major medical school affiliation ($r = .14$). Moreover, community size has a positive effect on the stability of the hospital as a teaching institution (the correlation with the number of changes in teaching accreditation from 1951 to 1960 is $r = -.16$), similar to the effect of hospital age on stability ($r = -.21$), as noted in Chapter 5. We also find that the larger the community, the smaller the rate of managerial succession, i.e., the turnover rate of top administrators,

Table 39

Simple Correlations Between Size of Community and Six Organizational Characteristics: Organizational Size, Degree of Functional Specialization, Structural Coordination, Professional Coordination, Hierarchical Coordination, and Administrative Coordination, by Service, Teaching Status, and Control

Correlation between Size of Community and:	U.S. Hosp.	All 12 Groups	Voluntary				State and Local Governmental				Federal (V.A.)			
			Nonteaching		Teaching		Nonteaching		Teaching		Nonteaching		Teaching	
(N)	6,825	3,544	Psy 30	Gen 1,507	Psy 13	Gen 467	Psy 139	Gen 956	Psy 91	Gen 185	Psy 23	Gen 56	Psy 17	Gen 60
Organizational Size	.37	.43	.22	.30	.13	.47	-.04	.29	-.02	.63	-.11	.31	.41	.40
Functional Specialization	.40	.51	-.03	.31	.50	.00	.16	.25	.07	.55	.12	.43	-.27	.00
Structural Coordination	.31	.40	.03	.18	.31	.33	.18	.13	.15	.42	.16	.25	-.29	.29
Professional Coordination	-.05	-.06	-.06	.07	.18	-.25	.21	.08	.00	-.23	.00	.02	-.42	-.01
Hierarchical Coordination	-.19	-.24	.25	-.16	.07	-.19	-.11	-.11	-.01	-.38	.14	-.13	-.28	-.07
Administrative Coordination	.07	.10	.42	.11	-.41	-.06	.06	.09	.11	-.21	.07	-.07	-.20	.04

although the relationship is weak ($r = .06$), and significant only at the .05 level. We may conclude, however, that both age and environmental complexity favor the stability of complex organizations.

As a group, teaching hospitals also exhibit a growth pattern which shows the powerful influence of a professionalized labor force. If we take the percentage of payroll expenses in 1951 as a measure of the extent of investment in a professionalized labor force at Time 1 (the payroll percentage being itself positively related to the hospital's age), then this investment is a significant determinant of the hospital's growth experience during the subsequent 10 years, i.e., between Time 1 (1951) and Time 2 (1960). Thus, the correlation between the percentage of payroll expenses in 1951 and the growth rate of technical facilities between 1951 and 1960 is $r = .20$; for the growth in the number of accreditations, $r = .26$; for the growth of the total payroll expense, $r = .13$. The total payroll expense, in turn, is one of the most important determinants of total hospital expenses between 1951 and 1960 ($r = .77$). A high payroll percentage at Time 1 also increases the likelihood that a given hospital will have a major medical school affiliation at Time 2 ($r = .14$).

Although data on community size at Time 1 (1951) were not available, it is safe to assume that the percentage of payroll expenses is positively related to community size. In other words, the more urbanized and complex the hospital environment, the higher the skill level of the hospital labor force and the larger the percentage of payroll expenses, holding autonomy and task complexity constant.

In order to gauge the joint effect of "internal" and "external" complexity on the modes of coordination, let us examine the results of an analysis of variance and covariance, with the four modes of coordination given in Table 37 as the dependent variables. In this analysis, organizational autonomy and the complexity of the task structure (control, teaching, and service) are the independent variables, but we are now controlling also for five additional variables: size of community, average length of stay, personnel/patient ratio, organizational size, and degree of functional specialization (Table 40). These five variables may be viewed as a continuum between external environmental complexity (community size) and internal complexity (here I am using functional specialization in deliberate contrast to departmental specialization, which is used as a dependent variable).

Table 40 has two parts. Part A shows the three main effects on the dependent variables alone; Part B adds the controls of the five additional variables.

The major result of this analysis is that the 12 main effects of autonomy and task complexity on the four modes of coordination are significantly reduced in almost all cases when the five intervening variables are controlled. This means that most of the differences between the 12 hospital types can to a considerable extent be "explained" by the control variables. However, in only three of the 12 effects can we say that the respective differences are "explained away": the difference between teaching and nonteaching hospitals with respect to hierarchical coordination, and the difference between psychiatric and general hospitals with respect to both administrative and structural coordination.

The teaching/nonteaching difference with respect to administrative coordination is slightly increased by controlling for the five variables, and the differences between types of ownership and control remain highly significant regardless of the use of control variables.

The patterns of variation summarized in Table 40 suggest that professionalization and hierarchical coordination are relatively strongly influenced by internal structural factors (see the relatively high service effects when using the controls), whereas administrative coordination is influenced differentially by internal and external factors.[27] In studying the determinants and consequences of an organization's degree of administrative bureaucratization, it is therefore necessary to consider the demographic and political context within which the organization operates, in addition to the specific influences of task and internal structural complexity.

As to professional coordination, we see that the main effects are reduced in comparison to the univariate analysis (Table 40, row 5 vs. row 1), but they are still significant. In other words, professional coordination is strongly tied to complexity of task structure and autonomy, even though external factors play an important role. Finally, it should be noted that the effect of ownership and control on structural coordination also remains relatively powerful, suggesting once again that this mode of coordination may be seen as an administrative device which is built into the structure of the organization. It is plausible, therefore, to continue to assume that ownership and control, in addition to reflecting relative budgetary independence, also represents factors such as managerial decision-making and administrative rationality.

The specific relation between size of community and hospital organization can now be evaluated as follows. Earlier, it was shown that psychiatric hospitals tend to be located in communities somewhat larger than those in which general hospitals are found;

Table 40
Effects of Control, Teaching Status, and Service on the Four Modes of Coordination: A) Alone; and B) Controlling for Community Size, Average Length of Stay, Personnel/Patient Ratio, Organizational Size, and Functional Specialization

	Main Effects			Interactions			
				First Order			Second Order
	Control	Teaching	Service	Control X Teaching	Control X Service	Teaching X Service	Order
			F-Ratio[a]				
A. Dependent Variables Alone:							
1. Professional Coordination	456.34	141.69	1,291.25	.93	30.44	51.84	5.82
2. Hierarchical Coordination	86.62	236.04	62.60	6.70	8.70	.45	1.38
3. Administrative Coordination	469.19	3.48	167.22	4.64	15.69	2.61	.87
4. Structural Coordination	325.02	1,106.31	317.90	12.95	25.16	10.54	.27
B. With Controls:							
5. Professional Coordination	175.00	46.13	168.15	.80	16.86	29.63	3.44
6. Hierarchical Coordination	25.25	1.61	27.54	.83	4.56	5.44	5.56
7. Administrative Coordination	420.71	5.93	.84	4.16	16.71	9.61	.62
8. Structural Coordination	199.57	268.22	3.61	4.08	21.33	10.09	.09
df₁=	2	1	1	2	2	1	2

[a]F-Ratios needed for significance at the .01 level: 4.60 ($df_1=2$); 6.64 ($df_1=1$); $df_2=3,532$ (for all effects).

293

teaching hospitals gravitate toward metropolitan communities, in contrast to nonteaching hospitals (Table 3). Now we can go one step further and conclude that the degree of complexity of the hospital environment is positively related to the complexity of the internal structure of the organization, especially in the case of the general and teaching hospitals, as compared to the psychiatric and nonteaching types.

This conclusion implies that specialized, unifunctional organizations have a lower rate of exchange with the external environment; they are more self-contained and structurally independent than nonspecialized, "diffuse," multifunctional, and diversified organizations. As a theoretical footnote to this conclusion, it may be suggested here that specialization does not necessarily lead to interdependence on all levels of social organization. Where the community or other supra-organizational social system constitutes the unit of analysis, specialized organizations may maintain some form of structural-functional autonomy, as compared to nonspecialized units.

As to the public psychiatric hospitals, this relative structural-functional independence could be accounted for by the nature of the patient population, which imposes strict limitations on what could be called the organization's "adaptive behavior." But length of stay does not provide a full explanation, since teaching hospitals have a longer average length of stay than nonteaching hospitals. Besides, even in the "nonautonomous" V.A. hospitals, where the patient population is quite homogeneous in certain respects, we find community size to be associated with internal structural variables.

Even if these conclusions are limited to organizational specialization in hospitals, the theoretical implications are of considerable interest for the study of the relationship between large social structures and the still larger societal environment. I am suggesting here that the system-subsystem model of that relationship has limited empirical application. In other words, even if we analyze simple formal organizations as systems whose subsystems, in turn, provide a systemic environment for still smaller subsystems, it does not follow that the organizations themselves are functionally specialized parts of the larger social system, e.g., the community.

We may, of course, single out the functionally specific characteristics or "social responsibilities" of mental hospitals in terms of one overall goal and specific goal-components. Parsons has done so by defining the goal of mental hospitals as coping "with the consequences for the individual patient and for patients as a social group, of a condition of mental illness."[28] Parsons further identifies the goal-components as custody, protection, socialization, and therapy. Finally, under the heading of "external functions," Parsons discusses "the relations of the mental hospital to the wider community," identifying, again, four specific

> boundary processes . . . [namely] . . . 1) the *legitimation* of the operation of the hospital in the community; 2) the processes involved in dealing with the *recipients* of the hospital's services, the patients, and above all, their families; 3) the process of acquiring the *facilities* necessary for carrying out its functions and 4) the ways in which the hospital is *integrated into the community* in which it operates.[29]

In this discussion there is no indication of *how* the mental hospital is empirically or structurally integrated into the wider community, and how this integration contrasts with that of other types of hospitals, e.g., the general hospital.[30]

On the basis of these considerations, it appears that the distinctions between specialized and nonspecialized (as well as between diversified and nondiversified) types of organizations prove to be important ones in the analysis of organizational patterns. Because of their theoretical implications, these distinctions may be brought to bear on the question of functional specialization at the inter-organizational and larger societal level.

From the analysis of the relative importance of external and internal factors, we can conclude that although it may be useful to analyze simple organizations in terms of their systemic characteristics, the applicability of the system model to the relation between organizations and their environment must be questioned, particularly since "external" or environmental variables have a differential effect on the internal organizational structure.

Specialized organizations are likely to be more self-contained, structurally independent systems than nonspecialized and diversified organizations. The latter, in turn, although internally more differentiated and complex, nevertheless are engaged in a greater degree of interchange with their environment. This suggests that the analysis of inter-organizational and organization-environment relationships may be more fruitful if conducted in terms of social process categories such as competition, conflict, exchange, and coalition, rather than in terms of subsystem interchange and structural-functional differentiation.

The formal-structural nature of organizations lends itself to some extent to analysis in structural-functional terms. However, as organizations become more complex, they become more intimately tied to the complexities and processes of the larger environment with permeable boundaries and a growing openness to change.[31]

Summary and Conclusions

In this chapter I have analyzed the phenomenon of organizational coordination from three perspectives: the internal division of labor, the nature of the task structure, and the characteristics of the organizational environment. It is generally taken for granted that complexity, i.e., the multiplicity and diversity of elements and relations, generates the need for coordination insofar as the organization is viewed as an entity and as a "going concern." But what kind of coordination or how much coordination is needed are open, empirical questions. This study has been primarily concerned with the kinds of coordination associated with certain kinds of structure, rather than with the question of how much coordination. To answer the latter question requires the use of definite criteria of operating efficiency and effectiveness in relation to coordination. Since organizations may be over- or under-coordinated, it would be necessary to determine adequate levels of coordination. For hospitals, such criteria are difficult to establish short of a comprehensive analysis of community health systems.

But it is possible to answer the question of what kind of coordination is needed, especially if we analyze hospitals as special cases of complex, formal, professionalized work organizations. For the purposes of that analysis, I have found the distinction between bureaucratic and nonbureaucratic modes of coordination relevant and useful. The assumption that bureaucratic modes of coordination are the most prevalent form of integration of the elements of a complex division of labor has not only been challenged, but can be modified by isolating various aspects of bureaucratization. Thus, I have shown that the complexity of the task structure in hospitals favors the development of an administrative-clerical staff, but not that of a bureaucratic hierarchy. Where a hierarchy exists, it is characterized by an upper echelon concentration of authority in the simpler, unifunctional, specialized organizations, a phenomenon which I have described in terms of the bureaucratization of professionals. But in the more complex, multifunctional, diversified organizations, bureaucratic authority is extensively delegated to lower levels of the organization, especially to the professionalized operating level.

In this last chapter in particular, I have focused on the question of what other kinds of coordination besides bureaucratic ones are operative in hospitals, and how nonbureaucratic modes of coordination relate to the bureaucratic ones. For this purpose, I have redefined the concept of departmental specialization in terms of "structural coordination" and that of professionalization in terms of "professional coordination." I have shown that both departmental specialization and professionalization can be seen as intervening between the task structure and the bureaucratic modes of coordination. Thus, a high level of departmental specialization becomes itself a factor of coordination. Administrative and bureaucratic-hierarchical modes of coordination are gradually shifted from the organizational level to subunit levels, a phenomenon typical of processes of delegation and decentralization. A high level of departmental specialization will not only increase the interdependence among subunits, but will also generate new modes of lateral communication and interaction. It is likely that lateral transactions include such processes as competition and conflict as well as various forms of cooperation.

While the nature and rate of such transactions can be observed empirically, I have confined myself here to spelling out the logical implications of a high level of departmental specialization for lateral coordination. The Gini coefficient of concentration and similar indexes of structural characteristics are particularly well suited for studying the internal structural complexity of organizations within a comparative-quantitative framework.

The second nonbureaucratic mode of coordination intervening between task structure and bureaucratization is professionalization. I have shown that the degree of professionalization and of departmental specialization interact in conditioning the relation between the complexity of the task structure and bureaucratic-administrative coordination. Thus, Stinchcombe's hypothesis as to the coordinating function of professionalization of the labor force appears to hold under conditions of relatively low internal structural complexity. I have suggested that under these conditions, division of labor does not imply a high degree of functional specificity; professionals will tend to act as generalists and are likely to share at least some functions with others, with the result of some overlap of tasks. The generalist definition of professionalization is consistent with Stinchcombe's use of the term.

However, in organizations with a more complex internal structure (due to a more complex task structure and technology) the coordinating effect of professionalization disappears. The professionalization of the labor force is accompanied by an increasing specificity of functions, contributing to an increasing need for the administrative-regulatory coordination of professional specialists. This finding is inconsistent with Stinchcombe's hypothesis because of the changed nature and meaning of professionalization. Our data suggest, in general, that the nature of professional work is contingent on the organizational context, i.e., on the type and degree of division of labor. Under conditions of high departmental specialization, the nature of professional work is transformed by becoming itself more task-specific, differentiated, and specialized. Obviously, this idea can be proposed only in the form of a hypothesis which needs to be tested on the basis of specific operational distinctions between generalist and specialist forms of professionalization.

Further attempts to answer the question of what kind of coordination is prevalent in different types of organizational structure have led to the construction of an empirical classification of hospitals in terms of task structure, size, internal complexity, and modes of coordination. The resulting typology of hospital organization shows that simple organizational forms have fewer dominant modes of coordination, and that the dominant mode tends to be hierarchical coordination. The more complex organizational forms not only have a larger number of dominant modes of coordination, but they also tend toward the use of structural and administrative modes rather than hierarchical ones. Professional coordination emerges at a moderate level of internal complexity, but disappears in its generalist form at the higher levels where professionals as specialists generate new problems of coordination rather than contributing to their reduction or solution.

Finally, the conceptual and empirical contrast between simple and complex types of internal structure has suggested a distinction between organizations on the basis of the degree to which they approach the characteristics of a system. Coordination can be seen as a system requirement in the sense that there are mechanisms which maintain the adaptive capacity of the organization by compensating for input deficiencies and by absorbing stress, malfunctions, incompatibilities, and conflict. In this view, complexity is assumed to generate the need for coordination, and perhaps even to require the simultaneous performance of different coordinating mechanisms. By assuming some minimum of adaptive behavior on the part of the organization, the stage is set for further assumptions about functional substitutes and alternatives. Unfortunately, the hypotheses derived from such concepts and assumptions are difficult to prove and impossible to disprove.

Nevertheless, it is true that certain types of organizations display a relative maximum of internal dynamics, with a relative minimum of interdependence with the external environment, and with few external influences operating on internal organizational structure and processes. Moreover, if departmental specialization is seen as a form of process specialization, it is likely to represent the internal structure maximally where there are few or only one major purpose or objective, i.e., where there is a high degree of organizational specialization. Such organizational systems exhibit a low degree of interdependence with the environment by virtue of a low degree of interchange with other organizations, low turnover of clientele or inmates, or a relatively high degree of isolation from the larger society, as is the case with large custodial mental hospitals. By the same token, one finds a comparatively high level of internal interdependence among parts and subsystems insofar as they have become differentiated in such organizations.

Similarly, the structural differences between nondiversified and diversified organizations manifest themselves, among other things, in the higher degree of professionalization and functional specialization of the latter. Here, the distinctions among specialties and among skill levels accentuate and articulate the diversity or conflict between major objectives and carry it over to different organizational levels. It is, therefore, not surprising to find a lower degree of interdependence between internal structural factors and the modes of coordination in the diversified organizations, especially in the teaching general hospitals. In fact, it is in this type of hospital where we encounter a kind of heterogeneous, open, pluralistic structure. Its parts are neither consensually nor structurally fully integrated. Nevertheless, from the point of view of professional and technical services, the organization performs on a high level. Reader and Goss, although discussing hospitals in general, have suggested that "possibly, in order to achieve their diverse purposes, hospitals must contain an irreducible residue of contradiction and resultant strain which may be mitigated but not eliminated entirely."[32]

In nondiversified organizations, on the other hand, the differentiation of work functions within the limits of specialization imposed by the relatively homogeneous nature of tasks and objectives. In this sense, the small community general hospital and the voluntary psychiatric hospital exemplify, to some extent, the qualities of the natural system model, in contrast to the more rationally planned, diversified types of organization, such as a large teaching hospital or medical center.[33]

In the community general hospital, functional *specialization* does not necessarily imply a high degree of functional *specificity*, so that professionals are more likely to share at least some functions with other specialists (e.g., nurses and general practitioners, aides, technicians, etc.). It is in the nondiversified organizational system, then, that Durkheim's general hypothesis finds one of its major applications, because functional specialization can be assumed to imply, or at least be correlated with, functional interdependence.

It should be noted, however, that the idea of "organic solidarity" does not only have "natural system" implications. After all, Durkheim's analysis does provide for the emergence of rational rules and the exercise of coordinating functions by some central agency.

In sum, we may conclude that diversified organizations are found to possess a higher degree of interdependence with the external environment and with other organizations. In the case of teaching hospitals, this is evidenced by their dependence on a special patient population, on medical schools, and on service organizations responsible for the maintenance of complex equipment and facilities.

Finally, type of ownership and control has, by definition, certain implications for the degree of interdependence between the organizational system and the environment. The term "organizational autonomy" suggests a certain intensity of interchange between an organization and its environment. In this study I have found a somewhat higher degree of autonomy in the case of both voluntary and federal hospitals, and somewhat more "controlled" independence, i.e., less autonomy, in the case of state and local governmental hospitals. This conclusion, however, requires further support on the basis of an adequate operational distinction between de jure (legal-political) and de facto (economic) autonomy.

Notes

1. See Chapters 3 and 7.
2. Note that the within-group homogeneity is very high, as shown by the fact that all within-group correlations are higher than that for the total.

3. Note that in these correlations the respective structural components used (per cent of professional nurses, per cent of administrative-clerical staff) are removed from the Gini index so as to avoid spurious correlation.

4. This latter interpretation is supported by the fact that the structural measure of delegation discussed earlier (relative skewness across 4 hierachical levels in nursing) is positively related to departmental specialization, with r=.31 for all U.S. hospitals.

5. Stanley H. Udy, *Organization of Work* (New Haven, Conn.: Human Relations Area File Press, 1959), p. 40.

6. This phenomenon is, of course, what Durkheim refers to as "organic solidarity." The more rationally oriented theory of March and Simon refers to it as "coordination by plan" based on process specialization, while Coleman has described it in terms of the mitigating effects of social structure on community conflict, and Gouldner has dealt with it in terms of the need for functional autonomy. Emile Durkheim, *The Division of Labor in Society*, tr. George Simpson (Glencoe, Ill.: The Free Press, 1947), pp. 219-229; James G. March and Herbert A. Simon, *Organizations* (New York: Wiley, 1958), pp. 113-171; James S. Coleman, *Community Conflict* (Glencoe Ill.: The Free Press, 1957), pp. 21-23. See also Luther Gulick and L. Urwick, eds., *Papers on the Science of Administration* (New York: Institute of Public Administration, 1937), pp. 3-45 159-169; Henry C. Metcalf and L. Urwick, eds., *Dynamic Administration: The Collected Papers of Mary Parker Follet* (New York: Harper, 1940), pp. 30-49, 71-117; Chester I. Barnard, *The Functions of the Executive* (Cambridge, Mass.: Harvard University Press, 1962), pp. 82-95, 127-138; A. W. Gouldner," Reciprocity and Autonomy in Functional Theory," in Lewellyn Gross, ed., *Symposium on Sociological Theory* (Evanston, Ill.: Row, Peterson, 1959), pp. 241-270; Louis R. Pondy, "Organizational Conflict: Concepts and Models," *Administrative Science Quarterly*, 12 (1967), 296-320.

7. For a discussion of the Lorenz curve, see W. Allen Wallis and Harry V. Roberts, *Statistics* (Glencoe, Ill.: The Free Press, 1957), pp. 257-258. The calculation and graphic representation of the Gini coefficient was adapted from John K. Wright, "Some Measures of Distribution," *Annals of the Association of American Geographers*, 27 (1937), 177-211.

Useful discussions of the logic of the Gini coefficient and its application to income and other distributions are contained in: Mary Jean Bowman, "A Graphical Analysis of Personal Income Distribution in the United States," *American Economics Review*, 35 (1945), 608-628; Lee Soltow, "The Distribution of Income Related to Changes in the Distribution of Education, Age, and Occupation," *The Review of Economics and Statistics*, 42 (1960), 450-453; and James Morgan, "The Anatomy of Income Distribution," *The Review of Economics and Statistics*, 44 (1962), 281.

8. For a lucid discussion of the "study of logical implications," see James S. Coleman, *Introduction to Mathematical Sociology* (New York: The Free Press, 1964), pp. 479-491; see also Dorwin Cartwright and Frank Harary, "Structural Balance: A Generalization of Heider's Theory,"

Psychological Review, 63 (1956), 227-293; Richard E. Walton, "Theory of Conflict in Lateral Organizational Relationships," in J. R. Lawrence, ed., *Operational Research and the Social Sciences* (London: Tavistock, 1966), pp. 409-426; Richard E. Walton and Robert B. McKersie, *A Behavioral Theory of Labor Negotiations* (New York: McGraw-Hill, 1965); Russell L. Ackoff, "Structural Conflicts within Organizations," in J.R. Lawrence, ed., op. cit., pp. 427-438; and Dorwin Cartwright, "The Potential Contribution of Graph Theory to Organization Theory," in Mason Haire, ed., *Modern Organizational Theory* (New York: Wiley, 1959), pp. 254-271.

9. Albert F. Wessen, "Hospital Ideology and Communication between Ward Personnel," E. Gartley Jaco, ed., *Patients, Physicians, and Illness* (Glencoe, Ill.: The Free Press, 1958), pp. 453-458.

10. Amos Hawley, *Human Ecology, A Theory of Community Structure* (New York: Ronald Press, 1950), p. 220.

11. As I had indicated already in Chapter 3, the Gini index involves essentially the same logic as the Gibbs-Martin index, although the latter is calculated on the basis of squared percentages rather than cumulated percentages; see Jack P. Gibbs and Walter T. Martin, "Urbanization, Technology, and the Division of Labor," *American Sociological Review*, 27 (1962), 667-677, and Jack P. Gibbs and Harley L. Browning, "The Division of Labor, Technology, and the Organization of Production in Twelve Countries," *American Sociological Review*, 31 (1966), 81-92. The measure has since been used in a similar way by others; see, e.g., William A. Rushing, "Hardness of Material as Related to Division of Labor in Manufacturing Industries," *Aministrative Science Quarterly*, 13 (1968), 229-245; and "The Effects of Industry Size and Division of Labor on Administration," *Administrative Science Quarterly*, 12 (1967), 273-295. Basically, then, the Gibbs-Martin index is, like the Gini index, a measure of relative concentration, since it becomes zero when the total labor force is concentrated in only one category. Gibbs and Martin used the following formula: $1 - [\Sigma x^2 / (\Sigma x)^2]$, where x is the number of the economically active population in a given industry. This is summed over all industry categories, thus adding up to the total labor force. A limitation of the measure is that its maximum is always a function of the number of categories among which a given population is distributed. For example, Gibbs and Martin originally used nine industry categories; the maximum value the measure can attain is .8889, or 8/9, i.e., $\frac{n-1}{n}$, where n is the number of industry categories. In adapting this measure for the present study, two modifications were made. First, in order to have this measure range from zero to one, it was multiplied by the factor $\frac{n}{n-1}$ Clearly, if n is very large, the value of this factor approaches unity. For 39 occupational categories, for example, the maximum value would be 38/39, or .974. If multiplied by 39/38, or 1.026, the value is adjusted upward and approximates 1.000.

The second modification was made to simplify the computations for each individual hospital. Since the various occupational categories and components had been calculated as a percentage of the total hospital labor force, it was easy to calculate the measure on the basis of percentages rather than actual numbers, since the denominator $(\Sigma x)^2$, if expressed in per cent, becomes 1.0. The formula for the modified measure is $[1-(\Sigma p^2)] [\frac{n}{n-1}]$ or $\frac{n(1-\Sigma p^2)}{n-1}$ where p is the percentage of personnel in a given occupational category or component of the total hospital labor force.

For the hospitals, this measure of occupational-functional differentiation was computed twice, once on the basis of the 39 occupational categories, and once on the basis of seven major organizational components to be described below. If in a given hospital one occupational category is relatively large, while relatively less personnel is allocated to other positions, the index will be correspondingly lower. Since the measure involves the square of the respective percentages, it gives relatively more weight to the larger categories than to the smaller ones. If a category is zero, i.e., if there is no personnel allocated to it, the index will be lower since the factor $\frac{n}{n-1}$ remains constant.

The correlation between the Gini and the Gibbs-Martin indexes is high enough to make it plausible that both measure the same phenomenon ($r=.95$ for the 3,544 hospitals, as well as all 6,825 U.S. hospitals). In all fairness to Gibbs and his associates, it should be stressed that they explicitly rejected the interpretation of their index in terms of interdependence. While this limitation is probably justified, in general, and applies to the Gini index as well, I am arguing for such an interpretation on the grounds of the logical implications of structural balance for coordination, as well as of the specific assumption of an interdependent work process in hospitals. Sociologically, interdependence gives rise to various forms of cooperation and exchange, as well as strategies of competition and conflict to maximize autonomy of subunits. The indicators of the actual social processes involved may well be frequency and types of communication and contacts between departments, functions, or categories of personnel.

12. The evolutionary-developmental analogy implied in these statements must at this relatively modest "level" of general theoretical development in the social sciences be treated as largely heuristic, i.e., as a conceptual crutch rather than as an explanatory device.

13. The ideal-typical contradistinction between generalist and specialist professionalization can be no more than a heuristic device at this point since there was no clear-cut measure available for either. But it should be noted that these two forms of professionalization are not opposite poles of one continuum, but two separate variables. In other words, even though a high value for one will *tend* to be associated with a low value for the other, it is conceivable that organizations have, e.g., high levels of *both* generalist and specialist professionalization at the same time.

14. On the basis of similar findings by other students of organizations, one could further generalize that this alternative becomes relevant primarily under conditions of internal structural change, instability, and uncertainty. Thus, bureaucratic coordination may be required for the accomplishment of routine tasks under stable conditions, while novel, emergent situations might either provoke charismatic leadership or demand reliance on

generalist professional judgment. The innovative leadership, spirit of inquiry, or creativity of professionals can, of course, be viewed as a charismatic element.

15. It may be suggested that under these conditions, division of labor does not necessarity imply a high degree of functional specificity so that generalist professionals are likely to share at least some functions with others resulting in some overlap of tasks, i.e., in a more diffuse content of the division of labor. This overlap, in turn, makes it more likely for professionals to be oriented toward the needs and problems of the larger organization, i.e., it implies the "local" orientation of the home-guard among professionals.

16. Hughes has pointed out that an organizational setting provides both context and impetus for the increased specialization of professionals. Rossi has described the same phenomenon in relation to research organizations. Everett C. Hughes, "Professions," *Daedalus*, XCII (1963), 663; Peter H. Rossi, "Researchers, Scholars, and Policy-Makers: The Politics of Large-Scale Research," *Daedalus*, XCIII (1964), 1151-1153.

17. In his earlier as well as his recent concern with professionalization and new types and forms of professionalism, Wilensky suggests that professional and bureaucratic (organizational) elements tend to mix and interpenetrate. Although I question the utility of Wilensky's ideal-typical conception of professions and would rather assume a continuum of professionalization, I concur strongly with his view of newly emerging structural forms which combine elements from both the professional and bureaucratic models and which represent mixed forms of organizational control. Harold L. Wilensky, "The Professionalization of Everyone?" *American Journal of Sociology*, LXX (1964), 137-158; see also his *Intellectuals in Labor Unions: Organizational Pressure on Professional Roles* (Glencoe, Ill.: The Free Press, 1956), pp. 196-208. This conclusion is essentially shared by Louis C. Goldberg and his associates in their article "Local-Cosmopolitan: Unidimensional or Multidimensional?" *American Journal of Sociology*, 70 (1965), 704-710; see also Warren G. Bennis' conception of future organizations in his *Changing Organizations* (New York: McGraw-Hill, 1966), pp. 7-14.

18. If the administrative and the supervisory functions of bureaucratic professionals were measured independently, it could probably be shown that only the hierarchical element decreases with increasing departmental specialization and professionalization, but not the administrative functions of professionals, at least not to the same extent. Only highly valued professionals might be able to delegate most administrative functions to others, while they themselves become increasingly involved in consultation and policy-making.

19. See Parsons' conception of professions in terms of functional specificity relative to the larger social system: Talcott Parsons, "The Professions and Social Structure," in his *Essays on Sociological Theory* (Glencoe, Ill.: The Free Press, 1949), pp. 198-199.

20. See also Goldberg et al., loc. cit.

21. For critical discussions of the consequences of such technocracies, see Robert Boguslaw, *The New Utopians: A Study of System Design and Social Change* (Englewood Cliffs, N.J.: Prentice Hall, 1965); Jacques Ellul, *The Technological Society* (New York: Vintage Books, 1967). A more "tolerant" view is expressed in John K. Galbraith, *The New Industrial State* (New York: Signet Books, 1967).

22. For example, some of these phenomena have been documented for colleges and universities: Paul F. Lazarsfeld and Wagner Thielens, *The Academic Mind* (Glencoe, Ill.: The Free Press, 1958); Theodore Caplow and Reece McGee, *The Academic Marketplace* (New York: Basic Books, 1958); James A. Davis, *Great Aspirations* (Chicago: Aldine, 1964); Albert Somit and Joseph Tanenhaus, *American Political Science, A Profile of a Discipline* (New York: Atherton Press, 1964).

23. The hospital numbers used in Table 38 are given in the preceding table, where they appear below the N of each of the 12 hospital groups. The cutting points dividing each set of 12 means into "high" and "low" were established by identifying the two major ranges or clusters of "high" and "low" values among the 12 groups. The clusters and corresponding cutting points are as follows:

Cluster Values

Mode of Coordination	Low range	High range	Cutting point
Hierarchical	.10 - .18	.27 - .48	.25
Professional	.05 - .08	.12 - .27	.10
Structural	.43 - .52	.56 - .72	.55
Administrative	.06 - .09	.11 - 18	.10

Dividing the variables into three or more groups, rather than dichotomizing them, would yield essentially the same results, but would make the presentation much more complex.

24. See Hanan C. Selvin and Warren O. Hagstrom, "The Empirical Classification of Formal Groups," *American Sociological Review*, XXVIII (1963), 399-411.

25. See William G. Summer, *Folkways* (Boston: Ginn, 1907), p. 54; see also A. W. Gouldner, "Organizational Analysis," in Merton, *Sociology Today*, pp. 400-407.

26. In my initial definition of autonomy in Chapter 3 and in the context of my discussion of the "extent of external relations" in Chapter 5, I had pointed out that organizational autonomy must be seen in terms of both of these dimensions. The absence of an adequate operational distinction between these two aspects of autonomy in the present study should, obviously, not be construed as a case against its conceptual validity and empirical usefulness.

27. See also the differences among the R^2's for hierarchical and administrative coordination in Table 36, row 4 vs. row 8.

28. Talcott Parsons, "The Mental Hospital as a Type of Organization," in

Milton Greenblatt et al., eds., *The Patient and the Mental Hospital* (Glencoe, Ill.: The Free Press, 1957), p. 109.

29. Ibid., p. 112.

30. Parsons' analysis applies, of course, also to the general hospital with only minor modifications, and is therefore not particularly useful from the point of view of the distinction made here; cf. Talcott Parsons, *Structure and Process in Modern Societies* (New York: The Free Press, 1960), pp. 44-47.

31. The development of coordinating agencies and roof organizations such as the American Hospital Association itself is a case in point, although there are bound to be a variety of types of interorganizational relationships; see, e.g., Eugene Litwak and Lydia F. Hylton, "Interorganizational Analysis," *Administrative Science Quarterly*, VI (1962), 395-420; and Sol Levine and Paul E. White, "Exchange as a Conceptual Framework for the Study of Interorganizational Relationships," *Administrative Science Quarterly*, 5 (1961), 583-601.

Part IV: Epilogue

11

Uses and Limits of Bureaucracy

This study of hospitals as formal organizations has almost certainly contributed little to the understanding of the subjective experience of being a patient or a worker in a hospital. But I should like to hope it has contributed something to the understanding of hospitals as professional work organizations and as general types of organizational structure. To understand professional organizations, one could also have studied universities, welfare organizations, or research institutes. But the modern general hospital is probably more complex than any of these other types. Moreover, the range of variation in the complexity of the task structure and the internal division of labor, as well as in size and in the degree of professionalization, has made it possible to use a fairly broad comparative framework for the analysis of hospitals in terms of general organizational characteristics. For this reason, I am confident that many of the findings of this study can be used as working hypotheses in the study of other professional organizations. Insofar as the hospital is a prototype of modern work organizations, the findings and conclusions of this study may be applicable to a whole range of organizations, especially to those in which bureaucratic modes of coordination are gradually being replaced by non-bureaucratic ones (see also Appendix G). I shall briefly review the major findings and conclusions, suggest the outlines of an "optimal" rather than an "average" type of hospital structure, and finally, draw some inferences from this study for a new theoretical conception of organizations.

Major Findings and Conclusions

If the ownership and control of a hospital represents a significant aspect of the nature and amount of control over political and economic resources, and if teaching status and type of medical service indicate something about the complexity of the task structure of the hospital and its requisite technology, then we can safely conclude that both the institutional structure of the larger society as well as the level of medical technology are powerful determinants of a hospital's internal structure and operation. Let us look at the implications of this statement for a particular set of examples, namely psychiatric as compared to general hospitals.

Psychiatric hospitals are predominantly publicly controlled and operated organizations in the United States. Compared to the few private psychiatric hospitals, the state mental hospitals are large, understaffed, and technologically inferior. Such a comparative statement means that certain psychiatric hospitals do not *have* to be large and inadequately staffed; the fact that others are indicates that the majority of mental patients are not treated on the same level as medical-surgical patients, that the budgets allocated for mental hospitals are inadequate for the purpose of running them, and that most state legislatures and local governments do not deem it necessary to allocate more than a token portion of the tax dollar to certain types of health care. Thus, while a high level of technology, for example, is available and could potentially determine the structure of all mental hospitals both within and across different communities, it does not in fact do so because of the selective influence of social, political, and economic factors. In other words, the availability of an adequate technology or an adequate staff does not guarantee that they will in fact be chosen and utilized as instruments of public service and welfare.

While general hospitals have a comparatively more uniform structure suggesting the strong influence of task structure and technology, there are nevertheless differences which reflect the element of social choice in the allocation of resources, the use of technology, and the utilization of manpower. Therefore, technology, division of labor, and the use of specialized skills and knowledge are dependent variables in a larger sense, even though they do also constitute "independent" sources of variation for other aspects of an organization's internal structure.

In short, technological determinism provides an insufficient explanatory framework for analyzing variations in organizational structure. But by the same token, a one-sided ownership or management-oriented framework would be inadequate. Such a framework is likely to underestimate the dynamics of technological innovation which makes it possible, though not in itself necessary, to prolong life or prevent suffering. For example, it is often for technological reasons that hospitals cannot be run like a business since community and professional pressures to acquire a certain technical apparatus or to employ a specialist may not be justifiable on economic grounds.

In other words, to explain the variation in task structure, technology, division of labor, and coordination, one cannot appeal to the somewhat trite observation that all hospitals share the basic goal of patient care since they do so in various ways and to different degrees. Defined in such a general way, the goal itself becomes a constant and therefore is incapable of explaining structural variations *among* hospitals even though it may serve to distinguish *between* hospitals and other types of organizations.

Turning now to the question of coordination, we can draw the following conclusions from the analysis: the greater the degree of complexity of the task structure, the greater the likelihood that different modes of coordination will be prevalent, and that bureaucratic-hierarchical modes become less significant for overall integration and are at best shifted to the subunit level. This means, first of all, that different modes of coordination may coexist in the same organization, i.e., that they are complementary rather than merely alternatives. Secondly, this means that the administration of complex tasks does not require the development or exercise of hierarchical authority, but rather discourages it. Where hierarchical patterns of coordination persist under conditions of complexity, they must therefore be explained on the basis of factors other than complexity of task structure, technology, and division of labor. For example, it is conceivable that professional, i.e., semi-charismatic, authority structures maintain hierarchical forms of coordination where they are not technically or functionally required. Voluntary psychiatric teaching hospitals appear to be a case in point. These hospitals have a fairly rigid professional authority structure which is reflected in an unusually high administrative-supervisory ratio in nursing and a concentration of bureaucratic authority at the middle levels of the nursing hierarchy rather than in delegation to lower levels. It is perhaps not accidental that in these specialized organizations which do have an unusually high level of internal structural complexity, professional authority dominates the organizational control structure to a greater extent than in less professionalized and complex psychiatric hospitals, or in the multifunctional or diversified general hospitals. Obviously, professional and organizational concerns may coincide more fully in these organizations which are more specialized as a whole, but which are also comparatively more professionalized and complex than others.

In this particular case, task complexity and division of labor are quite limited in explaining the modes of coordination. In fact, the combination of internal complexity and high level of professionalization within a specialized organization points to the characteristics of "meritocracy," i.e., a system of rule on the basis of competence and excellence. Such a system is a special case of a bureaucracy in which rank is largely determined by expertise and ability rather than by the delegation and derivation of authority from one source of legitimate power at the top of the organization.

For all these reasons, the voluntary psychiatric hospital provides a form of negative evidence which strengthens the conclusions for the other hospital types.

To say that hierarchical forms of coordination disappear where structural ones develop is another way of saying that the whole organization becomes decentralized. Departmental specialization implies delegation of authority to the departmental and subunit level. But we do not know whether delegation continues downward *within* the departments. One may speculate on theoretical and empirical grounds that decentralization at the level of the organization may provoke a higher degree of centralization within the departments. In the analysis of medical technology, for example, we found that the delegation of technical functions from salaried physicians to medical technicians not only leads to a numerical increase in this latter category but also to the formation of a hierarchy of technical experts in which qualified technicians occupy an intermediate position between physicians and subprofessional technical personnel.

As to the relative size of the administrative-clerical staff, long used as a measure of internal bureaucratization, the present study demonstrates the strong influence of external bureaucratization (V.A. hospitals) and of the complexity of the task structure, particularly the number of major objectives. Contrary to the widely held stereotypes about bureaucracy, organizational size has generally a negative effect on internal bureaucratization. However, the effect is strongest for intermediate size categories. There is some evidence to suggest that in very small and in very large organizations the level of internal bureaucratization is somewhat higher, but probably for different reasons.

In small organizations, i.e., hospitals with fewer than 25 patients, it may not be possible to reduce the administrative overhead effectively, since certain basic functions of communication, administrative coordination, and accounting have to be performed. While both medium and large organizations undoubtedly benefit from economies of scale, it is conceivable that in the very large organizations new problems of communication and administration have to be dealt with so that a slightly larger administrative-clerical staff is required. However, the new problems of communication probably derive from geographical dispersion of physical and administrative units, i.e., from the influence of size on ecology, rather than from a larger number of relationships and interactions. Thus, very large hospitals tend to comprise various buildings, annexes, and units which are located at some distance from the "old" building or the administrative headquarters. The simultaneous geographical and administrative deconcentration therefore gives rise to new administrative staffs within subunits, thus breaking the effect of economies of scale.

On the whole, organizational size as measured in terms of task size is a much less important factor in coordination than the complexity of the task structure. Size becomes relevant in two ways: by its differential association with task complexity and autonomy and by its strong positive effect on technology and internal division of labor, especially the degree of functional specialization. Thus, increasing size contributes to the process of internal differentiation and change, especially in a heterogeneous, pluralistic setting, because here increasing size creates new possibilities and probabilities of interaction within, and interdependence between, subunits. Size therefore counteracts the forces of integration and control. In other words, the empirically negative relation between size and the four modes of coordination, especially the bureaucratic ones, suggests that increasing organizational size contributes to further fragmentation, heterogeneity, differentiation, and diversification. In general hospitals, this process implies (up to a point) increasing functional interdependence, setting in motion processes of lateral coordination. In psychiatric hospitals and in the diversified teaching and research hospitals, increasing size may generate new mechanisms of centralized control, hierarchical in the former, mechanical-automatic in the latter.

The redefinition of departmental specialization in terms of structural coordination (a form of coordination by plan) and professionalization (a form of coordination by feedback) has made it possible to study the relation between division of labor and coordination from a somewhat more complex perspective than has been the case in previous studies of organizations. In fact, I have attempted to explore this relation between complexity and control from several different perspectives simultaneously. I had hypothesized, following Anderson-Warkov and Stinchcombe, that the relative size of the administrative-clerical staff varies directly with the internal division of labor but inversely with the professionalization of the labor force. While sustained at the zero-order level, these hypotheses can be specified by a multivariate analysis where the *level* of the internal division of labor is itself controlled. On a low level of complexity, internal bureaucratization varies directly with the division of labor, but inversely with professionalization.

On a high level of complexity, both relations are reversed: bureaucratization varies directly with professionalization, but inversely with the division of labor. I have suggested that a theoretical explanation of these empirical generalizations rests on certain dialectical properties of the division of labor. Under conditions of low task complexity and correspondingly low division of labor (a likely though not necessary correspondence) significant aspects of the work process are performed and controlled by the general professional practitioner (or the highly skilled craftsman). Insofar as increasing division of labor requires administrative coordination, it will be performed in competition and even conflict with the domain of professional control. At high levels of task complexity and internal division of labor, professional skills are likely to be of a specialist nature which contribute to further division of labor, therefore requiring further administrative coordination. At the same time, the division of labor reaches a level of complexity where further increases of administrative coordination have negative effects on the division of labor if and insofar as the former remains essentially *external* to the work process. I am suggesting, then, that in hospitals the division of labor generates its own structural coordination at a point where a quantitative increase in occupational specialization implies a qualitative change in the character of professional work and in the nature of work coordination and control. In other words, if at high levels of task complexity coordination is not built into work process, external forms of coordination (here I mean both hierarchical and administrative specialization) are not only ineffective, but dysfunctional and "counterproductive."

I am, of course, assuming that the hospitals under study are functioning entities, at least at the time of data collection, and that their continued existence is evidence for some minimum viability. This assumption is strengthened by the fact that the twelve hospital groups comprise all hospitals in that category, not just a type case or a sample.

"Structural coordination," as used here, refers not to a mystical process of self-actualization of a latent structure, but to the interaction between subunits, departments, and groups in an organization in which competition is eventually regulated and conflicts are eventually resolved. Thus, modern organizations, including hospitals, find it increasingly useful to hire generalists of various kinds, persons skilled in the coordination of diverse elements of a given work process, so as to counteract the destructive potential of further and further specialization.

In spite of the assumption of the continued viability of very complex hospitals, it is entirely conceivable that this dialectical change in the division of labor terminates a hospital's capacity to provide comprehensive patient and medical care. For example, a hospital may degenerate into a loosely structured, unstable form of group medical practice where individual specialists (even general practitioners have now "achieved" the status of specialists in family medicine!) give care on an ad hoc basis, compete for patients, and use the hospital as an extension of their private practice.

Moreover, there is no reason why organizational change in hospitals may not take revolutionary forms, with various groups polarized so as to act with and against each other; for example, patients against staff, e.g., in large mental hospitals,[1] professional specialties and subspecialties against others,[2] professionals against administrators, generalists against specialists, teaching and research staff against service staff (or teaching-oriented students against research-oriented faculty in universities), unskilled personnel (kitchen workers or aides, for example) against skilled and professional personnel. One usually expects the rules of civil discourse and interaction to prevail in established institutions and organizations. But there is nothing to prevent us from transferring to hospitals the likelihood of unexpected events occurring in other contexts, such as internal opposition and protest in universities, professional associations, social work agencies, political parties (left, center, and right), and research institutes.

The possibility of group conflict among staff groups in hospitals, or between patients and staff signifies the transformation of hospitals from work organizations to voluntary associations. Work organizations, in their emphasis on productivity, output, efficiency, and discipline, are frequently seen as operating outside democratic rules and procedures. Bureaucratic and charismatic authority, in fact, are always ademocratic and usually anti-democratic, although both may, of course, be employed in the service of a democratic cause. Questioning the basis of legitimacy is one of the most effective challenges to established authority. It arises from the development of alternative bases of legitimacy which, in turn, are generated by new skills and departmental specialization, by internal incompatibilities and contradictions between specific and general goals, and by learning from the experiences, successes, and mistakes of other similar systems undergoing rapid transformation.

Insofar as task complexity is a factor in the development of internal structural complexity, it will contribute to such democratizing processes so that the most complex structures are most open to internal and external pressures toward change, and are also the ones most likely to undergo rapid change. Hospitals in transition to a larger, diversified organizational structure do probably have a much smaller margin of stability than either the large psychiatric hospitals or the small community general hospitals. Thus, it is perhaps only in the latter where Durkheim's organic solidarity based on functional interdependence is operative. The large teaching general hospitals and medical centers are, from this perspective, beyond the optimal stage of organically integrated systems.

One could argue that as structural coordination based on departmental specialization becomes itself an inadequate mode of coordination, as in highly diversified organizations, the internal stability is gradually superseded by an increasing interdependence and interpenetration of the organization with the external environment and with other organizations, e.g., through various forms of affiliation and association. Whether such interdependence with the environment is functional for the organization's adaptation or survival depends on the criteria used in defining organizational boundaries, as well as on the nature of adaptation. Thus, both rigid *and* flexible organizational boundaries may be functional for adaptation, a proposition difficult to prove or disprove. The available evidence from this study suggests that psychiatric hospitals tend to operate more as closed systems, whereas teaching general hospitals appear to have an open, pluralistic structure to which systems models of organizations are not easily applicable, even if compromise concepts such as "open system" or "dynamic equilibrium" are used. The complexity of the task structure, the internal division of labor, and the external organizational environment thus appear to converge in favoring a flexible organizational type with permeable boundaries and a sufficiently responsive control structure which allows for internal change, and which is amorphous enough not to be threatened by external change.

Let us now look at an optimal type of hospital structure in more quantitative terms, but focusing on certain aspects of quality. We will see that this model hospital is in some (though by no means all) respects approximated by that open, pluralistic cluster of specialized activities called a general teaching hospital or medical center.

The Model Hospital: A Structural Profile

The well-known common sense "logic" of not considering ends in themselves without a realistic assessment of the means has an old, venerable history in human affairs. The "radical" decision-makers have often been put on the defensive by the "gradualists" in that the latter have claimed they reached the same goals, or only marginally different ones, by small increments and, on the whole, by exerting less strenuous effort. While the incremental decision-makers have emphasized the attainment of given goals, the radicals have constantly asked the question "which goals?"; they have been concerned with "what is to be done?" rather than with "how is it done?"[3]

In this book, I have essentially considered the question of hospital organization in terms of "how is it done?", i.e., what are the dominant patterns and types, what are the structural variations, and what are the conditions of variation. Let us now look at the average pattern of hospital organization and use it as a baseline from which to project the structural profile of an optimum pattern; a model hospital. This comparison is more than the construction of an ideal type: it forces us to consider a sociological model in terms of social policy, i.e., a set of value judgments, and then to specify the conditions under which the model can be realized. Rather than focusing on the explanations of the current state of affairs reflected in the average, we consciously seek to create a future state of affairs by investigating how it can be brought about.[4]

The basic ingredients of comprehensive patient care can be defined as medical care, nursing care, medical technology, maintenance, coordination, and context. For purposes of operationalizing these six ingredients, let us reconsider the following indicators for each:

1. *Medical Care*
   a. the proportion of physicians employed by the hospital (of total labor force)
   b. the net autopsy rate
2. *Nursing Care*
   a. the proportion of graduate professional nurses (of total)
   b. the proportion of subprofessional nursing personnel (of total)
   c. the nurse/patient ratio
3. *Medical Technology*
   a. the proportion of technical personnel (of total)
   b. the proportion of qualified technical personnel (of 3 a)
   c. the proportion of salaried (technical) physicians (of total)
4. *Maintenance*
   a. the proportion of maintenance personnel (general maintenance, kitchen, housekeeping, laundry, etc.) (of total)
5. *Coordination*
   a. the proportion of administrative and clerical personnel (of total)
   b. the proportion of professional nurses in administration (of 2 a)
   c. the degree of departmental specialization (Gini coefficient)
6. *Context*
   a. task size (average daily patient census)
   b. personnel resources per task size (personnel/patient ratio)
   c. the proportion of occupational titles actually filled (the degree of functional specialization)
   d. medical school affiliation
   e. nursing school affiliation

For these 17 variables, let us now look at the difference between the average and the optimum. The average is defined by the mean value of a given variable for all 6,825 U.S. hospitals in 1960. The optimum represents an adjustment of the average (mean) values, based on the quantitative, structural variations found in the empirical data, as well as on qualitative considerations involving questions of social policy. The result of this comparison is given in Table 41.

It should be fairly obvious from s comparison that the optimum structural profile resembles closely that of the most advanced

Table 41

"Average And Optimum" Structural Profiles Of Hospitals: A Comparison Of The Years 1960 And 2000 (?)

Basic Components	Average (1960)	Optimum (2000?)
1. a. % physicians employed by hospital[a]	1.9%	8.0%
b. Net autopsy rate	.32	.80
2. a. % graduate professional nurses[a]	21.5%	22.0%
b. % sub-professional nursing personnel[a]	31.9%	22.0%
c. Nurse/patient ratio	.44	.77
3. a. % technical personnel[a]	9.4%	12.0%
b. % qualified technicians	33.9%	60.0%
c. % salaried (technical) physicians	1.0%	4.0%
4. a. % maintenance personnel[a]	23.9%	24.0%
5. a. % administrative-clerical personnel[a]	8.3%	12.0%
b. % professional nurses in administration	30.0%	15.0%
c. % degree of departmental specialization (Gini Coefficient)	.53%	.80
6. a. Size (average daily patient census)	193	500
b. Personnel/patient ratio	2.08	3.50
c. % occupational titles filled (functional specialization)	51.0%	90.0%
d. % hospitals affiliated with medical school	5.3%	25.0%
e. % hospitals affiliated with nursing school	15.9%	50.0%

[a] These components make up the total hospital labor force and are the basic components used in the calculation of the Gini coefficient (5 c). The "other" component (4.9%) for 1960 was omitted, since it should be zero under optimal conditions. The "optimal" Gini was calculated on the basis of 6 components rather than 7.

---

general teaching hospitals of today. Teaching hospitals have the reputation of having generally high levels of technical and medical care; the frequently heard complaint that the human side of medical and patient care is lacking in these hospitals may be a dysfunctional consequence of high technical quality and specialization. However, it may also be a consequence of the structural peculiarities of organizationally diversified hospitals, and therefore not necessarily inevitable. The comparison in Table 41 indicates that the ingredients of an optimal form of hospital organization can be adjusted so as to combine the best aspects of medical care, nursing care, and medical technology. In this way, the medical-technological superiority of the contemporary teaching hospital can be matched by certain factors assumed to imply good patient care, such as a high nurse/patient ratio, a high ratio of professional to subprofessional personnel in nursing, or freeing the nurse's work schedule from extrinsic administrative and medical tasks by shifting them to the respective specialists.

Few of the characteristics of the optimum structural profile are "unrealistic" or "utopian." For example, the suggested increase in the proportion of physicians to 8% of the hospital labor force is already the average among the 60 contemporary V.A. general teaching hospitals, although that proportion includes residents and interns. While many more hospitals today probably have an attending and consulting medical staff of 8% or more, the total aggregate of time spent by these physicians at the patient's bedside is likely to be far below that of a comparable contingent of hospital-employed, full-time physicians. Moreover, a higher proportion of hospital-based physicians would insure round-the-clock medical care, a condition which is as yet not required of hospitals, in contrast to the requirement of round-the-clock nursing care.

As to the increase in the average of the net autopsy rate, it will be argued that a high rate is necessary or desirable only in teaching hospitals. This argument carefully separates the standards of good medical practice from their application. If medical students and interns learn from autopsies, they do so presumably to improve their diagnostic acumen and to learn from past mistakes. Such a feedback of practical medical knowledge is indispensable to good practice, regardless whether the object is medical education or medical service.

As I indicated above, the balance between professional and subprofessional nursing personnel and the freeing of the nurse's work from extraneous commitments is probably more important than a mere increase in the proportion of graduate professional nurses. Accordingly, the most significant change toward an optimum pattern here is the reduction of the proportion of subprofessional nursing personnel to a level approaching a 1:1 ratio, a condition which exists already among the 467 voluntary general teaching hospitals. Other corresponding changes are the increases in the proportion of physicians and of the administrative-clerical staff. In the latter case, one might suggest an increase especially among higher level administrative personnel so as to relieve nursing supervisors and assistant directors of nursing of their nonnursing-related administrative loads.

Such a relief has been proposed also for head nurses by the introduction of ward managers. But one may wonder about the possible negative consequences of this staff-line separation for patient care. The head nurse is characteristically close to the patient care process so that one may wish to avoid organizational conflict at that level of the organization. Therefore, a generalist professional nurse with improved training in administrative-managerial skills as well as with greater formal authority to coordinate the patient care process may be a wiser solution to the dilemma of role conflict vs. organizational conflict, in contrast to the use of a specialized generalist, viz. a nonnursing ward administrator. However, nursing will also continue to become internally more specialized and differentiated so that various types of nursing specialists will be available. Such specialist professionals might receive expanded training and certification within medical specialties so as to bridge the gap in knowledge, power, and prestige that exists between physicians and nurses. Various types of clinical nursing specialties would thus parallel the medical specialties on the one hand and the more generalist role of managerial nursing on the other.

It will be noted that the nurse/patient ratio can be adjusted upward without increasing the proportion of graduate professional nurses. But by increasing the absolute number of personnel per hospital, and thus the personnel/patient ratio, the nurse/patient ratio is correspondingly increased. I am aware of the fact that an increase in nursing manpower does not guarantee an increase in actual patient care time, but neither does a decrease in nursing manpower. The problem is therefore, partially, one of the organization of nursing practice in relation to other facets of the hospital work process. Thus, even if an improved nurse/patient ratio is not in itself a sufficient answer to the problem of patient care, it is a necessary step in the right direction, especially when other barriers to the performance of nursing functions proper, such as administrative and clerical tasks, are also lowered at the same time.

The suggested slight increase in the proportion of technical personnel results mainly from the expected further increases in technical specialization. This process of technical innovation is more or less continuous so that one may assume new specialties to be included in this category over time. In 1960, most of the new specialties were contained in the residual category of "other" personnel.

The more important change is the suggested increase in the proportion of qualified technicians and technically specialized physicians to 60 per cent of the technical personnel. Today, only the V.A. hospitals, both psychiatric and general, approximate the high level of technological complexity reflected in this figure.

As to the relative size of the administrative-clerical staff, I have already indicated that an increase should imply a relief of professional nurses of administrative and supervisory positions, a change which is also reflected in the corresponding reduction in the proportion of that category. However, another set of factors leading to an increase in administrative-clerical personnel is their increased utilization on patient care units, within departments and subunits and, generally, for maintaining external relations and communication. At the same time, the reduction of subprofessional nursing personnel would also contribute to corresponding changes in the two aspects of bureaucratization: it would imply an increase in administrative-clerical personnel due to increasing heterogeneity and a decrease in the administrative-supervisory ratio due to a diminished need for hierarchical coordination and control.

The preceding adjustments in the distribution of personnel suggested for the optimal staffing pattern result in a striking increase in the level of departmental specialization, viz. from .53 to .80. Today there are only a few hospitals which operate at such a high level of internal complexity. It is here that the idea of an optimum is perhaps most significant, since a maximum Gini value of 1.00 would clearly result in imbalances in the hospital's work organization. Such a condition is sometimes found in proprietary hospitals, where it is generated by a disproportionately high level in the employment of medical and administrative personnel.

A Gini coefficient of .80 is not a magic number, however. Apart from the variations to be expected because of special conditions under which the hospital may be operating, the value of the Gini coefficient will also vary slightly with the number of basic categories used. But as I have shown repeatedly, a crucial factor in the compositional homogeneity or heterogeneity of the hospital labor force is the proportion of subprofessional nursing personnel. If the subprofessional component is balanced relative to the professional nursing component, these two groups together with the medical staff will still constitute a core of patient care personnel composing about 50 per cent of the hospital labor force. Given a personnel/patient ratio of 350 staff per 100 patients, one would have approximately 175 patient care personnel per 100 patients, a ratio approaching 2:1. The current average patient care personnel/patient ratio is only a little over 1:1, with the largest proportion of patient care personnel being aides and attendants.

As to hospital size, the optimum of 500 represents a compromise between two extremes: the hospital that is too small to operate *efficiently* while providing a high level of medical technology and care, and the hospital that is too large to deliver high quality services *effectively* with a minimum of administrative control involving the human problems of patient care. It should be noted here especially that the 500 patient limit applies to psychiatric hospitals as well. It is, of course, possible to structure large institutional complexes of five or ten thousand patients into smaller, relatively self-contained units. A radical reorganization and deconcentration of present arrangements would constitute a significant step in the direction of adjusting size to the requirements of human social organization, rather than adjusting the latter to the pressures of task size and resources.

In line with the suggested changes in size are the necessary changes in the number of personnel per 100 patients. Today, the most glaring difference in this respect exists between psychiatric and general hospitals, the former dropping in some cases to as low as 40 personnel per 100 patients. By contrast, the voluntary psychiatric hospitals have ratios ranging up to 350 personnel per 100 patients, the level suggested by the optimal structural profile. The voluntary teaching general hospitals have an average of 240 personnel per 100 patients but range up to 700, twice the ratio suggested by the optimum.

"Limited financial resources" is one of the most frequently heard, and also one of the weakest, arguments against a high average personnel/patient ratio. It is probably true that increasing personnel costs account for the bulk of today's skyrocketing hospital and medical costs. However, if public social policy would redefine needs and priorities, it would be possible to allocate larger resources to the training and remuneration of health manpower. Hence, many of the glaring deficiencies in health manpower production and distribution could be alleviated. However, this policy change will not come about as long as health is defined as a predominantly individual phenomenon, both in terms of causation and financial responsibility. One may hope that the recent upgrading of general practice to a specialty of family and community medicine will help to move the current structural pattern of hospitals toward an improved profile, if not to the optimum level.

Like the personnel/patient ratio, the proportion of occupational titles actually filled, i.e., the degree of functional specialization, is an indicator of the availability of trained personnel in hospitals. While the baseline of this measure is constantly changing because of the proliferation of new titles and specialties, the optimal profile should include a high proportion, assuming that an adequate baseline is periodically defined and redefined. Such a defining and appraising function was temporarily performed by the Hospital Administrative Services, at one time a division of the American Hospital Association. It is a function which was paid for by the participating hospitals, and which may well be performed eventually by the Public Health Service for all hospitals.

The last two items on the list of basic components in Table 41 are admittedly more utopian than any of the others. Their inclusion here is to serve two purposes: to emphasize that the quality of patient care in all of its complex aspects in demonstrably higher in hospitals which are affiliated with both medical and nursing schools and to stress the need for a drastic expansion of training programs and facilities for future physicians and nurses. The urgent need for these two categories of health manpower has repeatedly been demonstrated. But hospitals can no longer be treated as individual enterprises which serve a particularistic health market. They are part of larger community health systems, and therefore are vitally involved in the broader questions of the distribution and quality of health services, and of the training, recruitment, and allocation of health manpower.

Some of the problems and their potential solution pointed up by the gap between average and optimum profile are obvious. For example, hospitals may be well advised to employ more professionals, both generalists and specialists, i.e., to concentrate existing resources on restructuring the skill mix in favor of highly trained personnel as well as personnel with generalist abilities and characteristics. One may also want to give attention to areas of cross-specialty skills, such as medically trained nurses, administratively trained nurses, psychiatric and medical social workers, and occupational therapists. Particularly nursing, however, should be made more attractive by increasing the status, the formal responsibility, and even the pay of nurses.

Insofar as specialists are a sine qua non of complex task performance, one may as well accept the consequences of co-existence or even conflict among specialists and among diverse objectives and subunits. Except in those areas where potential confrontations directly interfere with the work process, such as in medical and nursing care, one may want to minimize role conflict. In general, one may want to maximize vertical and lateral delegation by subunit formation and departmental specialization, and permit and institutionalize conflict resolution at the subunit level.

Since diversification tends to articulate conflict and to counteract functional interdependence within organizations, it is necessary to have clear definitions of priorities, e.g., to what extent service should precede teaching even in teaching hospitals. The need for a clear definition of goals and priorities, in turn, suggests that planning be maximized in the establishment of new hospitals, so as to limit a hospital, for example, to a certain size and to minimize haphazard growth, dispersion, and diversification. The planning and standardization of V.A. hospitals reflected in their comparative uniformity has often been criticized for not allowing variety and flexibility; yet it may be precisely that element of central planning which builds into the V.A. hospitals a uniformly high level of quality.

One realistic solution to the problem of moving from an average to an optimum structural profile of hospitals is the mobilization of federal support, especially to state and local governmental hospitals and to the voluntary nonteaching general hospitals. The data on ownership and control show quite unequivocally that the local public hospitals have neither the legal nor the financial independence necessary for their adequate operation. Such a condition of de facto independence appears to be maximally present in the voluntary general teaching hospitals and in the federal V.A. hospitals. A Federal Health Commission could presumably be given independent powers to regulate both financial support and general standards of health care in the provision of health services. Today, the health professions have neither the power nor the interest to perform such a vital function alone; their separate efforts, however, would be greatly aided by the economic and political resources which such a Commission would have. Moreover, the increase in the external bureaucratization that can be expected to result from such an arrangement would be more than offset by the gains in the distribution and high quality of health care. That such beneficial uses of bureaucracy are possible is perhaps demonstrated best by the high quality of federal hospitals, whether they are part of the armed services or the Veterans' Administration.

I shall now turn briefly to the more general implications of this study for a new theoretical conception of organizations.

Pluralism, Federalism, and Democratization in Organizations

The study of hospitals, both on the level of the case-study and on the level of the comparative and quantitative analysis of organizations, suggests that the complex hospitals of today represent a post-bureaucratic form of organization which may well become the prototype of modern organizations in general. This generalization, together with the specific hypotheses of this study, requires further systematic empirical research involving a variety of different types of organizations, and specifically organizations other than hospitals. The following considerations appear to have some bearing on this approach.

Multifunctional, diversified organizations, such as general teaching hospitals and the various structures affiliated with them, e.g., specialized clinics, medical schools, research institutes, etc., transcend the complexity which is merely the result of functional specialization and structural differentiation. These organizations are loosely structured clusters of heterogeneous and semi-autonomous units, representing a multiplicity of interests and claims to power.

To the extent that such organizational clusters resemble modern polycentric communities, they can be said to be pluralistic structures.

The reality of modern organizations consists of a multitude of independent elements. This reality can no longer be apprehended in terms of a single, unitary principle of legitimacy and hierarchy, or in terms of a convergent social "substance" made up of individual motivation and social norms integrated by presumed consensus. Nor can we assume that modern complex organizations create their own internal control mechanisms under any and all conditions, especially under those of diversification and the development of multiple goals.

The problems of coordination generated by such organizational phenomena appear to transcend those that are typically dealt with by rational planning and administration alone. The results of this study suggest that the nature of coordination in complex formal organizations is influenced by inter-organizational and extra-organizational factors, i.e., relations which are difficult if not impossible to apprehend with a system model of organizational behavior. Among these factors are the historical development of a specific task structure, of a particular constellation of internal structural elements, and of the relative autonomy of the organization vis-a-vis other organizations. Other factors are the operation of processes such as competition, interdependence, and the maintenance of a balance of particularistic interests through countervailing power within and between organizations, as well as a certain surface tolerance for diversity. These and other elements of social process must be taken into account in the study of coordination in pluralistic structures.

Durkheim had formally begun with two bases of social cohesion: shared norms and value orientations among the members of a comparatively homogeneous, undifferentiated society, and interdependence between specialized functions and subsectors of society. But we have seen that functional interdependence implies, substantively, a whole set of coordinating factors. Besides the dependence of specialists on each other, i.e., a kind of forced reciprocity which may lead to regularized interchange or the scheduling of activities, we find cooperation, and "voluntary" coordination and self-regulation as well as the emergence of networks of interaction and the proliferation of new rules and shared norms, together with their regulation. Interdependence conceived in this way implies the laborious development of contracts and negotiated settlements and the more or less continuous operation of informal agreements and of specialized legal-regulative functions.[5] It is here that social, political, and economic forms of coordination interpenetrate.

The findings of this study suggest that the greater the degree of task complexity, the greater the likelihood that different modes of coordination will be simultaneously present, that relational, structural, and "economic" modes of coordination will be prevalent, and that bureaucratic-hierarchical modes of coordination will recede in importance. It is obvious that we cannot make statements about equivalent amounts of coordination provided by different modes of coordination. However, depending on the type and degree of task complexity we can say that the presence, absence, relative prevalence, or transformation of a given mode of coordination will have certain ramifications throughout the structure and, specifically, will have certain effects on other modes of coordination. The transformation of professionalization from a mechanism of coordination to an integral aspect of the division of labor itself is an instance where one can demonstrate an increased need for the coordination of specialized functions.

The findings suggest that in general hospitals this need is met by increased departmental specialization and by a relatively larger administrative staff. Thus both structural and administrative modes of coordination can be shown to be directly influenced by task complexity. But with increasing internal differentiation, the administrative staff itself becomes more differentiated and is more closely integrated with the functionally differentiated organization of work. Differentiation and decentralization within the administrative component mean primarily that each subunit develops its own clerical and decision-making unit, as well as procedures and mechanisms of functional supervision and control.

It is likely that such administrative elements as record-keeping, periodic horizontal communication, and filling out of report forms and questionnaires will increasingly become part of the work and production process itself, as is the case in automation where decentralization requires a greater degree of feedback. This would mean a shift and dispersion of administrative processes to the work level, but at the same time increased centralization of information and potential control through automatic data processing and storage.[6] Essentially, such mechanisms amount to a form of pre-coordination of work which reduces decision-making discretion at the intermediate levels.

Certain aspects of this process of simultaneous administrative-supervisory decentralization and increased centralization of channels of communication and top-level decision-making have been reported for those organizations where operators and workers are increasingly engaged in report writing and other semi-administrative work, while the middle levels of management are reduced or eliminated.[7]

In the complex hospitals, the decrease of the administrative-supervisory component can be interpreted in terms of similar processes, since much administrative work is shifted to the work level of the organization, i.e., the patient care unit. While the application of data processing and feedback technology is obvious for such tasks as processing administrative and medical records and for facilitating diagnostic procedures, its implications for patient care are perhaps less conspicuous but of equal importance. Closed circuit television, monitoring systems, and two-way communication systems have greatly increased the centralization of nursing stations vis-a-vis patients, as well as their autonomy vis-a-vis the administrative hierarchy. Similarly, self-care units as well as general advances in medical technology serve to decentralize the hospital work process and lessen institutional controls, thus changing the processes of therapy and administration in the direction of the "therapeutic community" and away from the "total institution".

We must conclude from this discussion that with progressive differentiation of the goal structure and with further organizational diversification, even the natural system model implied by

Durkheim's theory of the division of labor appears to be of limited applicability.

It is here, then, that we may find a combination of structural and rational modes of coordination which supersede the operation of shared norms and values, legitimate authority, and direct controls. In other words, the relatively loose structure of multifunctional and diversified organizations approximates the differentiated, heterogeneous structure of the large modern society; organizational processes simulate the social processes of their environment. The structural parallelism suggested here is underscored by the high degree of interchange between these types of organizations and their environment, as I have shown.

The "openness" of diversified, complex organizations as well as their internal differentiation in terms of new specialties and skills constitute pressures which make the organization more accountable to the outside environment. At the same time, such pressures generate a form of democratic opposition to top level professional and bureaucratic authority within the organization. I have already indicated that such pressures toward co-determination and democratization gradually transform a bureaucratically organized, efficiency-oriented work organization into a more pluralistic type which has many characteristics of the voluntary association. Thus, pluralism in organizations can be seen as a transitory stage which contributes toward further diversification, the assertion of multiple bases of legitimacy, and the expression of various forms of vertical and lateral opposition. Pluralism ultimately generates, therefore, the need for regulation, co-determination, and especially representation of the public interest, not just that of the dominant groups. The high level of education and relative economic security of professional and technical groups may, indeed, constitute factors which make democratic participation and opposition to bureaucratic authority economically feasible and ideologically justifiable.

The pluralistic structure of modern organizations presupposes a certain autonomy of subunits. The greater the autonomy, the more will the normative, vertical, authoritative integration of the organization be reduced, and the more will new solutions be attempted, such as horizontal integration and structural balance, based on co-determination and the "voluntary" participation of, and interaction and interdependence among, subunits.

The characteristic weakness and failure of pluralistic structures is the formation of dominant centers of power bent on maintaining the status quo in the presumed interest of stability, order, and effective goal-attainment. The deterioration of structural balance based on diverse units is possible whenever these units are not truly equal or autonomous. This condition is as likely to obtain within organizations as between them.

The first and foremost task, therefore, of any rational attempt to maximize horizontal integration is to redistribute and regulate resources, inputs, and power among the respective units. Thus, even if there is disagreement over problems, causes, and methods of patient care, but some minimum agreement over the preferred outcome, it may be possible to arrive at decisions which favor the common interest of both staff and patients.[8]

The problem here is clearly to avoid "turning problems of politics into problems of administration," a favorite method of bureaucratic conservatism.[9] Applied to hospitals as pluralistic organizational structures, this means that the multiplicity of claims, i.e., the definition of legitimate interests arising from patient groups, technical and professional specialties, and unskilled or otherwise under- or unrepresented groups, must be taken into account in defining the common interest and preferred outcomes. This, at least, is one way in which the particularistic claims of specific group interests can be transcended. It is also a way of maximizing the voluntary "association" and federation of diverse units for specific, agreed-upon purposes.

The stability and effectiveness of an organization or a cluster of organizations lies therefore not so much in the adequacy of bureaucratic hierarchical control and manipulation, or the legitimacy of its dominant elites, or the consensus and harmony among dominant interests, but in the *representativeness of the goals* themselves, and thus in the adequacy of the definition of tasks, functions, methods, and performance from the perspective of all participants and groups.

In short, hospitals must serve the collective interests of the community, rather than merely particular patient groups or individual patients isolated from their social matrix. Modern hospitals should therefore *not* differ according to the social, demographic, cultural, and economic characteristics of their patient populations, the particularistic interests of professional practitioners, and the impersonal exigencies and so-called "imperatives" of technology, budgets, and administration.

In other words, modern hospital systems share problems and require decisions which are formally if not substantively similar to those of public school systems, public welfare systems, correctional systems, and other public service systems. It is for the reasons stated above that such systems require public, specifically federal, support and regulation.

However, in the long run, the process of collective decision-making must follow successive steps of *upward delegation* of powers, starting with relatively autonomous units which enter into forms of voluntary association and cooperation for specific purposes. The creation of new community health care units, mixtures of hospital, clinic, and group practice, is a case in point. Coordination within and among such units becomes a continuous process in which emergent goals, objectives, and tasks set the stage for new forms of planning and regulation. The unit or the system potentially emerging from this process, whether a single organization or a network of organizations, is secondary to the specific cluster and sequence of activities in which different functional groups participate. Such "freedom on the level of planning"[10] means that the needs of clients, and the interests of participants as well as the judgment of experts determine the goal and task structure of an organization insofar as it is, like the hospital, designed to serve the whole community. It means that technological and administrative considerations are sub-ordinated to or coordinated with—rather than super-ordinated to—the definition of human needs and the realization of social goals.

Notes

1. See the "collective disturbances" in mental hospitals, as described in William Caudill, *The Psychiatric Hospital as a Small Society* (Cambridge, Mass.: Harvard University Press, 1958), pp. 87-130.
2. See, e.g., Rue Bucher and Anselm Strauss, "Professions in Process," *American Journal of Sociology*, 66 (1961), 325-334.
3. See, e.g., Charles Lindblom, "The Science of 'Muddling Through,' " *Public Administration Review*, 19 (1959); and Wolf V. Heydebrand, "Administration of Social Change," *Public Administration Review*, 24 (1964), 163-165.
4. See also Johan Galtung, *Theory and Methods of Social Research* (New York: Columbia University Press, 1967), p. 488.
5. An example of a social-psychological description of these processes is Anselm Strauss et al., "The Hospital and Its Negotiated Order," in Eliot Friedson, *The Hospital in Modern Society* (New York: The Free Press, 1963), pp. 147-169.
6. See, e.g., Kaufman's observation that the periodic reports of forest rangers constitute a form of control, in Herbert Kaufman, *The Forest Ranger* (Baltimore: Johns Hopkins Press, 1960).
7. Frederick L. Richardson and Charles R. Walker, *Human Relations in an*

Expanding Company (New Haven, Conn.: Labor and Management Center, Yale University, 1948); Floyd C. Mann and R. Hoffman, *Automation and the Worker* (New York: Holt, Rinehart, and Winston, 1960); Robert Blauner, *Alienation and Freedom: The Factory Worker and His Industry* (Chicago: University of Chicago Press, 1964. C. Edward Weber suggests that middle management tends to be retained but assumes new functions derived from increased output of information as provided by automated data processing. See his "Change in Managerial Manpower with Mechanization of Data-Processing," *The Journal of Business*, XXXII (1959), 151-163.

8. See, e.g., the idea that under such conditions majority judgment in a collegial structure, i.e., in an essentially egalitarian setting, will obtain; James D. Thompson and Arthur Tuden, "Strategies, Structures, and Processes of Organizational Decision," in James D. Thompson, ed., *Comparative Studies in Administration* (Pittsburgh, Pa.: Pittsburgh University Press, 1959), pp. 198-204.

9. Karl Mannheim, *Ideology and Utopia* (New York: Harcourt, Brace and Co., 1936), p. 118.

10. Cf. Karl Mannheim, *Man and Society in an Age of Reconstruction* (London: Routledge & Kegan Paul, 1940), pp. 180-225; also Manfred Kochen and Karl Deutsch, "A Rational Theory of Decentralization," *American Political Science Review*, Sept., 1969.

Appendixes

Appendix A

Quality of the Data

Certain questions may be raised concerning the quality and usefulness of indices, survey, and registration data collected by organizations and institutions not primarily oriented toward social science research. For example, such data may be limited by the fact that definitions used may differ from those most useful for the investigation at hand. Standards of reliability and accuracy may be low or unknown.[1] Angell and Freedman, in particular, write:

> The completeness of registration data coverage varies from time to time with the efficiency of data collection, the nature of the data, and the incentives which the population has to record the event involved.... Because data are collected as an incident of administrative processes, they may suffer from their particular context.[2]

The following points will indicate what is known about the data used in this study. First of all, there is no reason to suspect that the data are systematically biased because of any particular motivation on the part of hospital administrators, or because of any built-in source of distortion. The fact that the questionnaires were distributed by the A.H.A. in its official capacity suggests that no special outside or additional authority had to be involved in order to get accurate and complete returns.

Secondly, surveys have been conducted annually by the A.H.A. since 1946, and by the American Medical Association since 1923. The surveys can therefore be considered a relatively routine procedure for most hospitals.

A questionnaire detailing occupational categories similar to the 1959 questionnaire had been used in 1958. If this experience can be assumed to have had any effect on the reliability of returns, one could argue that it increased the awareness and the expectation to keep more detailed records and to routinize and rationalize this aspect of data collection on the part of administrators.

It is perhaps more important to note that much of the information derives from records which are maintained regardless of the annual survey by the A.H.A. Routine data collection for various purposes has become a permanent feature of hospital administration. Not only is it stressed in the training of hospital administrators as a basis for informed decision-making;[3] data collection and the maintenance of statistical records is also required by the provisions of federal legislation, such as the Federal Hospital Survey and Construction Act (P.L. 725) of 1946, the "Hill-Burton Act." In addition, various planning agencies, such as state governments and state and regional hospital associations, frequently require or ask the hospital to provide information of the kind required by the national root organization, the A.H.A.[4]

Aside from the business-administrative orientation of boards and administrators, there are numerous legal requirements which constrain hospitals to maintain operating statistics.[5] Morbidity and mortality statistics, patient censuses, and medical records, as well as financial and payroll records, can also be assumed to contribute to an increasingly accurate system of data collection and maintenance in hospitals.

Finally, there is the question as to what extent definitions and terms are standardized and shared. Although this is a source of error which affects all types of surveys, there is reason to believe that despite its organizational diversity, the hospital universe shares definitions to the same, if not a greater, degree than other industries or statistical populations. Hospitals have used the widely distributed *Uniform Chart of Accounts and Definitions for Hospitals*[6] which supersedes the 1950 edition of the *Handbook on Accounting, Statistics, and Business Office Procedures for Hospitals*,[7] as well as earlier editions of a similar reference guide going back as far as 1922.[8]

Since questionnaire data may reflect conditions in the hospital which affect its status regarding accreditation and eligibility as a teaching hospital, it could be that a bias is introduced in the reporting of those aspects of hospital operation which reflect on its quality, performance, efficiency, and effectiveness, e.g., the autopsy rate, length of stay, and per cent occupancy. It is quite possible that some hospitals report inaccurately because they overrate themselves, or because there is an interest in retaining or increasing previous budgets. Biased reporting may occur for a variety of reasons and may operate in opposite directions.

Clearly, accuracy of reporting cannot be checked from hospital to hospital, and since there is no reason to assume that biased representation by some hospitals on a few selected items affects the reliability of the data as a whole, we have to accept them at face value.

In regard to the autopsy rate, care has been taken to eliminate factors which would unduly increase the rate (see Chapter 3 for a description and definition of the "net autopsy rate").

Generally, it may be held that while the data cannot be considered as free from errors, such errors are sufficiently random and will, therefore, not distort the findings significantly. Thus the quality of the data is considered adequate for the purposes of the present study.

Notes

1. Robert C. Angell and Ronald Freedman, "The Uses of Documents, Records, Census Materials, and Indices," in Leon Festinger and Daniel Katz, eds., *Research Methods in the Behavioral Sciences* (New York: Dryden, 1953), pp. 309-326; Claire Sellitz et al., *Research Methods in Social Relations* (rev. ed.; New York: Holt, Reinhart, and Winston, 1960), pp. 316-323; Mildred B. Parten, *Surveys, Polls, and Samples* (New York: Harper, 1950), pp. 383-402; E. S. Marks and W. P. Mauldin, "Response Errors in Census Research," *Journal of the American Statistical Association,* XLV (1950), 424-438.
2. Festinger and Katz, op. cit., p. 319, 320.
3. See, e.g., Ray E. Brown, ed., *Graduate Education for Hospital Administration* (Chicago: Graduate Program for Hospital Administration, University of Chicago, 1958).
4. See, e.g., "Illinois State Survey and Plan for the Construction of Hospitals and Medical Facilities" (14th rev. ed.; State of Illinois: Department of Public Health, Bureau of Hospitals, Springfield, 1962), which is published annually as part of the Illinois Hospital and Medical Care Facility Planning and Construction Program; Medical and Nursing Licensures of the Illinois State Department of Registration and Education; the Chicago Hospital Council; the Blue Cross and Blue Shield Plans; and various other medical and nurses' associations. Countless listings of similar organizations for other states and cities can be found in the Membership Directory of the A.H.A., which is published annually as part of the Guide Issue. See in this connection also: Elliott H. Pennell, et. al., "Business Census of Hospitals, 1935," Supplement No. 154 to the *Public Health Reports,* Washington, D.C.: U.S. Government Printing Office, 1939; Paul M. Densen, "The Development and Use of Statistical Practices in Hospital Work," Biometrics, III (1947), 109-118.
5. Emanuel Hayt et al., *Law of Hospital, Physician, and Patient* (2nd ed.; New York: Hospital Textbook Co., 1952).
6. Chicago: American Hospital Association, 1959.
7. Chicago: American Hospital Association, 1950.
8. See also Malcolm T. McEachern, *Hospital Organization and Management* (Chicago: Physicians' Record Co., 1946).

Appendix B

Transforming the Raw Data into Variables

A crucial step in preparing this type of data for analysis is the transformation of the raw data into variables. Here I want to describe the basic operations involved in this transformation.

The original A.H.A. data were punched on cards, partly coded, but mostly in raw form, i.e., the actual numerical values were punched on the cards. Moreover, the data were recorded on a set of twelve cards for each hospital, often in such a way that part of a given composite measure was on one card, while the rest was on another. For example, in calculating the percentage of selected technical personnel of the total full-time equivalent personnel, the following operations had to be performed, involving the selection of data from several cards:

1. Calculate the number of full-time personnel by summing over all full-time personnel categories, including residents and interns, excluding volunteers, students, and other categories of unpaid, nonregular personnel.

2. Calculate the number of part-time personnel by summing over the corresponding part-time personnel categories.

3. Add the part-time personnel categories, except salaried physicians, at the ratio of 1/2 to the respective full-time categories; add part-time physicians at the ratio of 1/3, and form a full-time equivalent total of all personnel.

4. Calculate the number of full-time and part-time selected technical personnel, and form a full-time equivalent technical personnel total.

5. Divide the total technical personnel by the full-time equivalent total personnel.

Similar operations had to be performed for other personnel groups. Considering the amount of time necessary to complete the various calculations, to generate the variables, and to prepare them for the statistical analysis, it was decided to reduce the number of cards to ten per hospital by transferring the information from two cards onto the others, and also to use a computer for the transformation of raw data into variables.

Thanks are due to the following persons who were involved in various phases of the processing of the data.

A special program had to be written for the IBM 7094, which had the function of computing the various measures and transforming the raw data into fifty-eight variables per hospital. This program was written by Sanford Abrams in March, 1963, and I am indebted to him for advice and help on many technical details concerning this phase of the analysis.

The actual card-to-tape operation was done at the Biological Sciences Computation Center at the University of Chicago. The transformation of the raw data was performed on the IBM 7094 under the auspices of the Center. The variable data tapes were screened and subgroup means were substituted for missing information through a special program written for the IBM by David Kleinman.

The first exploratory analysis was performed by means of the BIMD 29 Multiple Regression and Correlation Program No. 3. In this connection, I am indebted to Professor Paul Meier, Chairman, Department of Statistics, and Director, Biological Sciences Computation Center, University of Chicago, for substantive advice as well as generous support of this project; to Professor David Wallace, Department of Statistics, for valuable comments and suggestions, and to David Kleinman and Warren Davis, of the Biological Sciences Computation Center, for their equally generous help and extensive advice on the data processing phase.

A final tape with identification codes and fifty-eight variables on each of the 6,825 hospitals served as the basis for the input tape. For purposes of the subsequent analyses, additional tapes were created from the basic data tape, containing the twelve selected hospital groups with a number of selected variables on each hospital. I am indebted to Ron Skirmont and Marjorie Schultz, of the University of Chicago Computation Center, for writing various special programs and subroutines in connection with these operations, and for preparing the data tapes for input to the MESA 83 Multiple Regression and Correlation Program and the MANOVA Multivariate Analysis of Variance Program. I am particularly grateful to Allen Herzog, of the Illinois Department of Mental Health, formerly of the Department of Education, University of Chicago, for making his modified version of the MANOVA program available to me and for his generous advice on various aspects of this program.

Finally, I gratefully acknowledge the support of the National Science Foundation which provided funds for machine time on the IBM 7094, made available under the auspices of the Division of Social Sciences, and its coordinator, Professor Benjamin Wright. I would also like to express my gratitude to Mr. A. B. Addleman,

Operations Manager of the Computation Center, University of Chicago, for the active and continued support he has given to the "Hospital Organization Project," in addition to coordinating a complex organization in its own right.

Appendix C

Size of Community

This variable refers to the size of the Standard Metropolitan Statistical Area (SMSA) in which the hospital is located.

The variable (the new code) represents a scale involving multiples of about 25,000 and based on the median city size corresponding most closely to the mid-point of the A.H.A. size definitions. It is adjusted on the basis of the 1960 Census rank order of SMSA's. (See *U.S. Census of Population,* 1960, U.S. Summary, "Number of Inhabitants," Table 36, p. 117.)

	A.H.A.	Hospital Bureaucracy Study		
Card Code	Size Definition	New Code	Size Rank	Median Size
00	NonSMSA Areas	1		25,000
11	Under 100,000 Population	3	191-212	81,000
12	100,000-199,999	6	123-190	141,000
13	200,000-299,999	10	82-122	250,000
14	300,000-399,999	14	61-81	340,000
15	400,000-499,999	18	54-60	457,000
21	500,000-599,599	21	43-53	525,000
22	600,000-699,999	26	33-42	660,000
23	700,000-799,999	30	31-32	750,000
24	800,000-899,999	33	27-30	819,000
25	900,000-999,999	37	25-26	932,000
31	1,000,000-1,999,999	48	11-24	1,190,000
41	2,000,000 and over	131	1-10	3,273,000

Appendix D

Classification of Hospital Occupations

For the present study, the following A.H.A. classification of occupational titles was augmented by two categories: salaried physicians, and residents and interns, thus bringing the total number of categories to thirty-nine.

Classification

a. Graduate Professional Nurses

1) Superintendent and assistant superintendent of hospital
2) Director and assistant directors of nursing and/or nursing school
3) Instructors
4) Nurse anesthetists
5) Operating room: supervisors and assistant supervisors
6) Operating room: head nurses and assistant head nurses
7) Operating room: staff nurses (general duty)
8) Patient care units (general medical-surgical, obstetrics, orthopedics, pediatrics, psychiatry, tuberculosis): supervisors and assistant supervisors
9) Patient Care units: head nurses and assistant head nurses
10) Patient Care units: staff nurses (general duty)
11) Nurses not specified

b. Practical Nurses and Auxiliary Nursing Personnel

1) Practical nurses
2) Nursing aides and/or attendants
3) Orderlies
4) Other auxiliary nursing personnel

c. Selected Technical Personnel

1) Medical technologists registered by ASCP
2) Other medical technologists and laboratory technicians
3) X-ray technicians registered by ARXT
4) Other X-ray technicians

5) Registered medical record librarians (RRL)
6) Accredited medical record technicians (ART)
7) Other medical record personnel
8) Registered occupational therapists (OTR)
9) Other occupational therapists
10) Registered physical therapists (ARPT)
11) Other physical therapists
12) Dietitians (members ADA)
13) Other dietitians
14) All other dietary personnel
15) Medical social workers with master's degree
16) Other medical social workers
17) Pharmacists (R. Ph.)

d. All Other Personnel

1) Laundry personnel
2) Housekeeping personnel (includes floor maids)
3) Maintenance personnel
4) Administrative personnel (business and clerical)
5) All other personnel

Appendix E

Accreditation: Principles and Criteria

The following basic principles and criteria will give some insight into the type of minimum requirement that a general hospital applying for accreditation is expected to fulfill. This material is taken from *Hospital Accreditation References.* This 148-page booklet specifies in detail the minimum standards implied by the basic principles and criteria. One detail of some importance is that the minimum autopsy rate on hospital deaths is expected to be at least 20 per cent.

Basic Principles

The following basic principles must be followed in order for a hospital to be accredited by the Joint Commission on Accreditation of Hospitals.

I. Administration

A. Governing Body
The governing body must assume the legal and moral responsibility for the conduct of the hospital as an institution. It is responsible to the patient, the community, and the sponsoring organization.

B. Physical Plant
The buildings of the hospital must be constructed, arranged, and maintained to insure the safety of the patient; and must provide facilities for diagnosis and treatment and for special hospital services appropriate to the needs of the community.

C. The following facilities and services must be maintained:
1. Dietary
2. Medical records
3. Pharmacy or drug room
4. Clinical pathology and pathological anatomy
5. Radiology
6. Emergency care for mass casualties
7. Medical library

II. Medical Staff
   There must be an organized medical staff which is responsible
   to the patient and to the governing body of the hospital for the
   quality of all medical care provided patients in the hospital and
   for the ethical and professional practices of its members.

III. Nursing
   There must be a licensed, graduate, registered nurse on duty at
   all times and graduate nursing service must be available for all
   patients at all times.

Basic Criteria

For a hospital to qualify for a survey for accreditation, the following
criteria must be met:

1. The hospital shall have at least 25 adult beds.
2. The hospital shall have been in operation for at least 12 months.
3. The hospital shall be listed by the American Hospital
   Association. The American Hospital Association has set the
   following requirements for listing:

   a. The hospital shall have at least six beds for the care of patients
      who are nonrelated, who are sick and who stay on the average in
      excess of 24 hours per admission.

   b. The hospital shall be licensed in those states and provinces
      having licensing laws.

   c. Only doctors of medicine or doctors of osteopathy shall practice
      in hospitals listed by the American Hospital Association. (This
      requirement is not intended to eliminate dental and similar
      services from the hospital. Patients admitted for such services,
      however, must have an admission history and a physical
      examination done by a physician on the staff of the hospital, and
      a physician on the staff of the hospital shall be responsible for
      the patient's medical care throughout his stay.)

   d. Duly authorized bylaws for the staff of physicians shall be
      adopted by the hospital.

e. The hospital shall submit evidence of regular care of the patient by the attending physician and of general supervision of the clinical work by doctors of medicine.

f. Records of clinical work shall be maintained by the hospital on all patients and shall be available for reference.

g. Registered nurse supervision and such other nursing service as is necessary to provide patient care around the clock shall be available at the hospital.

h. The hospital shall offer services more intensive than those required merely for room, board, personal services, and general nursing care.

i. Minimal surgical or obstetrical facilities (including operating or delivery room), or relatively complete diagnostic facilities and treatment facilities for medical patients, shall be available at the hospital.

j. Diagnostic X-ray services shall be regularly and conveniently available.

k. Clinical laboratory services shall be regularly and conveniently available.[2]

As to psychiatric hospital standards, the rules are similar to those that apply to general hospitals.

As far as psychiatric medical records are concerned, the rules, with a few flexible interpretations, are the same as for short-term general hospitals. The general components of the chart are the same. The psychiatric portion of the patient's history is stressed.

The physical examination should be adequate and complete. The Commission believes long-term cases should have at least a yearly physical examination.

Progress notes on new admissions, acute cases, and intensive therapy cases should be written frequently and regularly. Progress notes on chronic and domiciliary cases should be written as needed, but preferably at least monthly.[3]

Notes

1. *Hospital Accreditation References* (Chicago: American Hospital Association, 1961).
2. Ibid., pp. X-XI.
3. Ibid., p. 37.

Appendix F

The Assumptions of Normality and Equality of Variance and the Transformation of Scales

Before the actual statistical analysis of the data was begun, the mean, standard deviation, skewness, kurtosis, and minimum and maximum values of the distribution of each variable were computed. Examination of these values confirmed the impression that some of the variables, especially the size variables and the ratios, had large standard deviations and a generally high degree of skewness.[1]

Since the assumptions of homoscedasticity and normality are crucial for both the analysis of variance and multivariate correlation analysis, it was decided to transform the variables so as to improve the stability of the variance and to approximate more closely a normal distribution of the variables. The logarithmic scale was used for the ratios and the size variables, and the angular (arcsin) transformation for the proportions.[2]

After the variables had been transformed, the mean, standard deviation, skewness, and kurtosis were again computed for each variable. The comparison of the characteristics of the distributions before and after the transformation showed that the degree of skewness had been significantly reduced in all variables, while the standard deviation had been reduced in most cases, although in a few instances it had not changed appreciably.

Although these operations do not create "ideal" distributions in the sense described by Bartlett and Kendall, they do increase confidence in the validity of the assumptions necessary for the statistical analysis.

Notes

1. The following sources were useful in this context: Henry Scheffé, *The Analysis of Variance* (New York: Wiley, 1959), pp. 331-334; Churchill Eisenhart, "The Assumptions Underlying the Analysis of Variance," *Biometrics*, II (1947), 1-21; William G. Cochran, "Some Consequences When the Assumptions for the Analysis of Variance are Not Satisfied," *Biometrics*, II (1947), 22-38.
2. Cf. M. S. Bartlett, "The Use of Transformations," *Biometrics*, III (1947), 43-47; M. S. Bartlett and D. G. Kendall, "The Statistical Analysis of Variance: Heterogeneity and the Logarithmic Transformation," *Journal of the Royal Statistical Society*, Supplement 7, 1946, 128; Scheffé. op. cit., pp. 364-368; C. R. Rao, *Advanced Statistical Methods in Biometric Research*

(New York: Wiley, 1952), pp. 210-214 on the arcsin transformation; John W. Tukey, "One Degree of Freedom for Non-Additivity," *Biometrics*, V (1949), pp. 323-342; Helen M. Walker and Joseph Lev, *Statistical Inference* (New York: Holt, Rinehart, and Winston, 1953), pp. 423-425. For the angular transformation, the formula $\phi = 2 \arcsin \sqrt{p}$, offered by Walker and Lev, was used.

Appendix G

Systematic List of Findings (Empirical Generalizations) Concerning Structural Differences Between and Relationships Within Organizational Types

The findings or empirical generalizations concerning structural differences are based on the analysis of variance and covariance; those on structural relationships within types are based on multiple and partial correlation analysis. These findings represent the relationships between the major variables and are derived from the original tables.

Although these empirical findings have been presented in the main text and are integrated into the theoretical discussion and interpretation, they are listed here in summary form to facilitate orientation and to provide easy reference.

Empirical Generalizations Concerning Structural Differences

11.1 Professionalization is directly related to the complexity of the task structure (number and diversity of major objectives) when the influence of size and the subprofessional component is controlled.

12.1 The administrative-supervisory ratio (hierarchical coordination) is inversely related to the complexity of the task structure.

12.11 The relationship in 12.1 holds when the joint influence of size, the professional component, and the subprofessional component is controlled.

13.1 The proportion of qualified technical personnel is directly related to the number of major objectives (general hospitals) when the influence of size is controlled.

13.2 The proportion of qualified technical personnel is directly related to the diversity of major objectives (teaching hospitals) when the influence of the proportion of salaried physicians is controlled.

14.1 Functional specialization is directly related to the complexity of the task structure.

14.11 The relationship in 14.1 holds when the influence of size is controlled.

15.1 Departmental specialization is directly related to the complexity of the task structure.
15.11 The relationship in 15.1 holds when the influence of size, the influence of functional specialization, and their joint influence is controlled.
16.1 The administrative-clerical component is directly related to the number of major objectives.
16.2 The administrative-clerical component is directly related to the diversity of major objectives when the influence of size is controlled.
16.3 The administrative-clerical component is directly related to the complexity of the task structure when the joint influence of size and functional specialization is controlled.
16.4 The administrative-clerical component is not related to the diversity of major objectives when the joint influence of the professional and subprofessional components is controlled.

Empirical Generalizations Concerning Structural Relationships
21.1 Functional specialization is directly related to organizational size.
22.1 Departmental specialization is directly related to size in multifunctional organizations (general hospitals), but inversely in unifunctional organizations (psychiatric hospitals).
22.11 The relationships in 22.1 are stronger in the respective diversified types.
22.12 Departmental specialization tends to be inversely related to size when the influence of functional specialization is controlled.
22.13 The relationship in 22.12 is stronger in unifunctional organizations.
22.2 Departmental specialization is directly related to functional specialization.
22.21 The relationship in 22.2 is stronger when the influence of size is controlled.
23.1 Professionalization is inversely related to size.
23.11 The relationship in 23.1 is stronger in unifunctional organizations.
23.2 Professionalization tends to be directly related to departmental specialization.
23.31 The relationship in 23.3 is stronger in unifunctional organizations when the influence of size is controlled.
24.1 Hierarchical coordination (administrative-supervisory ratio) is inversely related to size.

24.11 The relationship in 24.1 is stronger in multifunctional organizations.
24.2 Hierarchical coordination is inversely related to functional specialization.
24.21 Relationship in 24.2 is stronger in unifunctional organizations.
24.3 Hierarchical coordination is inversely related to departmental specialization.
24.31 The relationship in 24.3 is stronger in multifunctional organizations.
24.4 Hierarchical coordination is inversely related to professionalization.
25.1 The administrative-clerical component tends to be inversely related to organizational size.
25.11 The relationship in 25.1 is stronger in unifunctional organizations.
25.12 The relationship in 25.1 is stronger in diversified organizations.
25.13 The relationship in 25.1 tends to hold when the influence of functional specialization is controlled.
25.2 The administrative-clerical component tends to be inversely related to functional specialization in unifunctional, diversified organizations (psychiatric teaching hospitals).
25.21 The administrative-clerical component tends to be directly related to functional specialization in nondiversified organizations when the influence of size is controlled.
25.3 The administrative-clerical component tends to be directly related to departmental specialization in unifunctional organizations.
25.31 The relationship in 25.3 is reversed in organizations with a high level of departmental specialization.
25.4 The administrative-clerical component tends to be inversely related to professionalization when the joint influence of size and the subprofessional component is controlled.
25.41 The relationship in 25.4 is stronger in unifunctional organizations.
25.42 The relationship in 25.4 is reversed in organizations with a high level of departmental specialization when the joint influence of size and departmental specialization is controlled.
25.5 The administrative-clerical component tends to be inversely related to hierarchical coordination in unifunctional organizations with a high level of departmental specialization when the joint influence of size, functional specialization, departmental specialization, and professionalism is controlled.

26.1 The proportion of technical personnel is inversely related to organizational size.

26.2 The proportion of qualified-technical personnel tends to be directly related to size.

26.3 The proportion of salaried physicians tends to be directly related to size.

26.4 The subprofessional component is directly related to size in unifunctional organizations.

26.41 The relationship in 26.4 is reversed in multifunctional organizations.

27.1 Professionalization tends to be directly related to the proportion of qualified-technical personnel.

27.2 Professionalization tends to be inversely related to the proportion of salaried physicians.

28.1 Hierarchical coordination tends to be inversely related to the proportion of qualified-technical personnel.

28.2 Hierarchical coordination tends to be inversely related to the proportion of salaried physicians.

29.1 The administrative-clerical component tends to be directly related to the proportion of qualified technical personnel.

29.2 The administrative-clerical component tends to be directly related to the proportion of salaried physicians.

Index